# Textbook of
# DENTAL ANATOMY,
# PHYSIOLOGY AND OCCLUSION

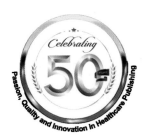

# Textbook of
# DENTAL ANATOMY, PHYSIOLOGY AND OCCLUSION

## Second Edition

**Rashmi GS Phulari** BDS MDS (Oral Path)
Professor and Head
Department of Oral Pathology and Microbiology
Manubhai Patel Dental College, Hospital and Oral Research Institute
Vadodara, Gujarat, India

**JAYPEE BROTHERS MEDICAL PUBLISHERS**
*The Health Sciences Publisher*
New Delhi | London | Panama

**Jaypee Brothers Medical Publishers (P) Ltd**

**Headquarters**

Jaypee Brothers Medical Publishers (P) Ltd
4838/24, Ansari Road, Daryaganj
New Delhi 110 002, India
Phone: +91-11-43574357
Fax: +91-11-43574314
Email: jaypee@jaypeebrothers.com

**Overseas Offices**

J.P. Medical Ltd
83 Victoria Street, London
SW1H 0HW (UK)
Phone: +44 20 3170 8910
Fax: +44 (0)20 3008 6180
Email: info@jpmedpub.com

Jaypee-Highlights Medical Publishers Inc
City of Knowledge, Bld. 235, 2nd Floor, Clayton
Panama City, Panama
Phone: +1 507-301-0496
Fax: +1 507-301-0499
Email: cservice@jphmedical.com

Jaypee Brothers Medical Publishers (P) Ltd
Bhotahity, Kathmandu
Nepal
Phone: +977-9741283608
Email: kathmandu@jaypeebrothers.com

Website: www.jaypeebrothers.com
Website: www.jaypeedigital.com

*Textbook of Dental Anatomy, Physiology and Occlusion*

*First Edition*: 2014

Second Edition: **2019**

ISBN: 978-93-5270-568-9

*Printed at: Samrat Offset Pvt. Ltd.*

# Dedicated to

*The fond memories of my dad and brother…*
*(Late Siddarajaiah K and Late Chidananda S)*

# And

*My mom and sister*
*Premakumari YR and Sushma GS*

*My parents-in-law*
*Subhashchandra and Shivalingamma Phulari*

*My beloved husband*
*Dr Basavaraj Subhashchandra Phulari*

*My little sons*
*Yashas and Vrishank*
*for their love, trust and encouragement*

# Contributors

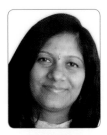

**Rashmi GS Phulari**
BDS MDS (Oral Path)
Professor and Head
Department of Oral Pathology and Microbiology
Manubhai Patel Dental College, Hospital and Oral Research Institute
Vadodara, Gujarat, India

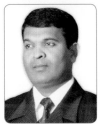

**Basavaraj Subhashchandra Phulari**
BDS MDS (Ortho TSMA-Rus) FRSH FAGE
Former Faculty
Department of Orthodontics and Dentofacial Orthopedics
Mauras College of Dentistry and Hospital
Mauritius

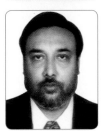

**Rajendrasinh Rathore**
BDS MDS (Oral Path)
Chairman and Professor
Department of Oral and Maxillofacial Pathology
Manubhai Patel Dental College
Hospital and Oral Research Institute
Vadodara, Gujarat, India

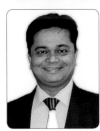

**Srinivas S Vanaki**
BDS MDS (Oral Path)
Principal
PM Nadagouda Memorial Dental College and Hospital
Bagalkot, Karnataka, India

# Preface to the Second Edition

It has been heartening to have the first edition so well received by the faculty and students alike. Every effort has been made in the second edition as well to bring out a comprehensive, engaging, easy-to-grasp and recall textbook that enhances the learning experience theory as well as practical aspects of dental anatomy.

The text has been thoroughly revised and edited although the basic format of the book is retained. The order of sections has been reorganized to allow discussion of the fascinating aspects of dental anatomy such as *Evolution, Dental anthropology, and Forensic odontology* to appear early on, so as to infuse interest and curiosity in the minds of young readers. Differences in morphology of various teeth, i.e. the *Class, Arch and Type Traits of Teeth* are tabulated in the respective tooth chapters rather than as a separate section for better correlation while reading. A new section on *Oral Physiology* is added that discusses functions of teeth, mastication, deglutition and phonation.

A picture is worth a thousand words, especially true while learning subjects such as anatomy. Thus, numerous high resolution pictures are incorporated throughout the book and they make narration of the text more like an atlas. New improved graphic illustrations of teeth, with important features labelled on each of the five aspects make understanding the anatomy much easier. Images of numerous extracted natural teeth, segregated as right and left specimens are given to lend good support to the text.

Numerous clinical photographs throughout the text demonstrating common anatomic variations, related anomalies and clinical relevance of tooth morphology in dental practice make the subject interesting. Unique and innovative flow charts listing the anatomic landmarks and a brief summary of major anatomic features of each tooth help students in revision during examination preparation.

Primary teeth, often neglected, are given due significance with a separate chapter, complete with detailed description of each tooth.

Few interesting fun facts are interspersed with the text in each chapter that makes for an engaging reading.

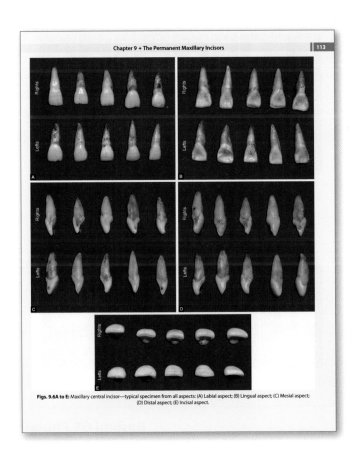

**Figs. 9.6A to E:** Maxillary central incisor—typical specimen from all aspects: (A) Labial aspect; (B) Lingual aspect; (C) Mesial aspect; (D) Distal aspect; (E) Incisal aspect.

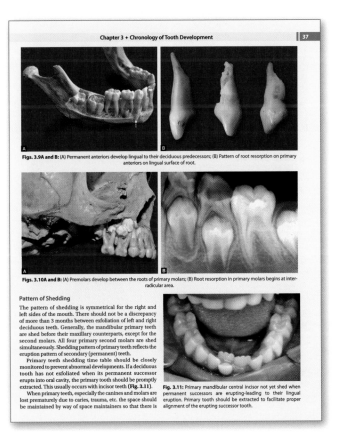

**Figs. 3.9A and B:** (A) Permanent anteriors develop lingual to their deciduous predecessors; (B) Pattern of root resorption on primary anteriors on lingual surface of root.

**Figs. 3.10A and B:** (A) Premolars develop between the roots of primary molars; (B) Root resorption in primary molars begins at inter-radicular area.

### Pattern of Shedding

The pattern of shedding is symmetrical for the right and left sides of the mouth. There should not be a discrepancy of more than 3 months between exfoliation of left and right deciduous teeth. Generally, the mandibular primary teeth are shed before their maxillary counterparts, except for the second molars. All four primary second molars are shed simultaneously. Shedding pattern of primary teeth reflects the eruption pattern of secondary (permanent) teeth.

Primary teeth shedding time table should be closely monitored to prevent abnormal developments. If a deciduous tooth has not exfoliated when its permanent successor erupts into oral cavity, the primary tooth should be promptly extracted. This usually occurs with incisor teeth **(Fig. 3.11)**.

When primary teeth, especially the canines and molars are lost prematurely due to caries, trauma, etc. the space should be maintained by way of space maintainers so that there is

**Fig. 3.11:** Primary mandibular central incisor not yet shed when permanent successors are erupting-leading to their lingual eruption. Primary tooth should be extracted to facilitate proper alignment of the erupting successor tooth.

The chapter on tooth carving that explains the rationale, armamentarium, basic principles and step-by-step carving procedure is revamped with graphic illustrations to depict the steps. Carving technique for different types of teeth is made self-explanatory using life size high resolution images of actual wax blocks in different stages of carving. *Video demonstrations* of carving procedure for various teeth are given as separate online-link that can be accessed by students to learn the procedure at their own pace.

Multiple choice questions (MCQs) form an important part of question paper format in most of the universities. Thus, MCQs are given at the end of each chapter in the textbook along with additional set of MCQs given as a separate online-link to aid the students in revision and preparation for viva voce and competitive examinations.

It has been a formidable endeavor to put together this edition with meticulous attention to details and I regret any deficiencies that might have crept in despite my best efforts. Any comments and suggestions for further improvement of the book are welcome and it is hoped that our sincere efforts will enhance and render dental anatomy learning experience more exciting and enjoyable.

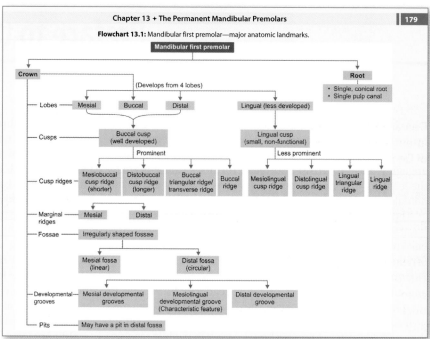

Flowchart 13.1: Mandibular first premolar—major anatomic landmarks.

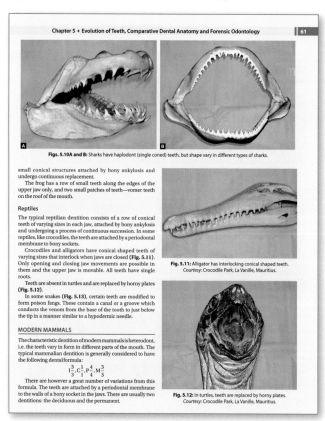

Figs. 5.10A and B: Sharks have haplodont (single coned) teeth, but shape vary in different types of sharks.

small conical structures attached by bony ankylosis and undergo continuous replacement.

The frog has a row of small teeth along the edges of the upper jaw only, and two small patches of teeth—vomer teeth on the roof of the mouth.

**Reptiles**

The typical reptilian dentition consists of a row of conical teeth of varying sizes in each jaw, attached by bony ankylosis and undergoing a process of continuous succession. In some reptiles, like crocodiles, the teeth are attached by a periodontal membrane to bony sockets.

Crocodiles and alligators have conical shaped teeth of varying sizes that interlock when jaws are closed **(Fig. 5.11)**. Only opening and closing jaw movements are possible in them and the upper jaw is movable. All teeth have single roots.

Teeth are absent in turtles and are replaced by horny plates **(Fig. 5.12)**.

In some snakes **(Fig. 5.13)**, certain teeth are modified to form poison fangs. These contain a canal or a groove which conducts the venom from the base of the tooth to just below the tip in a manner similar to a hypodermic needle.

**MODERN MAMMALS**

The characteristic dentition of modern mammals is heterodont, i.e. the teeth vary in form in different parts of the mouth. The typical mammalian dentition is generally considered to have the following dental formula:

$$I\frac{3}{3}, C\frac{1}{1}, P\frac{4}{4}, M\frac{3}{3}$$

There are however a great number of variations from this formula. The teeth are attached by a periodontal membrane to the walls of a bony socket in the jaws. There are usually two dentitions: the deciduous and the permanent.

Fig. 5.11: Alligator has interlocking conical shaped teeth.
*Courtesy: Crocodile Park, La Vanille, Mauritius.*

Fig. 5.12: In turtles, teeth are replaced by horny plates.
*Courtesy: Crocodile Park, La Vanille, Mauritius.*

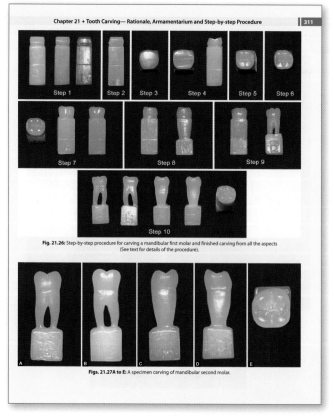

Fig. 21.26: Step-by-step procedure for carving a mandibular first molar and finished carving from all the aspects (See text for details of the procedure).

Figs. 21.27A to E: A specimen carving of mandibular second molar.

**Rashmi GS Phulari**

*rashugs@rediffmail.com*

# Preface to the First Edition

Dental anatomy forms the basis for all the fields of dentistry. *Textbook of Dental Anatomy, Physiology and Occlusion* is an attempt towards meeting the enormous challenge of providing an all comprehensive, yet simple-to-understand coverage of Dental anatomy, Physiology and Occlusion.

Detailed morphology of deciduous and permanent teeth is narrated in a pointwise and systematic manner which is easier to understand and recall. Apart from the images of typical teeth specimen, numerous clinical photographs are added to demonstrate common variations, anomalies and practical relevance of tooth morphology. Numerous tables, boxes and flowcharts throughout the text make understanding and recalling easier. The morphology of each permanent tooth is summarized using flowcharts that give the major anatomic landmarks of that tooth and a brief summary of the major features on all five aspects of that tooth.

Separate chapters are dedicated to tooth notation systems, chronology of tooth development, differences between primary and permanent dentitions, pulp morphology, temporomandibular joint and occlusion. Dental students are introduced to the fascinating aspects of dental anatomy such as forensic odontology, evolution of teeth, dental anthropology and comparative dental anatomy.

A separate chapter on tooth carving is included that explains the rationale, armamentarium, basic principles and step-by-step carving procedure. Carving technique for different types of teeth is made self-explanatory using life size high resolution images of actual wax blocks in different stages of carving. The ancillary DVD-ROMs contain visual demonstration of carving procedures for various teeth.

Numerous high quality photographs and professionally done graphic illustrations with informative legends make the text easy to grasp. Incorporation of numerous tables, flowcharts and boxes throughout the textbook will give the reader a convenient summary of the key features and also make reviewing easier.

Multiple choice questions (MCQs) given at the end of each chapter in the textbook and the additional MCQs in ancillary DVD-ROMs aid the students in revision and preparation for viva-voce and competitive examinations.

It is hoped that the concepts of dental anatomy, physiology and occlusion presented in a simple and logical style in the book will benefit all the undergraduate and postgraduate students of dental sciences and dental auxiliaries.

**Rashmi GS Phulari**
*rashugs@rediffmail.com*

# Acknowledgments

With profound sense of gratitude and respect, I express my heartfelt thanks to Dr Rajendrasinh Rathore, Chairman, and Dr Yashraj Rathore, Vice-Chairman and Head of Operations, Manubhai Patel Dental College, Hospital and Oral Research Institute, Vadodara, Gujarat, India, for all the support and encouragement shown during this endeavor and in all my academic pursuits.

I would like to extend my sincere thanks to Dr Sonali Kapoor, Dean, Professor and Head, Department of Conservative Dentistry and Endodontics, Manubhai Patel Dental College, Hospital and Oral Research Institute, Vadodara, Gujarat, India, for being a constant source of encouragement and guidance during compilation of the book.

It is my pleasant privilege and honor to express my sincere gratitude and respect to all my revered teachers who have made me what I am today. In particular, I would like to thank Dr Rajiv S Desai, Professor and Head, Department of Oral Pathology and Microbiology, Nair Dental College, Mumbai, Maharashtra, India, my postgraduate guide, for igniting the fire to seek academic excellence. I owe an immense debt of gratitude to my postgraduate teachers Dr Srinivas S Vanaki, Dean, and Dr RS Puranik, Professor and Head, Department of Oral Pathology and Microbiology, PM Nadagouda Memorial Dental College and Hospital (PMNMDCH), Bagalkot, Karnataka, India, for their constant encouragement throughout my academic career.

I would also like to thank all the faculty members of the institution and all the colleagues and postgraduate students at the Department of Oral and Maxillofacial Pathology, Manubhai Patel Dental College, Hospital and Oral Research Institute, Vadodara, Gujarat, India.

I thank my beloved husband Dr Basavaraj Subhashchandra Phulari, an author himself of several well-received books in the field of Orthodontics, for being there, helping me at every step of this project right from the text layout to final proofs. I fondly acknowledge my little sons Yashas and Vrishank for their patience, love and for being the source of inspiration to set and reach new goals in life.

My heartfelt gratitude goes to Shri Jitendar P Vij (Group Chairman), Mr Ankit Vij (Managing Director), Mr MS Mani (Group President), Ms Pooja Bhandari (Production Head), Ms Sunita Katla (Executive Assistant to Group Chairman and Publishing Manager), Dr Madhu Choudhary (Head Publishing–Education), Ms Samina Khan (Executive Assistant to Publishing Head–Education), Mr Rajesh Sharma (Production Coordinator), Dr Astha Sawhney (Development Editor), Ms Seema Dogra (Cover Visualizer), Mr Deepak Saxena (DTP Operator), Mr Binay Kumar (Proofreader) and Mr Rajesh Ghurkundi (Graphic Designer), and staff of M/s Jaypee Brothers Medical Publishers (P) Ltd, New Delhi, India, whose exceptional efforts made the production of this book possible.

Above all, I thank, the Almighty for all the kindness showered upon me…

# Contents

# 1 SECTION

# Introduction and Nomenclature

## Section Outline

1. Introduction to Dental Anatomy
2. Tooth Notation Systems

# Introduction to Dental Anatomy

---

> ### 🔦 Did you know?
> 🖎 **Tooth enamel** is the hardest part of our body. It is half as scratch resistant as a diamond.
> 🖎 Teeth decay easily in life. However, after death they are the most durable and well preserved structures of the body even up to thousands of years.

## INTRODUCTION

The field of dental anatomy is dedicated to the study of teeth including their development, eruption, morphology, classification, nomenclature, and function. Dental occlusion deals with the contact relationship of the teeth in function as in mastication, and also the static morphological tooth contact relationship as at rest. The knowledge of dental anatomy, physiology, and occlusion forms a firm basis for all the fields of clinical dentistry and is essential for rendering appropriate treatment to various dental problems. A brief overview of dental anatomy and the related basic terminologies are discussed in this chapter.

## DENTITIONS IN HUMANS

Humans, like most mammals, have two sets of teeth, the *deciduous or primary dentition* and the *permanent or*

*secondary dentition*. Such a condition where two generations of teeth are present in a lifetime is called "diphyodonty". Furthermore, humans have more than one type of teeth, i.e. incisors, canines, premolars, and molars; and such a dentition in which the teeth are regionally specialized into classes, is known as "heterodont dentition". Most submammalian vertebrates are *polyphyodonts* with many successions of teeth necessary to compensate for continual loss of teeth. Teeth in these animals are directly attached to the jaw bone and thus are frequently broken and lost during normal function. Most lower animals have teeth of same shape, i.e. *homodont dentition*.

A limited succession of teeth still occurs in most mammals including humans—not to compensate for continual loss of teeth, but to accommodate the growth of the face and jaws. In childhood, the smaller jaws carry few teeth of smaller size—the deciduous dentition. Later, an increase in the size of jaws occurs with growth necessitating larger teeth. They are thus replaced by a set of larger and greater number of teeth—the permanent dentition.

### Deciduous or Primary Dentition (Figs. 1.1A and B)

The primary dentition is called so since they are the first set of teeth to appear in the oral cavity. The term *deciduous* implies

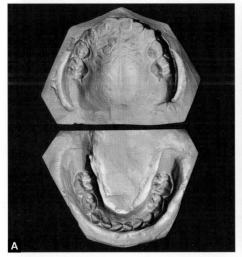
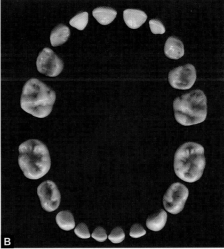

**Figs. 1.1A and B:** Deciduous or primary dentition: (A) Cast specimen; (B) Human extracted primary teeth arranged in arches in their respective positions.

that they are shed or fallen off naturally similar to the leaves of a deciduous forest tree. The primary teeth are sometimes also referred to as *milk teeth or baby teeth or lacteal teeth.* These terms are unfortunate and inappropriate since they imply a lack of importance to the first dentition. The terms "deciduous" and "primary" are more appropriate and are used interchangeably throughout the text.

The primary dentition consists of a total of 20 teeth, 10 in each jaw. The primary teeth begin to emerge into the oral cavity at about 6 months of age and a child would have the complete set of primary teeth by 2½ to 3 years. *Primary dentition does not have premolars and third molars.*

### Permanent or Secondary or Succedaneous Dentition (Figs. 1.2A and B)

There are a total of 32 teeth in the permanent dentition, 16 in each jaw. The permanent teeth are also called as *succedaneous teeth or secondary teeth* since they replace or succeed the primary teeth. However, the permanent molars erupt posterior to the primary molars and do not replace any primary teeth. *Therefore, in strict sense, the permanent molars are not succedaneous teeth.* They are called as *accessional teeth* as they do not have predecessors.

The permanent teeth begin to emerge at 6 years of age and gradually replace the smaller primary teeth. The eruption process is completed by 12–13 years except for the posterior most teeth, the four 3rd molars which erupt around 18–25 years of age.

### Arrangement in the Dental Arches (Figs. 1.3A and B)

The teeth making up each dentition are arranged in two arches, one in each jaw; *the maxillary* and *mandibular dental arches.* The teeth in the upper jaw, the maxilla, are called the *maxillary or upper teeth.* The teeth in the lower jaw, the mandible, are called the *mandibular or lower teeth.*

There are equal number of teeth in both the arches, 10 in primary and 16 in permanent dentition. Teeth in each arch are arranged symmetrically on either side of the median plane. The median plane divides each dental arch into left and right quadrants. Thus, there are four quadrants in oral cavity, namely the *upper right, upper left, lower left, and lower right quadrant* in a clockwise direction. The corresponding teeth in left and right side of each dental arch are mirror images, with similar size and form.

### Classes of Teeth (Table 1.1 and Fig. 1.4)

All the teeth in human dentitions are not of same shape, i.e. humans are *heterodonts.* Depending on the form and function,

**Table 1.1:** Classes of teeth in human dentitions.

| Permanent dentition | Primary dentition |
| --- | --- |
| Incisors | Incisors |
| Canines | Canines |
| Premolars | No premolars in primary dentition |
| Molars | Molars |

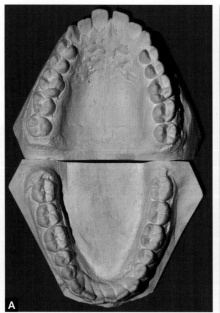 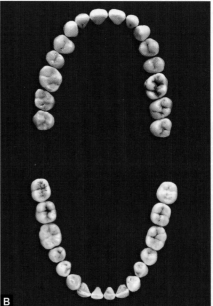

**Figs. 1.2A and B:** Permanent or secondary dentition: (A) Dental cast specimen; (B) Human extracted permanent teeth arranged in their respective positions.

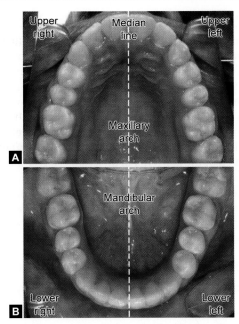

**Figs. 1.3A and B:** Teeth in maxillary and mandibular dental arches are arranged symmetrically on either side of the median plane (Note that the third molar has not erupted yet).

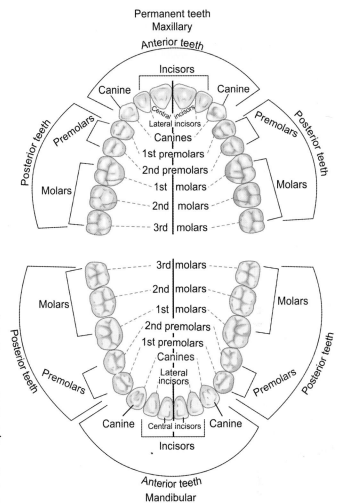

**Fig. 1.4:** Different classes and types of teeth in human permanent dentition.

there are four classes of teeth in permanent dentition: *the incisors,* the *canines, the premolars,* and the *molars.* Premolars are found only in the permanent dentition; there are no primary premolars. Therefore, the *primary dentition consists of only three class of teeth; the incisors, the canines, and the molars.*

The incisors and canines are collectively known as the *anteriors,* while the premolars and molars are collectively referred to as the *posteriors.* The etymologies (etymology = origin of words) of these dental terms are from the Latin **(Box 1.1)**.

### Types of Teeth (Table 1.2 and Fig. 1.4)

Within each class, the teeth may be subdivided into two or three types depending on their traits. The incisors are further divided into *central* and *lateral incisors.* Among premolar and molar classes, there are *first* and *second premolars* and *first, second,* and *third molars.* The molar class in the deciduous dentition has only two teeth, the *first* and *second molars.*

## TRAIT CATEGORIES OF TEETH

While describing the anatomy of a tooth, its morphologic characteristics are compared with that of the other teeth, so that any similarities and differences can be noted. *A trait is a distinguishing characteristic, quality or attribute.* The tooth traits are categorized as follows:

---

**Box 1.1: Etymology of names of teeth.**

- *Incisors (incidere in Latin = to cut into)*: Called so because their function is of incising and nipping; incisors are the "cutting teeth"
- *Canines (canis in Latin = dog, hound)*: The canine teeth derive their name from the prominent, well-developed corner teeth in the canidae (dog) family. These teeth in carnivorous animal are mainly used for prehension of their prey. However their value for prehension has been considerably diminished in humans where the canine teeth function essentially as incisors. They are also referred to as "cuspids" since these teeth consists of one large primary cusp
- *Premolars (premolars = before molar teeth)*: The term "premolars" merely recognizes the anatomical portion of these teeth that is in front of the molars. They are also sometimes referred to as "bicuspids" since these teeth commonly (but not always) have two cusps
- *Molars (molaris in Latin = millstone)*: The term molars refer to the grinding, triturating function of these teeth with their wide occlusal surfaces

**Table 1.2:** Types of teeth in human dentitions.

| Classes | Types of teeth | |
|---|---|---|
| | Permanent dentition | Primary dentition |
| Incisor class | Central and lateral | Central and lateral |
| Canine class | (Single type) | (Single type) |
| Premolar class | First and second | (No premolars) |
| Molar class | First, second, and third | First and second |
| | | (No third molars) |

## Set Traits

Set traits or dentition traits distinguish the teeth in the primary dentition from the permanent dentition. For example:
- Primary teeth have bulbous crowns and constricted necks
- Permanent teeth are darker in color, whereas the primary teeth are more whitish.

## Arch Traits

Arch traits distinguish maxillary from mandibular teeth. For examples, maxillary molars have three roots, while the mandibular molars have two roots.

## Class Traits

Class traits distinguish the four classes of teeth, namely—incisors, canines, premolars, and molars. For examples:
1. Incisors have straight incisal ridges efficient for cutting
2. Canines have single, pointed cusps for piercing food
3. Premolars have two or three cusps for shearing and grinding
4. Molars have 3–5 flattened cusps ideal for crushing food.

## Type Traits

Type traits differentiate teeth within one class, such as differences between central and lateral incisors, between first and second premolars, or between first, second, and third molars. For example, maxillary central incisor has a straight incisal ridge while that of the lateral incisor is curved with rounded incisal angles.

## NOMENCLATURE OF TEETH

Teeth are named by their set, arch, class, type, and side. The name of a specific tooth would include information whether it belongs to primary (deciduous) or permanent set, maxillary (upper) or mandibular (lower) arch, which class and type it belongs to, and whether it is of left or right side of the mouth. For example:
- Primary maxillary right lateral incisor
- Permanent mandibular left first molar.

Tooth notation systems are used to simplify the nomenclature of teeth. This facilitates communication and record keeping. The various tooth notation systems are discussed in detail in Chapter 2.

## DENTAL FORMULAE IN HUMANS

The number and type of teeth present in a dentition can be expressed in the form of a dental formula. The dental formulae are used to differentiate the human dentitions from that of the other species. The dental formula is different for primary and permanent dentitions.

Since the left and right halves of the dental arches are exact mirror images, the dental formulae include the teeth present in one side of the mouth only. Different classes of teeth are represented by the first letter in their name, e.g. *"I" for incisors, "C" for canine, "P" for premolars, and "M" for molars*. Each such letter is followed by a horizontal line. The number above the horizontal line represents such type of teeth present in the maxillary arch while the number below the line represents such type of teeth present in the mandibular arch.

### Dental Formula for Primary or Deciduous Dentition

The primary dentition has the following dental formula:

$$I\frac{2}{2}C\frac{1}{1}M\frac{2}{2} = \frac{5}{5} = 10 \,(\text{on each side})$$

(Expressed as 2 : 1 : 2, i.e. two : one : two).

Each quadrant in primary dentition has five teeth; beginning from the midline they are the central incisor, the lateral incisor, the canine, the first molar, and the second molar. There are 10 teeth on each side of the midline and thus adding to a total of 20 teeth in deciduous dentition.

### Dental Formula for Permanent Dentition

In permanent dentition, the premolars are present in addition to incisors, canines, and molars; the number of molar teeth is increased to three. The dental formula for permanent dentition is as follows:

$$I\frac{2}{2}C\frac{1}{1}P\frac{2}{2}M\frac{3}{3} = 16 \,(\text{on each side})$$

(Expressed as 2 : 1 : 2 : 3, i.e. two : one : two : three)

Each quadrant in permanent dentition has eight teeth. The teeth present in each quadrant from the midline are: central and lateral incisors, canine, first and second premolars, followed by first, second, and third molars.

## STAGES OF DENTITIONS IN HUMANS

Traditionally, three stages or periods of dentitions are recognized in humans. They are the *deciduous dentition period, mixed (transitional) period,* and the *permanent dentition period.*

### Deciduous Dentition Period (6 Months to 6 Years)

- The deciduous dentition stage begins from the time of eruption of first primary tooth, usually the mandibular central incisor at around 6 months of age. It lasts until the emergence of the first permanent tooth around 6 years of age.

- During this period there are only deciduous teeth present in the oral cavity.
- Oral motor behavior and speech are established during this period.

### Mixed Dentition Period (6–12 Years)

- Mixed dentition stage is a transition period when primary teeth are exfoliated in a sequential manner, followed by the eruption of permanent teeth.
- This stage lasts from 6 years to 12 years of age. Both primary and permanent teeth are present during this period.
- The mixed dentition period begins with the eruption of permanent first molars and mandibular central incisors. It is completed when the last primary tooth is shed.
- During this period, the primary incisors are replaced by the permanent incisors; the primary canines by the permanent canines; and *the primary molars by the permanent premolars.*
- It has to be noted that the successors of primary molars are the permanent premolars and not the permanent molars.
- Significant changes in occlusion occur during mixed dentition period due to growth of jaws and replacement of 20 primary teeth by their permanent successors.

### Permanent Dentition Period (12 Years and Beyond)

- Permanent dentition period is well established by about 13 years of age with the eruption of all the permanent teeth except the third molars that erupt late in life (around 18–21 years).
- The permanent molars (six in each jaw; three in each quadrant) have no deciduous predecessors. In other words, the permanent molars do not replace any primary teeth, but erupt distal to the last primary tooth on the dental arch. They extend the dental arches at the back of the mouth as the jaws increase in size with growth.

### PARTS OF TOOTH

Any tooth has two main parts:
1. Crown
2. Root.

The crown is the portion of the tooth that projects above the gum line into the oral cavity; while the root is that portion of the tooth that is embedded in the jaw bone and anchors the tooth. The crown and root portions are joined at the neck or cervical area. The junction between the crown and root portion is marked by a distinct line the *cervical line.*

*Anatomic crown* (**Fig. 1.5**)*:* Anatomic crown is defined as the part of the tooth that is covered by enamel.

*Anatomic root* (**Fig. 1.5**)*:* Anatomic root is that portion of the tooth that is covered by cementum. The cervical line that signifies the *cementoenamel junction* separates the anatomic crown from anatomic root. The cervical line can be clearly

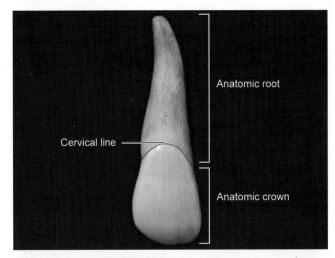

**Fig. 1.5:** An extracted tooth showing anatomic crown and root separated by the cervical line.

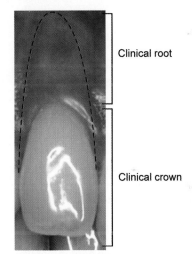

**Fig. 1.6:** Clinical crown and clinical root.

observed on an extracted tooth. This relation does not change with age.

*Clinical crown and clinical root* (**Figs. 1.6 to 1.8**)*:* Clinical crown is the part of a tooth that is visible in the oral cavity and is limited by the gingival margin or gums (**Fig. 1.6**). Clinical crown is smaller than the anatomic crown in a newly erupted tooth, where cervical part of the anatomic crown is still covered by gingiva (**Fig. 1.7**). On the other hand, clinical crown may become longer with age, as some part of the anatomic root also gets exposed to oral cavity due to gingival recession (**Fig. 1.8**).

Clinical root is that part of a tooth which is covered by gingiva and is not exposed to oral cavity. It is longer than the anatomic root on newly erupted teeth as the unexposed part of the crown is considered to be a part of the clinical root (**Fig. 1.7**). In an older person with considerable recession of gingiva, the

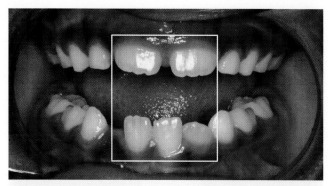

**Fig. 1.7:** Clinical crown smaller than the anatomic crown in a newly erupted tooth. Here clinical root is longer than the anatomic root.

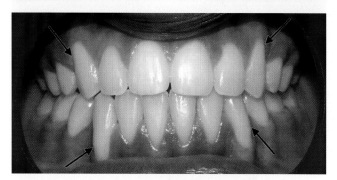

**Fig. 1.8:** Clinical crown longer than the anatomic crown due to gingival recession. Here clinical root is shorter than anatomic root.

clinical root is shorter than the anatomic root, as the portion of the root that is exposed to oral cavity is considered to be a part of the clinical crown **(Fig. 1.8)**.

## STRUCTURE OF TOOTH (FIG. 1.9)

The tooth is composed of three hard mineralized tissues, the *enamel,* the *dentin,* and the *cementum;* and one soft tissue component, the *pulp.* Enamel is ectodermal in origin while all other tissues of the tooth are mesodermal in origin.

### Enamel

Enamel is the hardest substance in the human body consisting of more than 96% inorganic material. It forms a protective covering over the crown portion of the tooth. Enamel is not present in the root portion. Although hard in nature, enamel is extremely brittle due to its high mineral content. Unlike dentin, cementum or bone, the enamel does not show a continuous formation throughout life. Once the crown formation is complete, no more enamel is deposited. The enamel develops from the enamel organ of the tooth germ (ectodermal in origin).

### Dentin

Dentin forms the major bulk of the tooth. It is present in both crown and root portions. It is not normally exposed on the

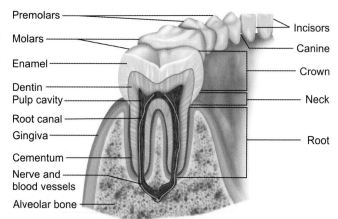

**Fig. 1.9:** Schematic diagram showing various components of a tooth.

surface of the tooth, unless the tooth is badly worn out. Dentin is more resilient owing to its collagenous organic content. It supports the enamel and compensates for its brittleness. It develops from *dental papilla* (mesodermal in origin).

### Cementum

Cementum is a hard avascular tissue that covers the roots of teeth. It gives attachment to the *periodontal ligament* that binds the tooth to the alveolar bone. Cementum develops from *dental sac* (mesodermal in origin).

### Pulp

Dental pulp is the specialized connective tissue that carries blood and nerve supply to the tooth. It is housed in the pulp cavity present at the core of the tooth. The pulp is well protected by the rigid dentin walls all around it. The portion of the pulp in the crown is called the *pulp chamber* and the portion of pulp in the root is called the *pulp or root canal.* Pulp develops from the *dental papilla* (mesodermal origin). Many functions are attributed to pulp including formative, sensory, and defensive functions.

## BASIC TERMINOLOGIES IN DENTAL ANATOMY

### Surfaces of Teeth (Figs. 1.10A and B)

Five surfaces can be recognized on the crowns of all the teeth. The fifth surface on the crowns of anterior teeth (incisors and canines) is a ridge (linear elevation) to begin with, when the tooth is newly erupted. However, it soon becomes a flattened surface due to wearing (attrition). The surfaces are named according to their positions. These five surfaces are shown in **Table 1.3**.

#### Labial or Buccal Surface

In the anterior teeth, the surface towards the lips is called the *labial surface.* The term *buccal surface* is used for the surface of posterior teeth toward the cheeks.

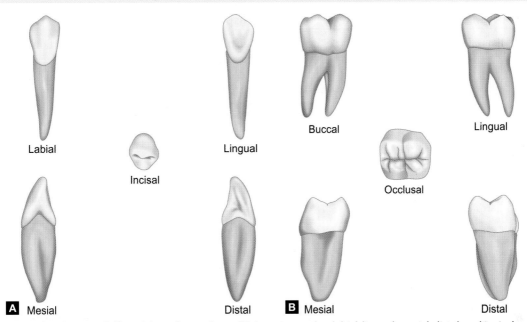

**Figs. 1.10A and B:** Crowns of all teeth have five surfaces: (A) Anterior teeth—labial, lingual, mesial, distal, and incisal surfaces; (B) Posterior teeth—buccal, lingual, mesial, distal and occlusal surfaces.

**Table 1.3:** Surfaces of teeth.

| In anterior teeth (Fig. 1.10A) | In posterior teeth (Fig. 1.10B) |
| --- | --- |
| 1. Labial surface | 1. Buccal surface |
| 2. Lingual or palatal surface | 2. Lingual or palatal surface |
| 3. Mesial surface | 3. Mesial surface |
| 4. Distal surface | 4. Distal surface |
| 5. Incisal surface | 5. Occlusal surface |

*Facial surface* is a collective term for referring to both labial and buccal surfaces of the anteriors and the posteriors.

### Lingual Surface

The surface of a tooth facing toward the tongue is called the *lingual surface.* It is used for both maxillary and mandibular teeth. In case of maxillary teeth, the term *palatal surface* is sometimes used interchangeably with the term *lingual surface.*

### Mesial and Distal (Proximal) Surfaces

The surfaces of the teeth facing toward the adjacent teeth in the same dental arch are called the *proximal surfaces.*

*Mesial surface* is the surface of the tooth that is nearest to the median line. The surface away from the median line is called the *distal surface.* The mesial surface of a tooth contacts with the distal surface of its adjacent tooth. This arrangement is true for all the teeth except the maxillary and mandibular central incisors, where their mesial surfaces contact each

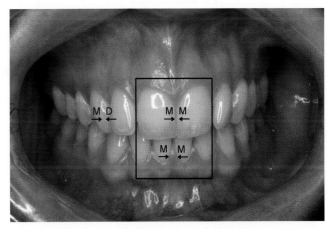

**Fig. 1.11:** Maxillary and mandibular central incisors are the only teeth in which mesial surfaces face each other. In all other teeth mesial surface is in contact with distal surface of the adjacent tooth.

(M: mesial surface; D: distal surface)

other **(Fig. 1.11)**. The distal surfaces of permanent third molars and primary second molars do not have contact with any surface as there are no teeth distal to them.

### Incisal and Occlusal Surface

The surfaces of teeth that come in contact with those in the opposing jaw during mastication are called the *incisal surface* in case of anterior teeth and *occlusal surface* in case of posterior teeth.

## ANATOMIC LANDMARKS ON TOOTH SURFACE

**Flowchart 1.1** lists all the anatomic landmarks on tooth surface.

## Cusp (Figs. 1.12A and B, Table 1.4)

Cusp is an elevation on the crown portion of a tooth making up a divisional part of the occlusal surface. Cusps are present

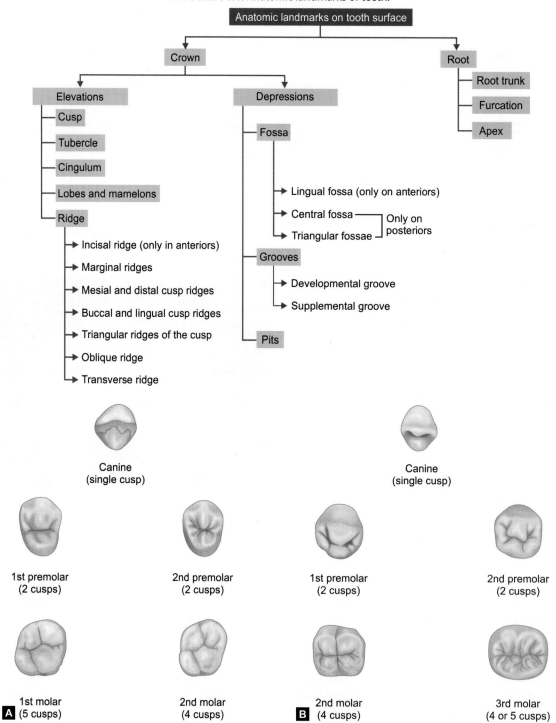

**Flowchart 1.1:** Anatomic landmarks of teeth.

**Figs. 1.12A and B:** Cusps are present in the canines and posterior teeth. Canine have a single cusp, premolars generally have two cusps and molars have 4–5 cusps: (A) Maxillary teeth; (B) Mandibular teeth.

**Table 1.4:** Number of cusps in different types of teeth.

| Tooth type | Maxillary arch | Mandibular arch |
|---|---|---|
| *Incisors* | 0 | 0 |
| *Canines* | 1 | 1 |
| *Premolars* | 2 | 2 in first premolar 3 or 2 in second premolar |
| *Molars:* | | |
| First molar | 4 + 1 accessory cusp (cusp of Carabelli) | 5 |
| Second molar | 4 | 4 |
| Third molar | 4 or 3 | 4 or 5 |

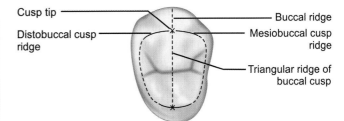

**Fig. 1.13:** Each cusp has a cusp tip and four ridges running down from the cusp tip. Cusp tip and four ridges of the buccal cusp of a premolar tooth are shown here.

in the posterior teeth and the canines. The number of cusps present in different types of teeth is listed in **Table 1.4**.

- Canine teeth have a single cusp; they are often called as the *cuspids.*
- Premolars generally have two cusps with an exception of the mandibular second premolar which frequently has three cusps. Premolars are therefore also called as the *bicuspids.*
- Maxillary and mandibular first molars have five cusps, while other molars generally have four cusps.

Each cusp is a gothic pyramid with four sides formed by four ridges that run down from the cusp tip **(Fig. 1.13)**:

- Mesial and distal cusp ridges
- Buccal or lingual cusp ridge
- Triangular ridge of the cusp

There are two cusp slopes on either side of the triangular ridge. In case of canines, there is a *labial ridge* analogous to the buccal ridge of posterior teeth; there is a lingual ridge analogous to triangular ridge of posterior teeth.

## Tubercle (Fig. 1.14)

It is a smaller elevation on some portion of the crown produced by an extra formation of enamel. A tubercle may be found on the lingual surface of a maxillary lateral incisor.

## Cingulum (Figs. 1.15A and B)

Cingulum (Latin word for "girdle") is a mound on the cervical third of the lingual surfaces of anterior teeth.

It develops from the lingual lobe of anteriors and makes up the major bulk of cervical third of the crown lingually.

Cingulum resembles a girdle encircling the lingual surface at the cervical third of the crown. It is present in all the anteriors and is most prominent on maxillary permanent canine.

### Anatomy

- The cingulum is smooth and convex both mesiodistally and cervicoincisally

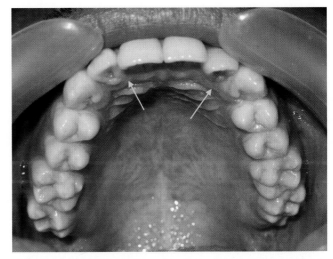

**Fig. 1.14:** Tubercle on lingual surface of the maxillary lateral incisor.

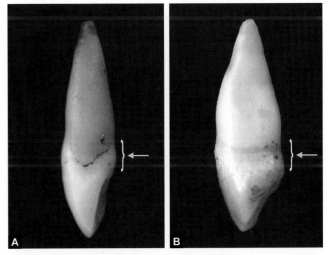

**Figs. 1.15A and B:** Cingulum is present only in anteriors and is most prominent on maxillary canine: (A) Maxillary central incisor; (B) Maxillary canine.

- It makes up the bulk of cervical third of the lingual surface
- Marginal ridges extend from cingulum forming the mesial and distal borders of the lingual fossa
- There is a concavity next to the cingulum incisally, called the *lingual fossa*
- Cingulum forms the cervical boundary of the lingual fossa
- Usually two developmental grooves extend from cingulum into the lingual fossa; especially on canines and maxillary incisors.

## Ridges

A ridge is any linear elevation on the surface of a tooth. It is named according to its location.

***Marginal ridge:*** All teeth have two marginal ridges; *mesial* and *distal.* These are rounded borders of enamel that form the mesial and distal margins of the occlusal surface of posterior teeth. In case of anteriors, the mesial and distal ridges form the mesial and distal margins of the lingual surfaces **(Fig. 1.16A)**.

***Buccal cusp ridge:*** It is a ridge on the buccal surface of a tooth that runs from the tip of a buccal cusp toward the cervical line. There is *labial ridge* in case of canines **(Fig. 1.16B)**.

***Lingual cusp ridge:*** It is a ridge on the lingual surface of a lingual cusp of premolar or molar tooth that runs from the cusp tip towards the cervical line. In case of canines, the lingual ridge runs on the lingual surface dividing the lingual fossa into two small fossae.

***Mesial and distal cusp ridges:*** Each cusp has mesial and distal cusp ridges on either side of its tip **(Fig. 1.16C)**.

***Triangular ridge:*** Triangular ridge is found on the occlusal surface of premolars and molars. It is the ridge that descends from each cusp tip towards the center of the occlusal surface of a posterior tooth **(Fig. 1.16D)**.

Triangular ridges are so named because the inclined planes on either side of the ridge resemble two sides of a triangle. They take the name of the cusp they belong to, e.g. triangular ridge of the buccal cusp of mandibular permanent first premolar.

***Transverse ridge:*** A transverse ridge is the union of two triangular ridges crossing the occlusal surface of a posterior tooth in a transverse (buccolingual) direction, e.g. transverse ridge between buccal and lingual cusps on premolar **(Fig. 1.16E)**.

***Oblique ridge:*** Oblique ridge is most prominent on permanent maxillary first molar **(Fig. 1.16F)**. It may be present on maxillary permanent second and third molars. It is also present in deciduous maxillary second molar.

***Cervical ridge:*** It is a ridge that runs mesiodistally on the cervical third of the buccal surface of the crown. Presence of cervical ridge is a characteristic feature of all primary teeth; most prominent on maxillary and mandibular primary first molars **(Fig. 1.16G)**. In permanent dentition, the cervical ridge is noticeable on the molar teeth.

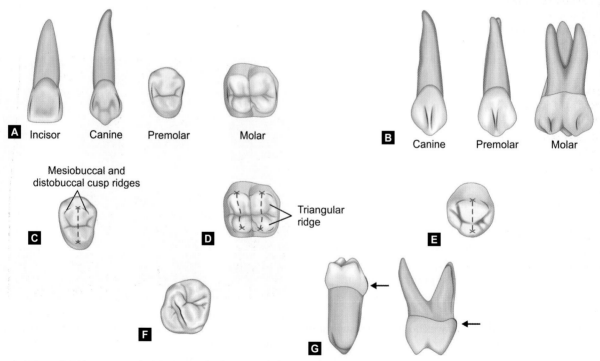

**Figs. 1.16A to G:** Ridges on teeth: (A) Marginal ridge; (B) Labial or buccal ridge; (C) Mesial and distal cusp ridge; (D) Triangular ridge; (E) Transverse ridge; (F) Oblique ridge; and (G) Cervical ridge.

## Lobe

A lobe is one of the primary sections of formation in the development of the crown. The minimum number of lobes involved in the development of a permanent tooth is four. All anterior teeth develop from four lobes; named as the *mesial, labial, distal,* and *lingual lobes* (**Fig. 1.17**). The lingual lobe forms the cingulum in these teeth.

All premolars except for the mandibular second premolar develop from four lobes; named as the *mesial, buccal, distal,* and *lingual lobes.* The mandibular second premolar often develops from five lobes; the *mesial, buccal, distal,*

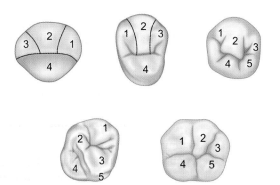

**Fig. 1.17:** All anteriors develop from 4 lobes. All premolars develop from 4 lobes, except mandibular second premolar which often develop from 5 lobes. Maxillary and mandibular first molars develop from 5 lobes. Other molars generally develop from 4 lobes.

**Table 1.5:** Number of lobes in different teeth.

| Tooth | No. of lobes | Names of lobes |
|---|---|---|
| Anteriors | 4 | Mesial, labial, distal, and lingual |
| *Premolars:* | | |
| Maxillary first and second premolar mandibular first premolar | 4 | Mesial, buccal, distal, and lingual |
| Mandibular second premolar | 5 | Mesial, buccal, distal, mesiolingual and distolingual |
| *Molars:* | | |
| Maxillary first molar | 5 | Mesiobuccal, distobuccal, mesiolingual, distolingual and fifth lobe |
| Maxillary second and third molar | 4 | Mesiobuccal, distobuccal, mesiolingual, and distolingual |
| Mandibular first molar | 5 | Mesiobuccal, distobuccal, distal, mesiolingual, and distolingual |
| Mandibular second and third molar | 4 | Mesiobuccal, distobuccal, mesiolingual, and distolingual (third molar can have 5 cusps from 5 lobes) |

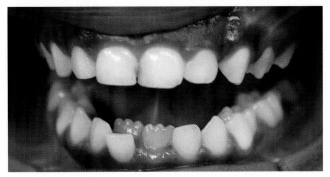

**Fig. 1.18:** Mamelons on erupting permanent incisor teeth. Primary incisors do not exhibit this feature.

*mesiolingual,* and *distolingual lobes.* The lingual lobe forms the lingual cusp in premolars.

The maxillary and mandibular first permanent molars develop from five lobes. All other molars develop from four lobes. Molar lobes are named same as the cusps. The tip of each cusp represents the primary center of formation of each lobe. The number of lobes in different teeth is listed in **Table 1.5.**

## Mamelons

Mamelons are the three rounded protuberances found on the incisal ridges of newly erupted incisor teeth (**Fig. 1.18**).

They represent the mesial, labial, and distal lobes of the incisor teeth. Mamelons soon disappear as the incisal ridges get worn away due to mastication. The mamelons are not seen in case of primary incisors.

## DEPRESSIONS ON THE TOOTH SURFACE

### Fossae

A fossa is a depression or concavity on the lingual surfaces of anteriors and occlusal surface of posterior teeth. A fossa is named according to its location or shape.

*Lingual fossa:* It is found on the lingual surfaces of anterior teeth (**Fig. 1.19A**). In case of canines, the lingual fossa may be divided into two small lingual fossae by the lingual ridge.

*Triangular fossae:* Found on the occlusal surface of all posterior teeth, mesial and distal to the marginal ridges (**Fig. 1.19B**). Base of the triangle is at the mesial or distal marginal ridge and the apex is at the mesial or distal pit.

*Central fossa:* It is found on the occlusal surface of molar teeth (**Fig. 1.19C**).

### Sulcus

A *sulcus* is a long depression or valley on the occlusal surface of the posterior teeth, the inclines of which meet at an angle.

*Developmental groove* is present at the bottom of a sulcus where the inclines meet.

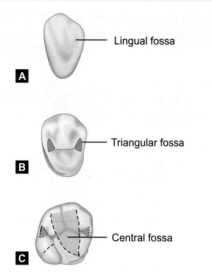

Figs. 1.19A to C: Fossae on various teeth: (A) Lingual fossa; (B) Triangular fossa; (C) Central fossa.

### Developmental Grooves

A developmental groove is a sharply defined groove or line separating the lobes or the primary parts of the crown or root, e.g. the *central developmental groove* running mesiodistally on the occlusal surface of a molar separates the buccal and lingual cusps **(Fig. 1.20)**.

A supplemental groove is a small irregular, less distinct line on occlusal surface of a tooth. It is supplemental to a developmental groove and does not mark the junction of primary parts of the tooth.

### Pit

Pits are small pinpoint depressions located at the junction of two or more developmental grooves or at the terminus of these grooves. They are named according to their location **(Fig. 1.21)**.

*Central pit:* It is a pit in the central fossa of molars where the developmental grooves meet.

*Buccal pit:* It is a pit on the buccal surface of a molar where the buccal developmental groove terminates.

*Lingual pit:* It is a pit on the lingual surface of a molar where the lingual developmental groove terminates. Lingual pit

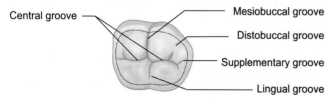

Fig. 1.20: Developmental grooves and supplementary grooves on occlusal surface of the teeth.

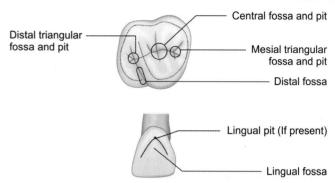

Fig. 1.21: Pits on occlusal surface of the teeth.

can also be seen on lingual surface of maxillary lateral incisors.

## LANDMARKS ON THE ROOT (FIG. 1.22)

### Root Trunk

Root trunk is present only in multirooted teeth. It is the undivided part of the root near the cervical line. Root trunk is very short and nearly absent in primary molars.

### Furcation

Furcation is the place on multirooted teeth where the root trunk divides into separate roots. Mandibular molars and maxillary first premolars are bifurcated while the maxillary molars are trifurcated.

### Apex of the Root

The apex of the root is the tip at the end of the root.

### Apical Foramen

The apical foramen is the opening at the apex of the root through which the nerves and blood vessels that supply the dental pulp enter the tooth. Thus it forms the channel

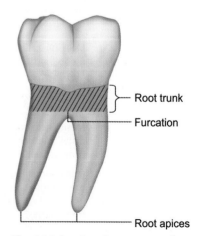

Fig. 1.22: Landmarks on root surface.

of communication between pulp and periodontal ligament space (*see* Chapter 14: Pulp Morphology in detail).

## ARBITRARY DIVISIONS OF CROWN AND ROOT INTO THIRDS (FIG. 1.23)

For descriptive purposes the surfaces of crowns and roots of teeth are arbitrarily divided into thirds. Such a division helps in describing the morphology of tooth.

### Divisions of Crown

The crown may be divided into thirds in three directions:
1. Mesiodistally
2. Cervico-occlusally or cervicoincisally
3. Faciolingually.

#### *Mesiodistally*

Mesiodistally, the crown is divided into:
- Mesial third

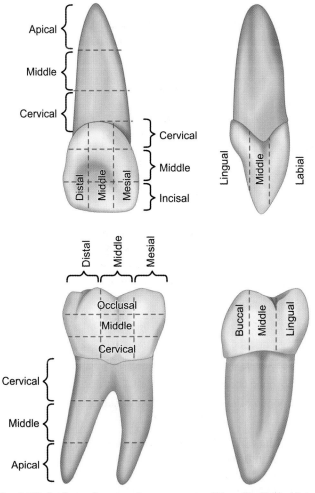

- Middle third
- Distal third.

#### *Cervico-occlusally or Cervicoincisally*

The crown is divided into:
- Incisal or occlusal third
- Middle third
- Cervical third.

#### *Faciolingually*

Faciolingually, the crown is divided into:
- Labial or buccal third
- Middle third
- Lingual third.

## DIVISIONS OF THE ROOT

Divisions of the root, mesiodistally and faciolingually, are exactly similar to that of the crown. Cervico-occlusally, the root may be divided into:
- Cervical third
- Middle third
- Apical third.

## LINE ANGLES AND POINT ANGLES ON THE CROWN

Most surfaces of the crown are spherical and no distinct angles can be made out on the tooth crown. The terms *line angle* and *point angle* are used for descriptive purpose to indicate a location and there are no actual angles on the crown.

Line and point angles can be understood easily by imagining a cube/box or a room. A line angle is formed where two walls meet and a point angle is formed where three walls meet.

### Line Angles (Figs. 1.24A and B, Table 1.6)

A line angle is formed by the junction of two surfaces. It is named from the combination of the two surfaces that join, e.g. the junction of mesial and buccal walls of a tooth is called the *mesiobuccal line angle*.

**Fig. 1.23:** Surface of root and crown are traditionally divided into thirds for descriptive purposes. It is a good practice to divide the wax block in thirds during carving exercises.

**Table 1.6:** Line angles.

| Line angles on anterior teeth | Line angles on posterior teeth |
| --- | --- |
| Mesiolabial | Mesiobuccal |
| Mesiolingual | Distobuccal |
| Distolabial | Mesiolingual |
| Distolingual | Distolingual |
| Labioincisal | Mesio-occlusal |
| Linguoincisal | Disto-occlusal |
| | Bucco-occlusal |
| | Linguo-occlusal |

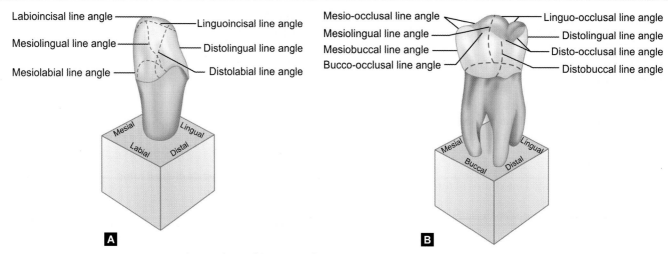

**Figs. 1.24A and B:** Line angles in: (A) Anterior; (B) Posterior teeth.

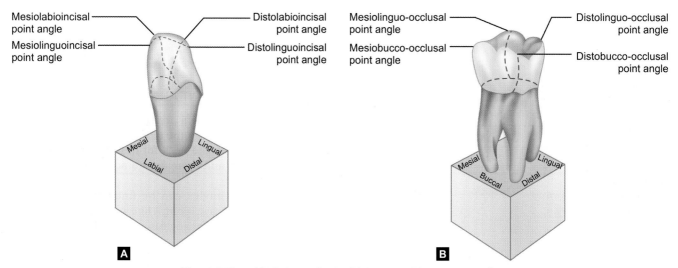

**Figs. 1.25A and B:** Point angles in: (A) Anterior; (B) Posterior teeth.

There are six line angles on an anterior tooth and eight line angles on a posterior tooth.

### Point Angles (Figs. 1.25A and B, Table 1.7)

A point angle is formed where three surfaces meet on the crown, and the name is derived from the same.

## MEASUREMENTS OF TEETH

The teeth are measured using eight calibrations for each tooth. Boley's gauge is used to measure various dimensions of a tooth such as crown length, root length, labiolingual diameter, and mesiodistal diameter of the crown, etc. The methods of measuring various dimensions of anterior and posterior teeth are given in **Boxes 1.2 and 1.3**.

**Table 1.8** Gives the average dimensions of permanent teeth. These average dimensions are used while caring the teeth.

**Table 1.7:** Point angles.

| Point angles on anterior teeth | Line angles on posterior teeth |
| --- | --- |
| Mesiolabioincisal | Mesiobucco-occlusal |
| Distolabioincisal | Distobucco-occlusal |
| Mesiolinguoincisal | Mesiolinguo-occlusal |
| Distolinguoincisal | Distolinguo-occlusal |

**Box 1.2: Methods of measuring anterior teeth.**

- Length of crown (labial)
  From—crest of curvature at cementoenamel junction
  To—incisal edge

- Length of root measurement
  From—apex
  To—crest of curvature at crown cervix

- Mesiodistal dimension of crown
  From—crest of curvature on the mesial surface (mesial contact area)
  To—crest of curvature on distal surface (distal contact area)

- Mesiodistal diameter of crown at cervix
  From—junction of crown and root on mesial surface
  To—junction of crown and root on distal surface

- Labiolingual diameter of crown
  From—crest of curvature on the labial surface
  To—crest of curvature on the lingual surface

- Labiolingual diameter of crown at cervix
  From—junction of crown and roof on the labial surface
  To—junction of crown and roof on the lingual surface

- Curvature of cementoenamel junction on mesial
  From—crest of curvature on cementoenamel junction an labial and lingual surfaces
  To—crest of curvature on cementoenamel junction on mesial surface

- Curvature of cementoenamel junction on distal
  From—crest of curvature on cementoenamel junction on labial and lingual surfaces
  To—crest of curvature on cementoenamel junction on distal surface

**Box 1.3: Methods of measuring posterior teeth.**

- Length of crown (buccal)
  From—crest of buccal cusp or cusps
  To—crest of curvature on cementoenamel junction

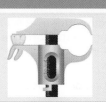

- Length of root
  From—crest of curvature at crown cervix
  To—apex of root

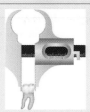

- Mesiodistal diameter of crown
  From—crest of curvature on the mesial surface (mesial contact area)
  To—crest of curvature on distal surface (distal contact area)

- Mesiodistal diameter of crown at cervix
  From—junction of crown and root on mesial surface
  To—junction of crown and root on distal surface

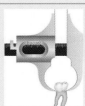

- Buccolingual diameter of crown
  From—crest of curvature on the buccal surface
  To—crest of curvature on the lingual surface

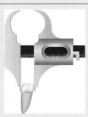

- Buccolingual diameter of crown at cervix
  From—junction of crown and root on buccal surface
  To—junction of crown and root on lingual surface

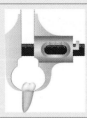

- Curvature of cementoenamel junction on mesial
  From—crest of curvature on cementoenamel junction on buccal and lingual surfaces
  To—crest of curvature on cementoenamel junction on mesial surface

- Curvature of cementoenamel junction on distal
  From—crest of curvature on cementoenamel junction on labial and lingual surfaces
  To—crest of curvature on cementoenamel junction on distal surface

**Table 1.8:** Measurements of teeth: Average dimensions for carving of teeth (in millimeters).*

| | Cervico-incisal length of crown | Length of root | Mesiodistal diameter of crown | Mesiodistal diameter of crown at cervix | Labiolingual diameter of crown | Labiolingual diameter of crown at cervix | Depth of curvature of cervical line on mesial | Depth of curvature of cervical line on distal |
|---|---|---|---|---|---|---|---|---|
| *Maxillary:* | | | | | | | | |
| Central incisor | 10.5 | 13.0 | 8.5 | 7.0 | 7.0 | 6.0 | 3.5 | 2.5 |
| Lateral incisor | 9.0 | 13.0 | 6.5 | 5.0 | 6.0 | 5.0 | 3.0 | 2.0 |
| Canine | 10.0 | 17.0 | 7.5 | 5.5 | 8.0 | 7.0 | 2.5 | 1.5 |
| First premolar | 8.5 | 14.0 | 7.0 | 5.0 | 9.0 | 8.0 | 1.0 | 0.0 |
| Second premolar | 8.5 | 14.0 | 7.0 | 5.0 | 9.0 | 8.0 | 1.0 | 0.0 |
| First molar | 7.5 | B-12 L-13 | 10.0 | 8.0 | 11.0 | 10.0 | 1.0 | 0.0 |
| Second molar | 7.0 | B-11 L-12 | 9.0 | 7.0 | 11.0 | 10.0 | 1.0 | 0.0 |
| *Mandibular:* | | | | | | | | |
| Central incisor | 9.0 | 12.5 | 5.0 | 3.5 | 6.0 | 5.3 | 3.0 | 2.0 |
| Lateral incisor | 9.5 | 14.0 | 5.5 | 4.0 | 6.5 | 5.8 | 3.0 | 2.0 |
| Canine | 11.0 | 16.0 | 7.0 | 5.5 | 7.5 | 7.0 | 2.5 | 1.0 |
| First premolar | 8.5 | 14.0 | 7.0 | 5.0 | 7.5 | 6.5 | 1.0 | 0.0 |
| Second premolar | 8.0 | 14.5 | 7.0 | 5.0 | 8.0 | 7.0 | 1.0 | 0.0 |
| First molar | 7.5 | 14.0 | 11.0 | 9.0 | 10.5 | 9.0 | 1.0 | 0.0 |
| Second molar | 7.0 | 13.0 | 10.5 | 8.0 | 10.0 | 9.0 | 1.0 | 0.0 |

*Compiled and modified from Ash MM, Nelson SJ (Eds). Wheeler's Dental Anatomy, Physiology and Occlusion, 8th edition. St Louis: Saunders; 2003.

## BIBLIOGRAPHY

1. Ash MM, Nelson SJ. Wheeler's Dental Anatomy, Physiology and Occlusion, 8th edition. Saunders: St Louis; 2003.
2. Brand RW, Isselhard DE. Anatomy of Orofacial Structures, 5th edition. CV Mosby: St Louis; 1994.
3. Kraus B, Jordan R, Abrams L. Dental Anatomy and Occlusion. Williams and Wilkins: Baltimore; 1969.
4. Sicher H, DuBrul EL. Oral Anatomy, 7th edition. CV Mosby: St Louis; 1975.
5. Woelfel JB, Scheid RC. Dental Anatomy: Its Relevance to Dentistry, 5th edition. Williams and Wilkins: Baltimore; 1997.

## MULTIPLE CHOICE QUESTIONS

1. The permanent teeth that are not succedaneous teeth in the strict sense are:
   a. Permanent incisors
   b. Permanent premolars
   c. Permanent canines
   d. Permanent molars
2. Dental formula for human deciduous dentition is:
   a. I2/2 C1/1 P2/2 M3/3
   b. I2/2 C 1/1 M3/3
   c. I2/2 C1/1 M2/2
   d. I2/2 C1/1 P1/1 M2/2
3. The only teeth that have their mesial surfaces facing each other are:
   a. Maxillary and mandibular third molars
   b. Maxillary and mandibular central incisors
   c. Maxillary and mandibular canines
   d. None of the above
4. The minimum number of lobes in the development of permanent tooth is:
   a. 5
   b. 3
   c. 4
   d. 2
5. The buccal cervical ridge is most prominent on:
   a. Permanent first molars
   b. Deciduous first molars
   c. Permanent second molars
   d. Deciduous second molars
6. The number of line angles and point angles on posterior teeth:
   a. 4 line angles and 4 point angles
   b. 6 line angles and 6 point angles
   c. 4 line angles and 6 point angles
   d. 6 line angles and 4 point angles
7. Which of the premolar teeth has two cusps of same height and width?
   a. Maxillary first premolar
   b. Maxillary second premolar

c. Mandibular first premolar
d. Mandibular second premolar

8. In maxillary permanent first molar, the cusp of Carabelli is located on:
   a. Mesiobuccal cusp
   b. Mesiolingual cusp
   c. Distobuccal cusp
   d. Distolingual cusp

9. Who and when described the cusp of Carabelli?
   a. George C Carabelli in 1842
   b. Carabelli Maxwell in 1800

c. Donald in 1900
d. Phillip in 1616

10. Cusp of Carabelli is a:
    a. Functional cusp
    b. Nonfunctional cusp
    c. Fifth cusp
    d. Both B and C

**Answers**

1. d    2. c    3. b    4. c    5. b    6. d    7. b    8. b
9. a    10. d

# Tooth Notation Systems

## INTRODUCTION

When one enters any new field of study, it is important to learn the particular language of that field. For more than 130 years, several systems for designating and encoding teeth have been in use. Tooth numbering systems have been developed in order to have a standard way of referring to particular teeth.

When identifying a specific tooth, one has to list the dentition, dental arch, quadrant and the tooth name. Listing all these information in words, while referring to each of 52 teeth (20 primary and 32 permanent) becomes cumbersome and time consuming.

For example, speaking, writing or typing permanent maxillary right central incisor (37 letters and 5 words) is more taxing than referring to the same tooth as "11" (one-one) in Federation Dentaire Internationale (FDI) numbering system. Tooth notation acts like a dental "short hand" providing a standard and an easy way of communication among dental professionals, students and care providers. It also gives a convenient method of record keeping in dental practice. It is important for anthropologists also to be familiar with the tooth-coding systems.

Although, there have been more than 32 different tooth notation systems, three systems are commonly in use and they are discussed in this chapter. It is necessary to be familiar with all the three popular systems so that communication between dental offices is efficient. However, it is important to stick to one notation system in a dental practice so as to avoid confusion. Also, it is important to specify which system is used.

For example, "# 11" (read as "eleven") in universal system refers to the permanent maxillary left canine. While 11 (read as "one-one") in FDI system refers to the permanent maxillary right central incisor.

The following are the three tooth notation systems that are in common use:
1. Universal numbering system

2. Zsigmondy-Palmer notation system
3. FDI system.

Universal system is widely used in United States. Zsigmondy-Palmer notation is the oldest system in use. Although superseded by the FDI system in most countries it continues to be used in UK and many parts of Asia. Internationally, the two-digit FDI system is widely used.

Some of the other tooth notation systems that were in use are listed here:
- The Dane or Haderup system
- The Reverse numeration system
- The Latin numeral system
- The Metcalf system
- The Bosworth system
- The Crow system
- The US army system
- The US navy system
- The Lowlands system
- The Holland system
- The South African system
- The French system
- The Dutch system
- The Cincinnati system.

Most of these numbering systems are of only historical value now. Among these, the Haderup system was popular in Norway, Sweden, Denmark, Finland and Ireland. It was practically the only system used in these countries for some decades after its introduction in 1891.

## UNIVERSAL NOTATION SYSTEM (BOX 2.1)

Universal numbering system was first proposed by *Parreidt* in 1882. It was officially adopted by the *American Dental Association (ADA)* in 1975. It is still widely used by dentists in USA and also endorsed by the *American Society of Forensic Odontology*.

Today the universal system for tooth-coding is an interesting misnomer, because it is only used in the United States. The universal system uses continuous numbers and letters to denote each tooth. Numbering is done clockwise beginning with the last tooth in the upper right quadrant and ends with the last tooth in the lower right quadrant.

**Box 2.1: Universal tooth notation system.**

*Permanent teeth*

Right                                                  Left

| 1 | 2 | 3 | 4 | 5 | 6 | 7 | 8 | 9 | 10 | 11 | 12 | 13 | 14 | 15 | 16 |
|---|---|---|---|---|---|---|---|---|----|----|----|----|----|----|----|
| 32 | 31 | 30 | 29 | 28 | 27 | 26 | 25 | 24 | 23 | 22 | 21 | 20 | 19 | 18 | 17 |

*Primary teeth*

Right                                                  Left

| A | B | C | D | E | F | G | H | I | J |
|---|---|---|---|---|---|---|---|---|---|
| T | S | R | Q | P | O | N | M | L | K |

*Examples:*
Upper right permanent central incisor = #8
Lower left primary second molar = #K

The numbers, 1–32 are used to denote the permanent teeth; English alphabets, A to T in upper case are used to denote the primary teeth.

## Universal Notation for Permanent Teeth (Figs. 2.1A and B)

Numbers 1–32 are used to denote teeth in permanent dentition.

The numbering begins from the posterior most tooth in the upper right quadrant, i.e. the maxillary third molar, which is designated as tooth "#1". Numbering goes in a clockwise direction.

The count continues along the upper teeth to the left side, so that left maxillary third molar is designated as "#16".

After descending down to mandibular third molar, tooth "#17", numbering continuous along the mandibular arch and ends at the last tooth in mandibular right quadrant, the mandibular right third molar as tooth "#32".

- One must remember that notation charts traditionally are printed in *dentist's view*. In other words, patient's right side corresponds to tooth chart's left side. To put it simply, *always visualize a patient's dentition in front of you while designating teeth in any system.*
- It helps to remember that "#1", "#16", "#17", "#32" are third molars and "#8", "#9", "#24" and "#25" are central incisors.

## Universal Notation for Primary Teeth (Figs. 2.2A and B)

The universal notation system for primary dentition uses upper case English letters for each of primary teeth. The maxillary teeth are designated as letters "A" through "J", beginning with right maxillary second molar.

- For mandibular teeth, letters "K" through "T" are used, beginning with the left mandibular second molar.
- It helps to remember that A, J, K, T are second molars (at distal ends quadrants) and E, F, O, P are central incisors.

## Advantages of Universal Numbering System

- Concept is very simple.
- Each tooth has a unique numerical or an alphabetical code.
- Left and right teeth of same type have different designations, e.g. permanent right maxillary 1st molar is "#3" while permanent left maxillary first molar is "'#14".
- It can be communicated verbally.
- It is compatible with computer keyboard and easy for typing.

## Disadvantages

- Difficult to memorize the notation of each tooth.
- Needs practice. Difficult to visualize graphically.

## ZSIGMONDY-PALMER SYSTEM/SYMBOLIC SYSTEM/QUADRANT SYSTEM/GRID SYSTEM/ANGULAR SYSTEM (BOX 2.2)

The Zsigmondy-Palmer notation system is the oldest method in use and the most popular system for much of the 20th century. The Zsigmondy-Palmer system was recommended

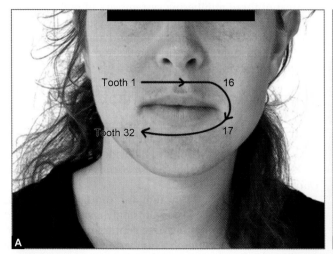

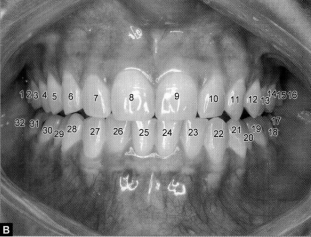

**Figs. 2.1A and B:** (A) Universal notation for permanent teeth; (B) The numbers from 1–32 are used in a clockwise manner beginning from upper right most tooth.

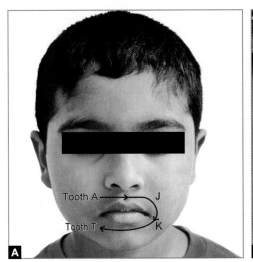

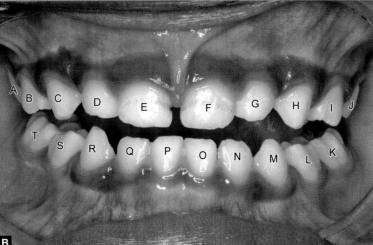

**Figs. 2.2A and B:** Universal notation for primary teeth. English alphabets from A to T are used in a clockwise direction.

**Box 2.2: Zsigmondy-Palmer tooth notation system.**

*Permanent teeth*

| Right | | | | | | | | | | | | | | | Left |
|---|---|---|---|---|---|---|---|---|---|---|---|---|---|---|---|
| 8 | 7 | 6 | 5 | 4 | 3 | 2 | 1 | 1 | 2 | 3 | 4 | 5 | 6 | 7 | 8 |
| 8 | 7 | 6 | 5 | 4 | 3 | 2 | 1 | 1 | 2 | 3 | 4 | 5 | 6 | 7 | 8 |

*Primary teeth*

| Right | | | | | | | | | | Left |
|---|---|---|---|---|---|---|---|---|---|---|
| E | D | C | B | A | A | B | C | D | E |
| E | D | C | B | A | A | B | C | D | E |

*Examples:*
Permanent upper right central incisor = 1⌋
Primary lower left second molar = |Ē

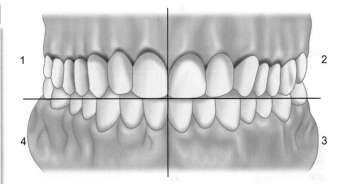

**Fig. 2.3:** Facsimile of a diagram by Palmer, 1891 showing the division of the dentition into four quadrants. The patient's quadrants are: 1. Upper right, 2. Upper left, 3. Lower left, 4. Lower right.

as the numbering system of choice by a committee at the ADA in 1947. However, with the move from written dental notes to electronic/computer records, difficulties were encountered in reproducing the "symbols" with standard computer keyboard. Thus, ADA later officially recommended universal notation system, which is still the widely used method in United States.

The symbolic notation system was originally termed the Zsigmondy system after the Hungarian (Vienna) dentist *Adolf Zsigmondy,* who developed the idea in 1861, using a *Zsigmondy cross* grid to record quadrants of tooth positions. He then modified the system for denoting primary dentition in 1874.

An Ohio dentist *Corydon Palmer* also invented the system independently in 1870. The system then, came to be known as Zsigmondy-Palmer system. However, it is simply called the Palmer system in most English speaking countries.

In this system, the mouth is divided into four sections called the *quadrants* **(Fig. 2.3)**. The system uses a unique "L" shaped symbol/grid, ( ⌐, ¬, ∟, ⌐ ) to depict in which quadrant

the specific tooth is found. These four symbols remain same for both permanent and deciduous dentitions. The vertical line segment of the "symbol" indicates the patient's midline and the horizontal line indicates the occlusal plane that separates the upper and lower arches. The numbers/letters indicate the position of the tooth from the midline.

The counting always begins at the midline and progresses backwards. Numbers 1 through 8 are used to denote the permanent teeth in each quadrant. For primary teeth the upper case English letters "A" through "E" are used.

**Table 2.1** gives the quadrant symbols and tooth codes used in Palmer system for both permanent and primary dentitions.

### Zsigmondy-Palmer Notation for Permanent Teeth (Figs. 2.4A and B)

- Permanent teeth are numbered 1–8 in each quadrant.
- The numbering begins from the midline and moves backwards. Thus, "1" is a central incisor, "3" is a canine, "4" and "5" are premolars and "8" is a third molar.

**Table 2.1:** Quadrant symbols and tooth codes used in Palmer system for permanent and primary dentitions.

| Quadrant symbols (same for both dentitions) | | Tooth codes | | | |
|---|---|---|---|---|---|
| | | Permanent teeth | | Primary teeth | |
| Upper right quadrant | ⌐ | 1 | Central incisor | A | Central incisor |
| Upper left quadrant | ⌐ | 2 | Lateral incisor | B | Lateral incisor |
| Lower right quadrant | ⌐ | 3 | Canine | C | Canine |
| Lower left quadrant | ⌐ | 4 | First premolar | D | First molar |
| | | 5 | Second premolar | E | Second molar |
| | | 6 | First molar | | |
| | | 7 | Second molar | | |
| | | 8 | Third molar | | |

- The symbol indicates the quadrant in which the specific tooth is found and the number indicates the position of the tooth from the midline.
- Individual teeth are represented by writing the specific tooth number inside the symbol of that quadrant.

### Zsigmondy-Palmer Notation for Primary Teeth (Figs. 2.5A and B)

The quadrant symbols are same as that used for the permanent dentition.

The upper case English letters A to E are used to represent the primary teeth in each quadrant.

Numbering begins at midline and progresses backward so that A is a central incisor, C is a canine and E is a second molar.

- Individual teeth are denoted by placing the letter of specific tooth inside the quadrant symbol.

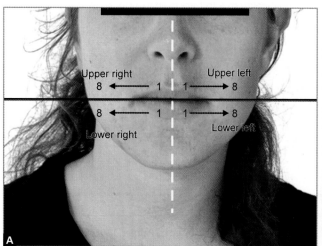
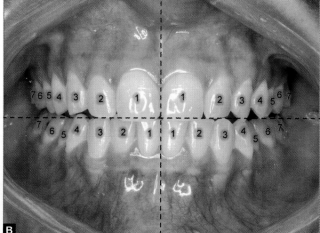

**Figs. 2.4A and B:** Zsigmondy-Palmer system for permanent dentition. Mouth is divided into four quadrants. Permanent teeth are numbered 1–8 in each quadrant beginning from midline proceeding backward.

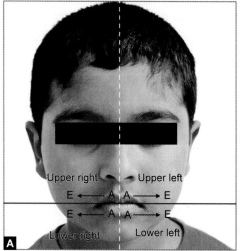
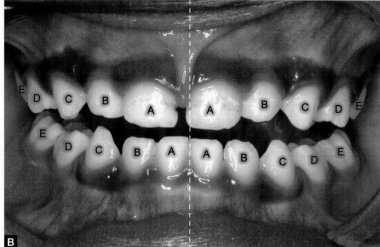

**Figs. 2.5A and B:** Zsigmondy-Palmer system for primary dentition. Mouth is divided into four quadrants. Primary teeth are given A to E in each quadrant beginning from midline proceeding backward.

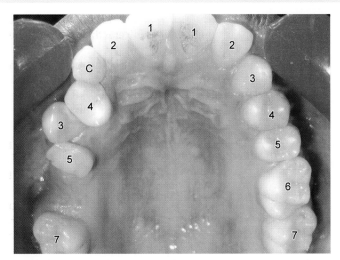

**Fig. 2.6:** A major advantage of Zsigmondy-Palmer system is that it permits graphical representation of any anomalies, missing teeth, etc. For example, 7 5 3 4 C 2 1 | 1 2 3 4 5 6 7
*Note:* Retained primary canine and buccally erupted permanent canine between premolars.

## Advantages

- One major advantage of Zsigmondy-Palmer notation is that, it produces a very graphical image, akin to a "map" of dentition. Thus, any anomalies like tooth transposition, edentulous spaces, can be easily represented using Zsigmondy cross **(Fig. 2.6)**.
- It is simple to follow and user friendly.
- Quadrant symbols are same for both the dentitions.

## Disadvantages

The major drawback of symbolic system is that, it is generally incompatible with computers and word processing systems. It is difficult to create the symbol using standard keyboard.

It is difficult to use this system for verbal communication. For instance, if one has to communicate "permanent maxillary right central incisor", it is not possible to verbally pronounce the tooth designation⌐1⌐.

Though the method is simple, there are more chances of error while designating the side of the tooth.

## FDI NOTATION SYSTEM/TWO-DIGIT SYSTEM/ISO NOTATION/INTERNATIONAL NUMBERING SYSTEM (BOX 2.3)

Since the above discussed methods did not comply with the requirements set by *FDI World Dental Federation,* the organization introduced its own two-digit system in 1970. This system was developed by a "Special Committee on Uniform Dental Recording" and passed as a resolution of the FDI General Assembly at its 1970 meeting in Bucharest, Romania.

---

**Box 2.3: FDI tooth notation system.**

*Permanent teeth*

| Right | | | | | | | | Left | | | | | | | |
|---|---|---|---|---|---|---|---|---|---|---|---|---|---|---|---|
| 18 | 17 | 16 | 15 | 14 | 13 | 12 | 11 | 21 | 22 | 23 | 24 | 25 | 26 | 27 | 28 |
| 48 | 47 | 46 | 45 | 44 | 43 | 42 | 41 | 31 | 32 | 33 | 34 | 35 | 36 | 37 | 38 |

*Primary teeth*

| Right | | | | | Left | | | | |
|---|---|---|---|---|---|---|---|---|---|
| 55 | 54 | 53 | 52 | 51 | 61 | 62 | 63 | 64 | 65 |
| 85 | 84 | 83 | 82 | 81 | 71 | 72 | 73 | 74 | 75 |

*Examples:*
Permanent upper right central incisor = 11, pronounced "one-one"
Primary lower left second molar = 75, pronounced as "seven-five"

---

While the FDI labeled, this *"Two-digit system"*, it became commonly known as the *"FDI system".* According to the FDI committee, five criteria are met by the two-digit system. They are:

1. Simple to understand and teach
2. Easy to pronounce in conversation of dictation
3. Readily communicable in print
4. Easy to translate into computer output
5. Easily adapted to standard charts used in general practice.

The FDI two-digit system is now being used internationally and is the most accepted method. The two-digit system has been adopted by the *World Health Organization (WHO)* and accepted by the other organizations such as the *International Association for Dental Research (IADR)*. It is the only method that makes visual, cognitive and computer sense.

The FDI committee combined the Zsigmondy-Palmer's tooth numbering system with the prefix number to denote the quadrant thereby removing the computer nonfriendly grid/symbol.

The FDI system uses *two-digit*s for each tooth—permanent and primary.

- *The first-digit always denotes the quadrant:* Each quadrant is assigned a number 1–4 for the permanent dentition and 5–8 for the primary dentition. The quadrant code denotes the dentition, arch and side in which the tooth is present.
- The second digit denotes the tooth (1–8 for permanent teeth and 1–5 for deciduous teeth). The teeth are numbered from midline to posterior. The two-digit combination of quadrant code and tooth code gives the notation of a specific tooth.

**Table 2.2** gives the quadrant and tooth codes used in FDI system for permanent and primary dentitions.

### FDI Notation for Permanent Dentition (Figs. 2.7A and B)

The mouth is divided into four quadrants. The first digit represents the quadrant. The quadrants in permanent

**Table 2.2:** Quadrant codes and tooth codes used in FDI system for permanent and primary dentitions.

| Quadrant codes (First digit) | | Tooth codes (Second digit) | |
|---|---|---|---|
| Permanent teeth | Primary teeth | Permanent dentition | Primary dentition |
| 1. Upper right | 5. Upper right | 1. Central incisor | 1. Central incisor |
| 2. Upper left | 6. Upper left | 2. Lateral incisor | 2. Lateral incisor |
| 3. Lower left | 7. Lower left | 3. Canine | 3. Canine |
| 4. Lower right | 8. Lower right | 4. First premolar | 4. 1st molar |
| | | 5. Second premolar | 5. Second molar |
| | | 6. First molar | |
| | | 7. Second molar | |
| | | 8. Third molar | |

dentition are numbered 1–4 in a clockwise manner such that, 1 is upper right, 2 is upper left, 3 is lower left, 4 is lower right quadrant.

The second digit represents the type of the tooth denoted in the quadrant. Each quadrant in permanent dentition has 8 teeth. They are designated with numbers 1–8, beginning from the midline such that, 1s are central incisors, 3s are canines, 6s are 1st molars, etc.

*Note that two digits are always pronounced separately.* For example, "16'" denoting permanent maxillary right first molar is spelt as "one-six" and not as "sixteen".

### FDI Notation for Primary Dentition (Figs. 2.8A and B)

The first digit designated as 5–8 indicates primary dentition quadrants in a clockwise manner.

Here, the second digit denoted by numbers 1–5 indicates teeth from the midline.

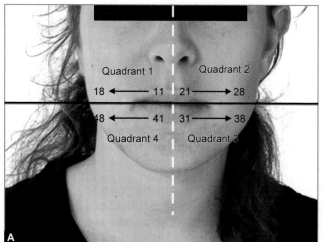

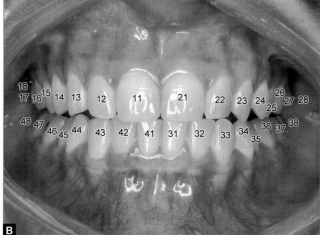

**Figs. 2.7A and B:** FDI notation for permanent dentition. The four quadrants are assigned the unique numbers. First digit 1–4 represents quadrant; second digit represents specific tooth in quadrant. (*Note:* Third molars are not visible in the image)

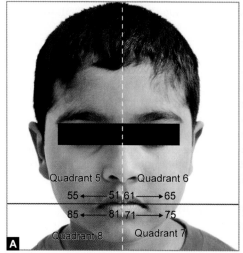

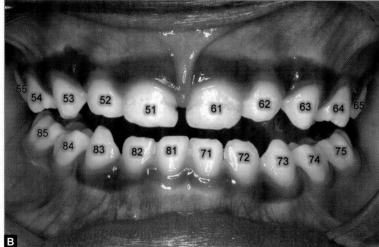

**Figs. 2.8A and B:** FDI notation for primary dentition. The four quadrants are assigned the unique numbers. First digit 5–8 represents quadrant; second digit 1–5 represents specific tooth in quadrant.

**Table 2.3:** Comparison of various tooth identification systems.

| | | Universal | | Zsigmondy/Palmer notation | | Federation Dentaire Internationale (FDI) | |
|---|---|---|---|---|---|---|---|
| | **Tooth** | **Right** | **Left** | **Right** | **Left** | **Right** | **Left** |
| Deciduous dentition — Maxillary teeth | Central incisor | E | F | A⌋ | ⌊A | 51 | 61 |
| | Lateral incisor | D | G | B⌋ | ⌊B | 52 | 62 |
| | Canine | C | H | C⌋ | ⌊C | 53 | 63 |
| | 1st molar | B | I | D⌋ | ⌊D | 54 | 64 |
| | 2nd molar | A | J | E⌋ | ⌊E | 55 | 65 |
| Deciduous dentition — Mandibular teeth | Central incisor | P | O | A⌉ | ⌈A | 81 | 71 |
| | Lateral incisor | Q | N | B⌉ | ⌈B | 82 | 72 |
| | Canine | R | M | C⌉ | ⌈C | 83 | 73 |
| | 1st molar | S | L | D⌉ | ⌈D | 83 | 74 |
| | 2nd molar | T | K | E⌉ | ⌈E | 85 | 75 |
| Permanent dentition — Maxillary teeth | Central incisor | 8 | 9 | 1⌋ | ⌊1 | 11 | 21 |
| | Lateral incisor | 7 | 10 | 2⌋ | ⌊2 | 12 | 22 |
| | Canine | 6 | 11 | 3⌋ | ⌊3 | 13 | 23 |
| | 1st premolar | 5 | 12 | 4⌋ | ⌊4 | 14 | 24 |
| | 2nd premolar | 4 | 13 | 5⌋ | ⌊5 | 15 | 25 |
| | 1st molar | 3 | 14 | 6⌋ | ⌊6 | 16 | 26 |
| | 2nd molar | 2 | 15 | 7⌋ | ⌊7 | 17 | 27 |
| | 3rd molar | 1 | 16 | 8⌋ | ⌊8 | 18 | 28 |
| Permanent dentition — Mandibular teeth | Central incisor | 25 | 24 | 1⌉ | ⌈1 | 41 | 31 |
| | Lateral incisor | 26 | 23 | 2⌉ | ⌈2 | 42 | 32 |
| | Canine | 27 | 22 | 3⌉ | ⌈3 | 43 | 33 |
| | 1st premolar | 28 | 21 | 4⌉ | ⌈4 | 44 | 34 |
| | 2nd premolar | 29 | 20 | 5⌉ | ⌈5 | 45 | 35 |
| | 1st molar | 30 | 19 | 6⌉ | ⌈6 | 46 | 36 |
| | 2nd molar | 31 | 18 | 7⌉ | ⌈7 | 47 | 37 |
| | 3rd molar | 32 | 17 | 8⌉ | ⌈8 | 48 | 38 |

## Advantages

- Internationally followed system in most parts of the world.
- It is the only method that makes visual, cognitive and computer sense.
- It can be used for verbal communication.
- Easy to type and print and it is suitable for computer processing. It can be easily incorporated into dental software.
- It helps to prevent errors when differentiating between right and left sides of mouth or between upper and lower dental arches.

The comparison of the tooth designation in all three systems is described in **Table 2.3**.

## BIBLIOGRAPHY

1. American Dental Association, Committee on Nomenclature: Committee adopts official method for the symbolic designation of teeth. J Am Dent Assoc. 1947;34:647.
2. Federation Dentaire Internationale. Two Digit system of designating teeth. Int Dent J. 1971; 34:312.
3. Keiser-Nielsen N. Two-digit system of designating teeth. Br Dent J. 1971;21:104-6.
4. Peck S, Peck L. A time for change of tooth numbering systems. J Dent Educ. 1993;57:643-7.
5. Zsigmondy A. A practical method for rapidly noting dental observations and operations. Br J Dent Sci. 1874;17:580.

## MULTIPLE CHOICE QUESTIONS

1. Who and when was the Universal tooth numbering system reported?
   a. Parreidt in 1882
   b. Dane in 1782
   c. Palmar in 1880
   d. Haderup in 1682

2. According to universal tooth numbering system, the alphabets used to designate teeth in deciduous dentition are:
   a. 1–32
   b. A–T
   c. I–XX
   d. All of the above

3. According to Universal tooth numbering system the tooth denote universal number by #1:
   a. Maxillary permanent right central incisor
   b. Mandibular permanent right central incisor
   c. Maxillary permanent right third molar
   d. Mandibular permanent right third molar

4. According to Universal tooth numbering system the tooth denote universal number #27:
   a. Maxillary permanent left second molar
   b. Mandibular permanent right canine
   c. Maxillary permanent left canine
   d. Mandibular permanent left second molar

5. According to Universal tooth numbering system, denote universal number #F:
   a. Maxillary deciduous left central incisor
   b. Maxillary deciduous second molar
   c. Maxillary deciduous right first molar
   d. Maxillary deciduous right central incisor

6. Who and when Zsigmondy-Palmer notation was reported:
   a. Adolph Zsigmondy in 1861
   b. Zsigmondy in 1850
   c. Palmer in 1870
   d. Both a and b

7. Numerical used for permanent dentition in Zigmondy-Palmer notation are:
   a. 1–8
   b. 9–16
   c. 17–24
   d. 25–32

8. According to Zsigmondy-Palmer notation teeth in deciduous dentition are represented by:
   a. 1–8
   b. A–E
   c. Both of the above
   d. None of the above

9. Which of the following is a major disadvantage of Zsigmondy/Palmer notation system?
   a. Difficult in verbal communication
   b. Tedious to write using computers
   c. More chances of errors
   d. Not commonly used system

10. In FDI system, first and second digit denotes:
    a. Quadrant and tooth
    b. Tooth and quadrant
    c. Both of the above
    d. None of the above

**Answers**

1. a    2. b    3. c    4. b    5. a    6. d    7. a    8. b
9. b    10. a

# 2

## SECTION

# Chronology of Tooth Development and Form and Function

### Section Outline

3. Chronology of Tooth Development
4. Form and Function of Orofacial Complex

# Chronology of Tooth Development

## INTRODUCTION

Humans have two sets of teeth namely, the primary/deciduous dentition and the secondary/permanent dentition, which contain 20 and 32 teeth respectively. In both the dentitions, not all the teeth are formed and appear in oral cavity at the same time. Some teeth are completed before others are formed, resulting in different times of eruption for different groups of teeth. Groups of teeth develop at specific rates so that the sequence of their appearance into oral cavity is well defined, although with few variations.

The enamel organ, dental papilla and dental sac together constitute a *tooth bud or tooth germ.* Ten such tooth germs arise in each dental arch to form the primary dentition. Tooth germs that give rise to permanent successors (i.e. the permanent incisors, canines and premolars) develop on the lingual aspect of their deciduous predecessors in the same bony crypt, by lingual proliferation of dental lamina called the *successional lamina.* The permanent molar tooth germs, which have no deciduous predecessors, develop from the *distal extension of the dental lamina/accessional lamina* when the jaws grow long enough **(Figs. 3.1A and B)**.

A thorough knowledge of development of teeth and timing and pattern of their eruption is essential for all clinical fields of dentistry. For example, an understanding of development of teeth, jaws and skull as a whole is essential for orthodontic treatment of malocclusions. It is imperative to know developmental chronology of secondary teeth so as to avoid injury to the developing tooth germs especially during the early surgical treatment of cleft palate.

It is also important to understand the effects of certain diseases and environmental factors on the development of teeth. For example, *amelogenesis imperfecta* **(Fig. 3.2A)** and *dentinogenesis imperfecta* **(Fig. 3.2B)** are genetic conditions that cause structural defects in teeth. Calcium deficiency and syphilis in expectant mothers causing congenital defects in the child's teeth are examples of environmental factors that affect development of teeth.

Ingestion of drinking water that contains excessive fluoride content during the formative years of teeth may lead to defective enamel formation. The affected teeth show yellow/brownish spots on teeth or pitted enamel, and the condition is known as *fluorosis* **(Fig. 3.3)**.

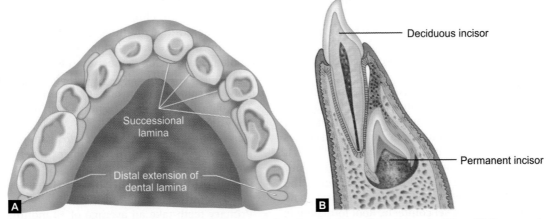

**Figs. 3.1A and B:** (A) Dental lamina gives rise to 10 teeth in each dental arch to form the primary dentition; (B) Permanent successors develop from successional lamina on lingual aspect of their predecessor teeth.

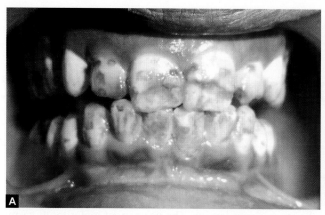 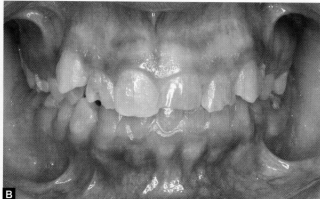

**Figs. 3.2:** (A) Amelogenesis imperfecta; (B) Dentinogenesis imperfecta.

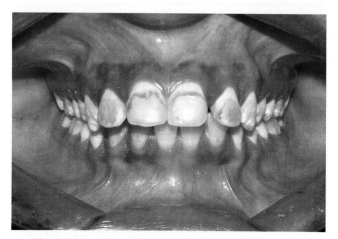

**Fig. 3.3:** Enamel mottling caused due to dental fluorosis.

## ERUPTION AND EMERGENCE OF TEETH

Tooth eruption is a developmental process in which, the tooth moves in an axial direction from its anatomical position within the alveolar crypt of the jaw into its functional position within the oral cavity. The term *"eruption"* has thus come to mean a continuous process of tooth movement from within its socket until it reaches the final functional position.

The actual *emergence* of the tooth into oral cavity, when it breaks through the gum, is only one phase of eruption. Tooth eruption is a continuous process while its emergence through the mucous membrane is a single event.

In the chronology charts and in discussions about dental age the term *"eruption"* is used interchangeably with the term *"emergence"*. The eruptive movement continues after the incidence of emergence, and eventually the tooth comes into occlusion with the teeth in opposite arch. Even then it continues to erupt to compensate for occlusal wear (attrition).

Eruption of tooth begins soon after completion of the crown. When the tooth reaches the functional occlusal plane the root development is not yet complete. Root formation is usually completed 1–3 years after the eruption of the tooth.

## CHRONOLOGY OF TOOTH DEVELOPMENT

Humans have three stages of dentition—primary, mixed/transitional and permanent. **Figures 3.4A and B** graphically depict the development of primary and permanent human dentitions.

The important developmental events that are recorded in the chronology chart are:
- First evidence of calcification
- Crown completion
- Emergence (eruption) through mucosa into oral cavity
- Root completion.

## PRIMARY DENTITION STAGE

Usually there are no teeth present in the mouth at birth. However, occasionally infants may be born with erupted mandibular incisors, which are called the *natal teeth*. Primary dentition stage begins at around 6 months of age when the first primary teeth, generally the mandibular central incisors erupt into oral cavity **(Fig. 3.5)**. Primary dentition stage lasts until the eruption of first permanent tooth around 6 years of age.

### Chronology of Primary Dentition

**Table 3.1** gives the chronology of primary teeth. It must be remembered that the times given in chronology table reflect approximate values since no two individuals will chronologically develop in precisely the same manner. Thus, considerable variation exists. Nonetheless, these tables are of immense value in diagnosing any abnormal development.

The following points may be noted from the chronology of primary dentition:
- *Development of primary teeth occurs both prenatally and postnatally*; whereas the development of permanent teeth is entirely postnatal
- Crowns of primary teeth begin to calcify between 4 months and 6 months of intrauterine life
- Primary teeth take an average of 10 months for crown completion

Deciduous dentition

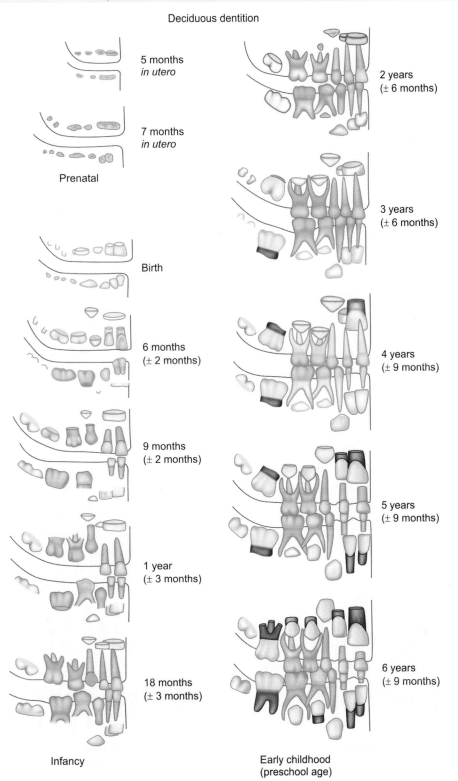

5 months
*in utero*

7 months
*in utero*

Prenatal

Birth

6 months
(± 2 months)

9 months
(± 2 months)

1 year
(± 3 months)

18 months
(± 3 months)

Infancy

2 years
(± 6 months)

3 years
(± 6 months)

4 years
(± 9 months)

5 years
(± 9 months)

6 years
(± 9 months)

Early childhood
(preschool age)

**Fig. 3.4A:** Development of human dentitions—primary dentition stage.
*Source:* Schour L, Massler M. The development of the human dentition. J Am Dent Assoc. 1941;28:1153.

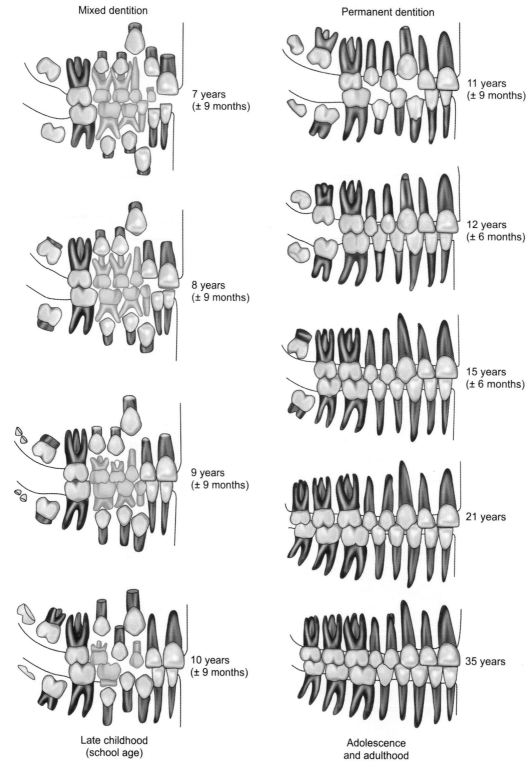

Mixed dentition

7 years (± 9 months)

8 years (± 9 months)

9 years (± 9 months)

10 years (± 9 months)

Late childhood (school age)

Permanent dentition

11 years (± 9 months)

12 years (± 6 months)

15 years (± 6 months)

21 years

35 years

Adolescence and adulthood

**Fig. 3.4B:** Mixed and permanent dentition stages

*Source:* Schour L, Massler M. The development of the human dentition. J Am Dent Assoc. 1941;28:1153.

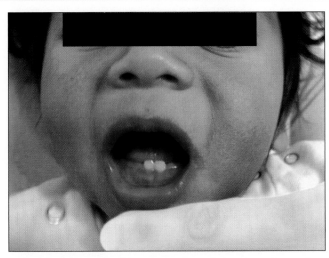

**Fig. 3.5:** Primary dentition stage generally begins at 6 months with emergence of mandibular central incisors.

- Primary teeth emerge into oral cavity some 6–8 months after the completion of their crown
- On an average, root completion occurs 1–2 years after the emergence of the crown
- Formation of primary teeth from initial calcification to root completion occurs in only 2–3 years (However, mineralization of permanent dentition takes about some 8–12 years, and is entirely postnatal).
- Emergence of primary dentition into oral cavity occurs between 6th and 30th month of age (postnatal)
- The mandibular central incisors are usually the first primary teeth to appear in mouth about 6 months of age
- It is followed by other incisors, so that by about 9–12 months, all the primary incisors have exposed

- Then the first primary molars emerge by about 12–16 months and establish contact with antagonistic teeth several months later, before the canines are fully erupted
- The primary canines emerge around at 16–20 months of age
- The last teeth to emerge are the maxillary second molars at the age of 20–30 months.

## Sequence of Emergence of Primary Teeth

Although some variation can occur, the predominant sequence of eruption of the primary teeth in each jaw is as follows:
- Central incisor (A)
- Lateral incisor (B)
- First molar (D)
- Canine (C)
- Second molars (E).

The lateral incisors, first molars and canines tend to erupt earlier in the maxilla than the mandible. The eruption sequence of primary dentition can be represented as follows:

$$\frac{AB \quad D \quad C \quad E}{A \quad B \quad D \quad CE}$$

## Primary Dentition Period

The primary dentition is considered to be completely established by about 30 months/2½ years of age or when the primary molars are in occlusion **(Fig. 3.6)**. All the teeth are in use from about 2 years to 2½ years until the age of 6–7 years, a total of up to 5 years. The primary molars and maxillary canines stay in the oral cavity up to 11–12 years. Premature loss or prolonged retention of primary teeth, especially that of the molars and canines often leads to development of malocclusion in the permanent dentition stage **(Fig. 3.7)**.

Although the primary teeth seem to serve for a relatively short period of time in one's life, they nevertheless are as

**Table 3.1:** Chronology of primary dentition.*

| Tooth | First evidence of calcification weeks in utero | Amount of enamel formed at birth | Crown completed | Eruption | Root completed |
|---|---|---|---|---|---|
| *Maxillary teeth* | | | | | |
| Central incisor | 14 | Five-sixths | 1½ months | 10 months | 1½ years |
| Lateral incisor | 16 | Two-thirds | 2½ months | 11 months | 2 years |
| Cuspid | 17 | One-third | 9 months | 19 months | 3½ years |
| 1st molar | 15½ | Cusps united | 6 months | 16 months | 2½ years |
| Second molar | 19 | Cusp tips still isolated | 11 months | 29 months | 3 years |
| *Mandibular teeth* | | | | | |
| Central incisor | 14 | Three-fifths | 2½ months | 8 months | 1½ years |
| Lateral incisor | 16 | Three-fifths | 3 months | 13 months | 1½ years |
| Cuspid | 17 | One-third | 9 months | 20 months | 3½ years |
| 1st molar | 15½ | Cusps united | 5½ months | 16 months | 2½ years |
| Second molar | 18 | Cusp tips still isolated | 10 months | 27 months | 3 years |

* Logan WHG, Kronfeld R. Development of the human jaws and surrounding structures from birth to the age of fifteen years. J Am Dent Assoc. 1933;20:379-427. (modified by McCall and Schour)

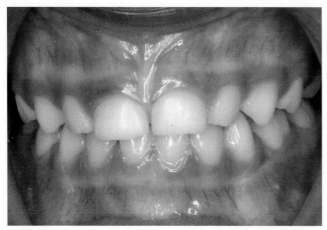

**Fig. 3.6:** Primary dentition is completely established when primary molars are in occlusion, generally by 30 months of age.

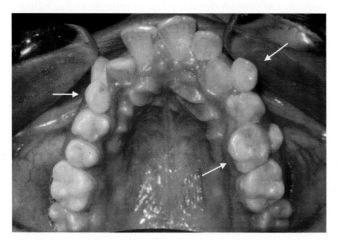

**Fig. 3.7:** Retained primary canines and second molars leading to malocclusion development.

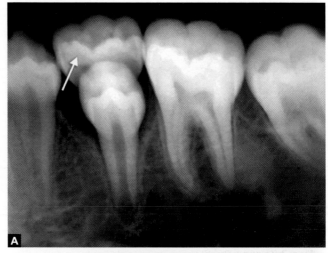

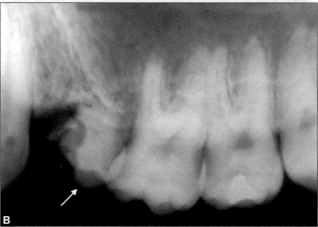

**Figs. 3.8A and B:** (A) Primary second molar root is completely resorbed. It is at the verge of exfoliation; (B) Shedding of primary second molar is delayed due to congenital absence of permanent second premolar.

important as the permanent teeth. Major physiological, psychological, cognitive and neuromuscular development, acquisition of masticatory skills including complex mandibular and tongue movements occur during the primary dentition stage.

Thus, it is equally important to care for primary teeth that play an important role in the maintenance of child's welfare during his/her first years of growth and development both physically and mentally.

### Shedding of Primary Teeth

Primary teeth are shed naturally when their permanent successor teeth are ready to erupt. Not all the primary teeth are lost at the same time; central incisors are lost early at 6–7 years while the canines and second molars are lost at around 12 years of age.

Exfoliation of primary teeth occurs due to physiologic resorption of their roots **(Fig. 3.8A)**. Only 3 years after the roots are completed they begin to resorb as the permanent successor teeth begin their occlusal migration. Pressure from erupting successional teeth plays a key role in shedding of the deciduous dentition. When a successional tooth germ is missing congenitally, shedding of its deciduous predecessor tooth is delayed **(Fig. 3.8B)**. However, the tooth is shed eventually.

Pattern of resorption is influenced by the position of the permanent tooth germ. For example, permanent anteriors develop lingually to the deciduous teeth and erupt in an occlusal and vestibular direction **(Fig. 3.9A)**. Thus, the resorption occurs on the lingual surface of roots in case of deciduous anteriors and these teeth are shed with much of their pulp chamber intact **(Fig. 3.9B)**.

Permanent premolars on the other hand, develop between the divergent roots of the primary molars and erupt in an occlusal direction **(Fig. 3.10A)**. Hence, resorption begins at inter-radicular area. Some resorption of pulp chamber, coronal dentin, and sometimes even enamel may occur **(Fig. 3.10B)**.

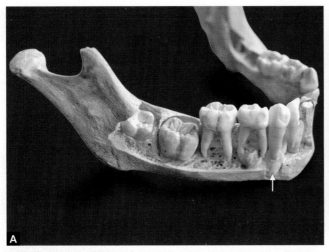 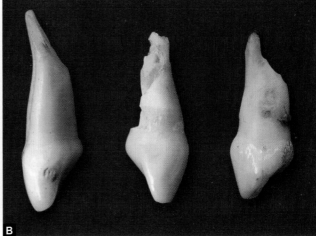

**Figs. 3.9A and B:** (A) Permanent anteriors develop lingual to their deciduous predecessors; (B) Pattern of root resorption on primary anteriors on lingual surface of root.

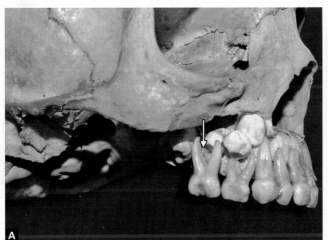 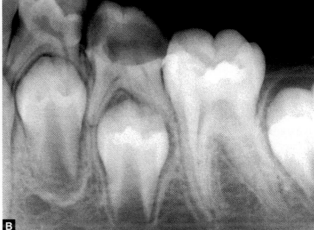

**Figs. 3.10A and B:** (A) Premolars develop between the roots of primary molars; (B) Root resorption in primary molars begins at inter-radicular area.

## Pattern of Shedding

The pattern of shedding is symmetrical for the right and left sides of the mouth. There should not be a discrepancy of more than 3 months between exfoliation of left and right deciduous teeth. Generally, the mandibular primary teeth are shed before their maxillary counterparts, except for the second molars. All four primary second molars are shed simultaneously. Shedding pattern of primary teeth reflects the eruption pattern of secondary (permanent) teeth.

Primary teeth shedding time table should be closely monitored to prevent abnormal developments. If a deciduous tooth has not exfoliated when its permanent successor erupts into oral cavity, the primary tooth should be promptly extracted. This usually occurs with incisor teeth **(Fig. 3.11)**.

When primary teeth, especially the canines and molars are lost prematurely due to caries, trauma, etc. the space should be maintained by way of space maintainers so that there is

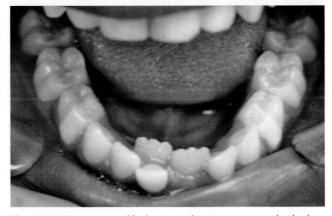

**Fig. 3.11:** Primary mandibular central incisor not yet shed when permanent successors are erupting-leading to their lingual eruption. Primary tooth should be extracted to facilitate proper alignment of the erupting successor tooth.

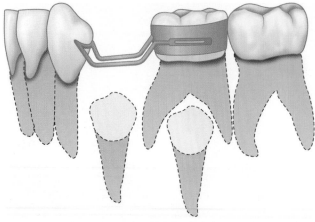

**Fig. 3.12:** A space maintainer designed to maintain space for the eruption of the permanent successor tooth at a later stage.

enough space in the arch when their permanent successor teeth are ready to erupt **(Fig. 3.12)**.

Premature loss of primary teeth and/or unrestored proximal caries resulting in loss of arch length **(Fig. 3.13A)**, prolonged retention of primary teeth are important causes of malocclusion development in the permanent dentition **(Fig. 3.13B)**.

## MIXED DENTITION STAGE

It is a transition stage between 6 years and 12 years of age, when primary teeth are exfoliated in a sequential manner, followed by the eruption of their permanent successors. In the *first transitional period*, eruption of permanent first molars and replacement of primary incisors by the permanent incisors occur. The *second transitional period* involves replacement of the primary molars and canines by the permanent premolars

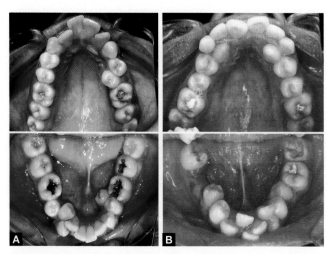

**Figs. 3.13A and B:** Development of malocclusion due to: (A) Premature loss of primary teeth and failure to maintain space; (B) Prolonged retention of primary teeth.

and canines respectively, and emergence of second permanent molars.

**Figure 3.4B** shows mixed dentition period.

## PERMANENT DENTITION STAGE

Permanent dentition stage is established by about 12–13 years excluding the third molars.

### Chronology of Permanent Dentition

The following observations can be made from the chronology table of permanent teeth **(Table 3.2)**:

- The permanent dentition begins to form at birth, at which time, initial calcification of permanent 1st molars becomes evident. Their crowns are completed by 3 years of age.
- Most of the anteriors begin to calcify between 3 months and 5 months and their crowns are completely formed by 5–7 years
- The premolars begin to calcify by 1½ to 2½ years. Crown completion occurs by 7 years of age
- The second molars begin to form by 2½ to 3 years and their crowns are completed by 7 to 8 years
- The last teeth to develop, the third molars begin to calcify by 7–10 years, and crowns are not completed until 12–16 years.
- Usually, the first permanent teeth to emerge are the 1st molars at around 6 years of age. They are, thus, also referred to as *6-year molars.*
- The mandibular central incisors emerge next around 6–7 years, which are closely followed by the mandibular lateral incisors
- The maxillary central incisors emerge next in the order about 7–8 years. The maxillary lateral incisors emerge about 1 year later
- The mandibular canine follows next at 9–10 years. However, the maxillary canine erupt late after one or both the maxillary premolars erupt around 11–12 years
- The premolars emerge between 10 years and 12 years
- The second molars erupt next, around 12 years of age; they are also called the *12-year molars.*
- The third molars do not erupt until 17–21 years. In many individuals, the third molars remain impacted or may even be completely absent.

### Eruption Sequence

- The mandibular permanent teeth tend to erupt before their maxillary counterparts.
- In addition, there are significant differences in the eruption sequences between the maxillary and the mandibular arches **(Fig. 3.14)**.
- It must be noted that there is a difference in the eruption timing of the upper and lower canine teeth.
- Thus, the maxillary canine often erupts buccally or palatally when the space is lost due to mesial migration of the already erupted premolars leading to crowding of teeth **(Fig. 3.15)**.

**Table 3.2:** Chronology of permanent dentition.*

| Tooth | First evidence of calcification | Amount of enamel formed at birth | Crown completed | Eruption | Root completed |
|---|---|---|---|---|---|
| *Maxillary* | | | | | |
| Central incisor | 3–4 months | - | 4–5 years | 7–8 years | 10 years |
| Lateral incisor | 10–12 months | - | 4–5 years | 8–9 years | 11 years |
| Cuspid | 4–5 months | - | 6–7 years | 11–12 years | 13–15 years |
| First bicuspid | 1½–1¾ years | - | 5–6 years | 10–11 years | 12–13 years |
| Second bicuspid | 2–2¼ years | - | 6–7 years | 10–12 years | 12–14 years |
| 1st molar | At birth | Sometimes a trace | 2½–3 years | 6–7 years | 9–10 years |
| Second molar | 2½–3 years | - | 7–8 years | 12–13 years | 14–16 years |
| 3rd molar | 7–9 years | - | 12–16 years | 17–21 years | 18–25 years |
| *Mandibular* | | | | | |
| Central incisor | 3–4 months | - | 4–5 years | 6–7 years | 9 years |
| Lateral incisor | 3–4 months | - | 4–5 years | 7–8 years | 10 years |
| Cuspid | 4–5 months | - | 6–7 years | 9–10 years | 12–14 years |
| First bicuspid | 1¾–2 years | - | 5–6 years | 10–12 years | 12–13 years |
| Second bicuspid | 2¼–2½ years | - | 6–7 years | 11–12 years | 13–14 years |
| 1st molar | At birth | Sometimes a trace | 2½–3 years | 6–7 years | 9–10 years |
| Second molar | 2½–3 years | - | 7–8 years | 11–13 years | 14–15 years |
| 3rd molar | 8–10 years | - | 12–16 years | 17–21 years | 18–25 years |

* Logan WHG, Kronfeld R. Development of the human jaws and surrounding structures from birth to the age of fifteen years. J Am Dent Assoc. 1933;20:379-427. (modified by McCall and Schour)

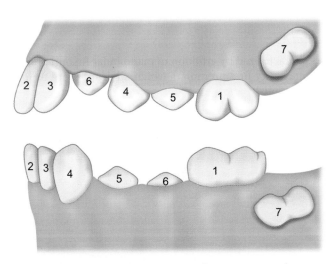

**Fig. 3.14:** Eruption sequence of permanent teeth.

Most common eruption sequence in maxillary arch:
6-1-2-4-3-5-7-8
or
6-1-2-4-5-3-7-8
Most common eruption sequence for mandibular arch:
(6-1)-2-3-4-5-7-8

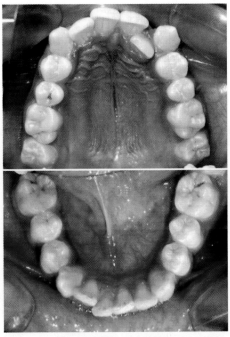

**Fig. 3.15:** Maxillary canine erupts after the eruption of premolars. Thus anterior crowding is a common problem in maxillary arch due to buccal/palatal eruption of maxillary canine.

## DENTAL AGE

Estimation of age is an important requisite in forensic, judicial and criminal proceedings. Circumstances where age assessment is required include—asylum seeker of unknown age, young people accused of criminal activities, convicted criminals whose age is claimed to be less than 18 years prior to sentencing and identification of subjects from mass disasters.

Apart from forensics and anthropology, dental age assessment has an important role in pediatric dentistry and orthodontics.

The chronological age (actual age from date of birth) of an unknown person with uncertain birth record can be predicted by correlating his/her physical, skeletal and dental development. Dental age is considered a better indicator of biologic maturity than physical, skeletal or sexual age since tooth formation is least affected by nutritional status and endocrinal disturbances.

Dental age can be assessed mainly by two methods:
1. Tooth eruption status, and
2. Tooth formation status

### Based on Tooth Eruption/Emergence Status into the Oral Cavity

This method takes into account the number of teeth that have emerged into the oral cavity and the last tooth to erupt. The method can only be an informed guess since tooth emergence through the mucous membrane is a single event for each tooth. Furthermore, local factors such as caries, tooth loss, ankylosis, and lack of space in the dental arch may affect emergence of teeth through gingiva.

Thus, chronologies of eruption of teeth are less satisfactory for dental age assessment than those based on tooth formation. However eruption status can be used in mixed dentition period to get a rough idea about the dental age.

**Figures 3.16 and 3.17** give examples of dental age assessment using eruption status of teeth in mixed dentition period.

The permanent teeth tend to erupt in groups and it is important to know the expected timing of these eruption stages. These eruption stages are used to calculate dental age, particularly during the mixed dentition period.

### Dental Age 6 (Fig. 3.18A)

The first stage of eruption of the permanent teeth is at age of 6 years. It is characterized by simultaneous eruption of the mandibular central incisors, maxillary first molars and mandibular first molars. The onset of eruption of this group of teeth characterizes dental age 6.

### Dental Age 7 (Fig. 3.18B)

In the second stage of eruption at dental age 7, the maxillary central incisors and the mandibular lateral incisors erupt.

### Dental Age 8 (Fig. 3.18C)

It is characterized by the eruption of the maxillary lateral incisors. After these teeth erupt there is a delay of 2–3 years before any further permanent teeth appear.

### Dental Ages 9 and 10 (Fig. 3.18D)

It is marked by the eruption of mandibular canines and is assessed by the extent of resorption of the primary canines and molars and the extent of root development of their permanent successors.

### Dental Age 11 (Fig. 3.18E)

It is characterized by eruption of mandibular first premolars and maxillary first premolars which all erupt more or less simultaneously.

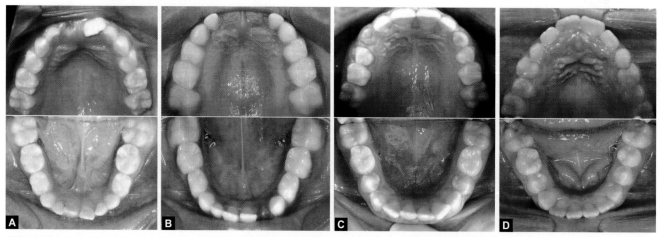

**Figs. 3.16A to D:** Dental age assessment using eruption status of teeth in mixed dentition period (Tooth notation in FDI system): (A) Last erupted tooth—21; approximate dental age = 7–8 years; (B) Last erupted tooth—31, 41; approximate dental age = 6–7 years; (C) Erupting teeth—13; approximate dental age = 11–12 years; (D) Erupting teeth—25 and 13; approximate dental age = 10–12 years.

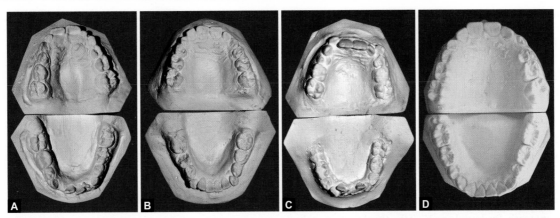

**Figs. 3.17A to D:** Dental age assessment using eruption status of teeth in mixed dentition period—cast specimen (Tooth notation in FDI system): (A) Erupted teeth-all first permanent molars, erupting teeth—32, 11, 21, 12, 22; approximate dental age 7–9 years; (B) Last erupted teeth—12 and 22; approximate dental age 8–9 years; (C) Erupting tooth—14; approximate dental age 10–11 years; (D) Erupting tooth—23; approximate dental age 11–12 years.

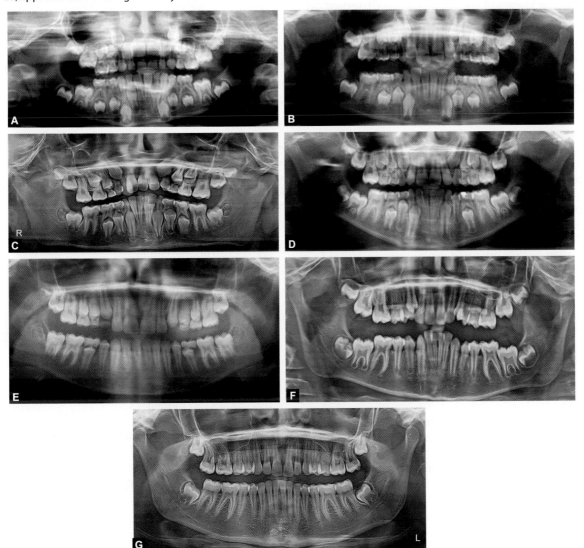

**Figs. 3.18A to G:** (A) Dental age 6; (B) Dental age 7; (C) Dental age 8; (D) Dental ages 9 and 10; (E) Dental age 11; (F) Dental age 12; (G) Dental ages 13 to 15.

At dental age 11, the only remaining primary teeth in oral cavity are the maxillary canine and second molar and mandibular second molar.

### Dental Age 12 (Fig. 3.18 F)

At dental age 12, the remaining succedaneous permanent teeth erupt, i.e. the maxillary canine; the maxillary and mandibular second premolars.

In addition, the second permanent molars in both the arches are nearing eruption.

### Dental Ages 13–15 (Fig. 3.18 G)

They are characterized by the extent of completion of the roots of permanent teeth. By dental age 15, if the third molar is going to form, it will be apparent on the radiographs and the roots of all other permanent teeth should be complete.

### Based on the Stages of Tooth Formation Observed on Radiographs

Tooth formation (calcification) is a continuous process occurring throughout the growth period from birth to adolescence, and can be divided into various stages that can be defined.

Dental age based on tooth formation is superior to that based on tooth emergence because emergence of a tooth is a fleeting single event and its precise time is difficult to determine. Whereas tooth calcification is a continuous process that can be assessed on permanent records such as radiographs.

Dental age is estimated by comparing the tooth development status in a person of unknown age with published reference dental development dataset prepared from a similar or a different population group.

Demirjian in 1973 proposed dental maturity scores from a French-Canadian population and this has served as a reference dataset for evaluation of age for various population groups.

Radiographic studies of tooth formation have used three basic stages:
1. First evidence of calcification
2. Crown completion
3. Root completion.

Nolla expanded the number of stages to 11 and Gleiser and Hunt to 13.

Morrees et al. defined 14 stages of permanent tooth formation (**Fig. 3.19**). The 14 stages are designated by abbreviations. Morrees et al. studied the development of mandibular canines and provided normative data.

### Abbreviations

- C: Cusp
- Cr: Crown
- R: Root
- Cl: Cleft
- A: Apex

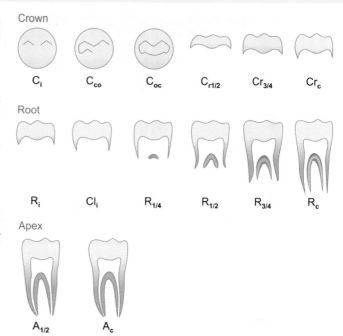

**Fig. 3.19:** 14 stages of permanent teeth formation as defined by Morrees et al.

### Subscripts

- i: Initiated
- co: Coalescence
- oc: Outline complete
- c: Complete

The 14 stages would be:
1. $C_i$: Cusp initiated
2. $C_{co}$: Cusp coalescence
3. $C_{oc}$: Cusp outline completed
4. $C_{r1/2}$: Crown half formed
5. $C_{r3/4}$: Crown three-fourth formed
6. $C_{rc}$: Crown completed
7. $R_i$: Root initiated
8. $Cl_i$: Cleft initiated
9. $R_{1/4}$: Root one-fourth formed
10. $R_{1/2}$: Root half formed
11. $R_{3/4}$: Root three-fourth formed
12. $R_c$: Root complete
13. $A_{1/2}$: Apex half formed
14. $A_c$: Apex complete

Clinicians can use such chronologies to avoid treatment that can damage developing teeth (age of attainment schedules), to assess an unknown age of a patient (e.g. age prediction in forensics), and to assess growth (maturity).

### BIBLIOGRAPHY

1. Demirjian A, Goldstein H, Tanner JM. A new system of dental age assessment. Human Biol. 1970;45:211-27.
2. Friel S. The development of ideal occlusion of gum pads and teeth. Am J Orthod. 1954;40:196-227.

3. Hughes TE, Bockmann MR, Seow K, et al. Strong genetic control of emergence of human primary incisors. J Dent Res. 2007;86(12):1160-5.
4. Massler M, Schour I, Poncher HG. Developmental pattern of the child as reflected in the calcification pattern of the teeth. Am J Dis Child. 1941;63:33-67.
5. Morrees CFA, Kent RL. A step function model using tooth counts to assess the developmental timing of the dentition. Am Hum Biol. 1978;5:55-68.
6. Morrees CFA, Fanning EA, Hunt EE. Age variation of formation stages for ten permanent teeth. J Dent Res. 1963;42;1490-502.
7. Nolla CM. The development of permanent teeth. J Dent Child. 1960;27:254-66.
8. Schour L, Massler M. The development of human dentition. J Am Dent Assoc. 1941;28:1153-60.

## MULTIPLE CHOICE QUESTIONS

1. Development of teeth in human begins:
   a. At birth
   b. Prenatally
   c. At 6 months
   d. At 1 years
2. Primary teeth begin to calcify at:
   a. Birth
   b. 6 months
   c. 6 weeks in utero
   d. 14 weeks in utero
3. First primary tooth to show its evidence of calcification (begin its development):
   a. Primary maxillary 1st molar
   b. Primary mandibular 1st molar
   c. Primary mandibular central incisor
   d. Primary mandibular lateral incisor
4. All primary teeth would have begun to calcify by:
   a. 14 weeks of intrauterine life
   b. 18–20 weeks of intrauterine life
   c. 6 months of gestation
   d. 6 months of age
5. The duration of time each primary tooth takes for its formation, from first evidence of calcification to root completion is:
   a. 3–4 months
   b. 2–3 years
   c. 5–6 years
   d. 1–2 years
6. The duration of time each permanent tooth takes for its complete formation is:
   a. 3–4 months
   b. 2–3 years
   c. 5–6 years
   d. 8–12 years
7. Mineralization of permanent teeth is:
   a. Entirely prenatal
   b. Entirely postnatal
   c. Occurs both prenatally and postnatally
   d. None of the above
8. Eruption of all the primary teeth would be completed by:
   a. 6 months
   b. 12 months
   c. 12 years
   d. 2½ years
9. Development of primary dentition is considered to be completed:
   a. At 6 months
   b. 30 months
   c. When second primary molars are in occlusion
   d. Both b and c
10. Transitional (mixed) dentition period begins at:
    a. 6 months
    b. 6–7 years
    c. When first permanent teeth erupts
    d. Both b and c

**Answers**

| 1. b | 2. d | 3. c | 4. b | 5. b | 6. d | 7. c | 8. d |
|------|------|------|------|------|------|------|------|
| 9. d | 10. d | | | | | | |

# 4

# Form and Function of Orofacial Complex

## INTRODUCTION

The phrase *"form and function"* is often used in the context of evolutionary science. Biologists often say form follows function meaning that, due to the evolutionary process the morphological features (e.g. teeth) of an organism's body are fitted to the activities of an organism. The concept of form and function explains the inter-relation of the shape of certain part and its function.

In the context of dentistry, this phrase is applied to the entire masticatory system, which acts as a highly coordinated functional unit. Form of each component of the masticatory system is closely related to its individual functions and to that of the whole system including mastication, deglutition, phonetics, esthetics, and maintenance. The idea that the form and function are inter-related has to be borne in mind in clinical practice, for instance while restoring teeth, treating malocclusion, etc.

The primary function of teeth is to prepare food for swallowing and to facilitate digestion. Different types of teeth with their respective form are adapted to incise, shear, and grind food. The teeth with their proper form and alignment protect the supporting periodontal tissues against trauma during mastication, facilitate the jaw movements, speech, and enhance the esthetic appearance of face.

In order to understand the form and function of teeth, the following aspects must be considered:
- Size of crown and root; root form
- Tooth form and jaw movements
- Interproximal spaces and protection of interdental gingiva
- Proximal contact areas
- Embrasures (Spillways)
- Facial and lingual contours of teeth: mesial and distal
- Curvature of the cervical line (cementoenamel junction)
- Occlusal curvatures.

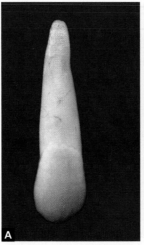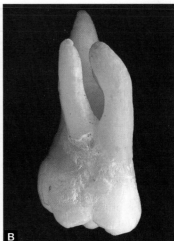

**Figs. 4.1A and B:** (A) Canine teeth have longest roots to withstand shear forces at corners of the mouth; (B) Tripod arrangement of maxillary molar roots provides excellent anchorage in the alveolar bone.

## SIZE OF CROWN AND ROOT

The crown and root should be proportional to each other and to the jaw size. Size and shape of roots reflect the function of respective teeth, e.g. the canine teeth located at the corners of the mouth have the longest roots **(Fig. 4.1A)**. The extra size and length of the root ensures enough anchorage and support for canine teeth that bear shear forces.

Maxillary and mandibular molars that perform the most part of trituration of food require multiple roots to withstand the masticatory forces. Trifurcated roots of maxillary molars give a tripod arrangement in the alveolar bone that provides excellent anchorage **(Fig. 4.1B)**. Developmental depressions on the lateral surfaces of the roots also enhance anchorage in the alveolar bone.

## TOOTH FORM AND JAW MOVEMENTS

Apart from comminution of food, the incisal and occlusal forms of the teeth have a direct influence on the jaw movements. The relation of tooth form and jaw relation can be understood by comparing human jaw movements with that of animals.

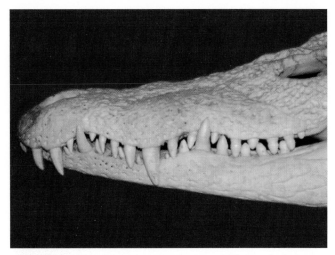

**Fig. 4.2:** Interlocking conical teeth in crocodile limit lateral jaw movements.

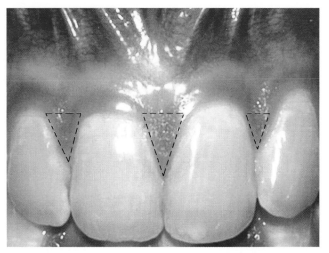

**Fig. 4.3:** Triangular-shaped interproximal spaces between adjoining teeth accommodate interproximal gingival tissue.

In many animals only simple opening and closing type of jaw movements are possible without lateral excursion.

This is because of their interlocking conical form of teeth, temporomandibular joint (TMJ) morphology, isognathic jaws (equal-sized jaws), and lack of muscles to carryout lateral movements. Conical form of teeth and equal-sized jaws permit limited lateral jaw movement. For example, crocodiles have interlocking conical teeth of different size **(Fig. 4.2)**.

Carnivores (wild boars, pigs, dogs) and primates have conical shaped cusps *(bunodont)*, equal-sized jaws, and very prominent canine teeth that limit lateral jaw movements. Extreme lateral movements are seen in cattle (herbivores) and may be attributed to their elongated flattened condyles, selenodont molars (molars with crescent-shaped cusps), and unequal jaw size.

In humans, however, maxillary and mandibular jaws are not perfectly equal sized. The maxillary arch overlaps the mandibular arch labially and buccally in horizontal plane. The TMJ is specialized in humans and the occlusal anatomy of teeth is complex. It can be observed that, increasing complexity of jaw movement is associated with increasing complexity of occlusal anatomy of teeth.

## INTERPROXIMAL SPACES AND PROTECTION OF INTERDENTAL GINGIVA

The teeth are narrower at the cervix mesiodistally than they are toward the occlusal surfaces. This arrangement creates a triangular or pyramidal shaped space between the approximating teeth just cervical to the contact area **(Fig. 4.3)**. The base of the triangle is at the alveolar process between the adjacent teeth; the sides of the triangle are formed by the proximal surfaces of the teeth and the apex of the triangle is at the contact area of the two teeth. These spaces accommodate and protect interproximal gingival tissue and are referred to as the *interproximal spaces*. The gingival tissue that fills the interproximal space is called the *gingival papilla or interdental papilla.*

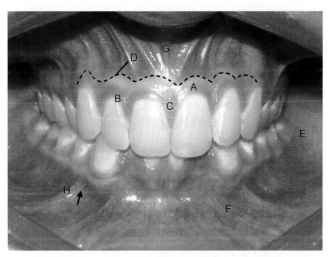

**Fig. 4.4:** Gingiva: A. Attached gingiva; B. Free or marginal gingiva; C. Interdental gingiva or papilla; D. Mucogingival junction; E. Buccal corridor or post-vestibular fornix; F. Anterior vestibular fornix or mucobuccal fold; G. Labial frenum; H. Buccal frenum.

The gingiva covers the alveolar process of jaw bones—*attached gingiva*, extends around the neck of tooth to form gingival crevice—*free or marginal gingiva,* and fills the interdental spaces—*gingival or interdental papilla* **(Fig. 4.4)**. The part of interdental gingival tissue that lies below the contact area and extends faciolingually is called the col. *Mucogingival line* marks the junction between attached gingiva and the alveolar mucosa.

Col is nonkeratinized and vulnerable to trauma during mastication and invasion by bacteria. Tight contacts and proper interproximal spaces between adjacent teeth help to protect the col and interproximal gingival tissue **(Fig. 4.5)**.

When viewed buccally or lingually, the roots of teeth taper from cervix to apices creating enough space between the roots of adjacent teeth. This allows sufficient alveolar bone between one tooth to another, so that the teeth are securely anchored

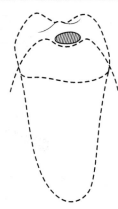

**Fig. 4.5:** Form of interproximal gingiva col in relation to contact area. Tight contact between adjacent teeth helps to protect the col and interproximal gingival tissue.

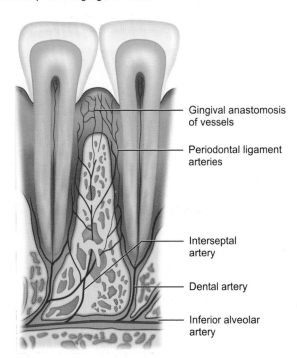

Gingival anastomosis of vessels

Periodontal ligament arteries

Interseptal artery

Dental artery

Inferior alveolar artery

**Fig. 4.6:** Conical tapering form of root allows sufficient anchorage in bone and provides adequate space for blood and nerve supply to the investing tissues of teeth.

in the jaws. The arrangement also ensures adequate space for blood and nerve supply to the supporting and investing tissues of teeth **(Fig. 4.6)**.

The form of interproximal space will vary with the proximal contours of adjacent teeth and their alignment. Proper contact and alignment of adjacent teeth is essential to provide enough interproximal space between them for normal bulk of the gingival tissue to be attached to the bone and teeth.

## PROXIMAL CONTACT AREAS

When a tooth erupts and takes its position in the dental arch, it comes in contact with two adjacent teeth of the same arch—

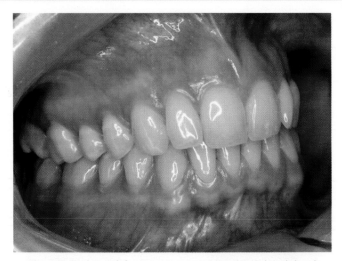

**Fig. 4.7:** Each tooth has two contact areas: Mesial and distal, except last molar which does not have distal contact.

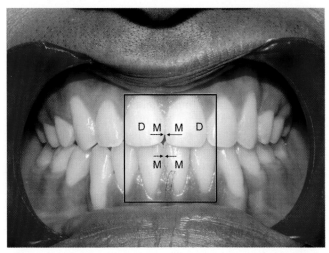

**Fig. 4.8:** The maxillary and mandibular central incisors are the only teeth which have their mesial surfaces facing each other.

one mesial and one distal to it. Thus, each tooth in a dental arch, except the last molars, has two contact areas—the mesial and the distal. The third molar or the second molar, when third molar is absent, is in contact only with the tooth mesial to it **(Fig. 4.7)**.

The mesial contact area of one tooth faces the distal contact area of the adjoining tooth except in case of central incisors. The maxillary and mandibular central incisors are the only teeth that have their mesial surfaces facing each other **(Fig. 4.8)**.

### Clinical Significance of Contact Areas

Adjacent teeth should have tight contact with each other **(Fig. 4.9)**. Proper contact relation between adjoining teeth is important due to the following reasons:

• Since adjacent teeth are in contact with each other, the whole dental arch functions as a single unit and masticatory forces are well distributed.

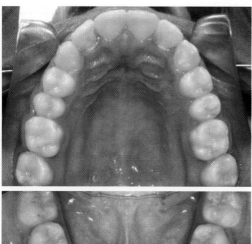
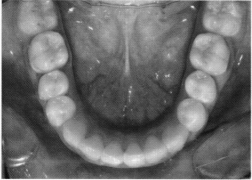

**Fig. 4.9:** Proper contact relation between the adjacent teeth.

- The combined anchorage of all teeth ensures occlusal stability.
- Proper contact prevents food impaction, which can lead to decay and periodontal problems.
- Tight contact between adjacent teeth helps to protect the interproximal gingival tissue by diverting or shunting food toward the buccal and lingual areas.
- If the contact between adjacent teeth is lost due to some reason (e.g. proximal caries, loss of a tooth, malocclusion, etc.), food is forced between the teeth and pathologic changes occur in interdental gingival tissue, leading to gingivitis.
- If unresolved, the inflammation may reach deeper periodontal structures with loss of interdental alveolar bone causing periodontitis.
- For these reasons, it is important to establish proper proximal contact during crown prosthesis **(Fig. 4.10A)**, proximal restoration of teeth **(Fig. 4.10B)**, and in treatment of malocclusion.

## Position of Contact Areas (Box 4.1)

Position of contact areas depends on the type and form of the crown and alignment of teeth.

Position of contact areas can be examined from two views:

1. *Facial (labial or buccal) view*: It shows the relative position of the contact areas cervicoincisally or cervico-occlusally.
2. *Incisal or occlusal view*: It shows the relative position of the contact areas labiolingually or buccolingually.

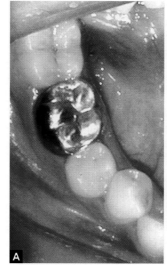
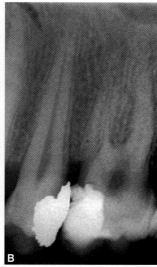

**Figs. 4.10A and B:** (A) Crown prosthesis with proper proximal contacts; (B) Improper proximal restoration causing interdental bone loss.

## Contact Area Location as Viewed Facially (Fig. 4.11)

*Generally, in all the teeth:*
- The height of the crown decreases as one moves from the central incisor to the last molar. Thus, the contact areas become more cervically positioned when moving away from the midline.
- Distal contact area is more cervically placed than the mesial contact area in all the teeth except:
  - In mandibular permanent first premolars where the mesial contact area is cervically located than the distal contact area.
  - In mandibular permanent central incisors where both mesial and distal contact areas are at the same level. This is because the mandibular central incisors are bilaterally symmetrical.

*In anteriors:*
- The mesial and distal contact areas are at dissimilar levels when compared to posterior teeth.

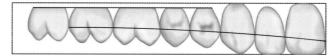

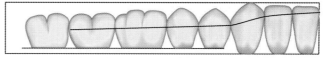

**Fig. 4.11:** Location of contact areas becomes more cervically placed as moved away from the midline. Distal contact area is more cervically placed than the mesial contact area.

- The contacts become more cervically placed when moving from incisors to distal of canines.
- Mesial contacts of the incisors are in the incisal third. The distal contacts are at or near the junction of incisal and middle thirds.
- The contacts are more incisally placed in mandibular incisors.
- Canines are the teeth in which the mesial and distal contacts are markedly at different levels. Their mesial contacts are at or near the junction of incisal and middle thirds. The distal contacts are in the middle thirds.

***In posteriors:***
- The mesial and distal contacts of posteriors are more nearly at the same level than for anterior teeth.
- The mesial and distal contacts of premolars are at/cervical to the junction of middle and occlusal thirds.
- The location of contacts in molars is more regular. Mesial and distal contacts are usually at the middle third of the crown.

## Location of Proximal Contacts as Viewed Occlusally (Figs. 4.12A to D)

***In anterior teeth:*** The contact areas are nearly centered labiolingually and are smaller.

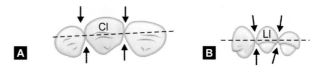
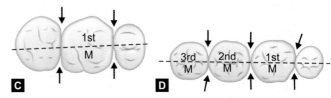

**Figs. 4.12A to D:** Buccolingual location of contact areas as viewed occlusally: (A and B) Maxillary and mandibular anterior teeth; (C and D) Maxillary and mandibular posterior teeth.

(CI: central incisor; LI: lateral incisor)

***In posterior teeth:***
- The contact areas are broader than that of the anterior teeth.
- The contact areas on posterior teeth tend to be placed buccal to the center of the crown buccolingually.
- Compared to maxillary teeth, the contact areas in mandibular teeth are more centered buccolingually.

**Box 4.1** gives the location of contact areas of different teeth both cervico-occlusally and buccolingually.

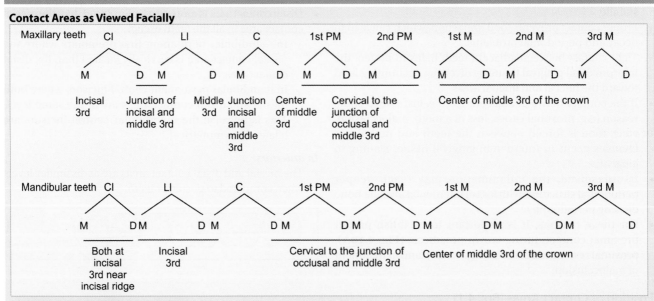

**Box 4.1: Location of contact areas of teeth.**

**Contact Areas as Viewed Facially**

| Maxillary teeth | | | | | | | |
|---|---|---|---|---|---|---|---|
| CI | LI | C | 1st PM | 2nd PM | 1st M | 2nd M | 3rd M |
| M    D | M    D | M    D | M    D | M    D | M    D | M    D | M    D |
| Incisal 3rd | Junction of incisal and middle 3rd | Middle 3rd    Junction of incisal and middle 3rd | Center of middle 3rd | Cervical to the junction of occlusal and middle 3rd | Center of middle 3rd of the crown | | |

| Mandibular teeth | | | | | | | |
|---|---|---|---|---|---|---|---|
| CI | LI | C | 1st PM | 2nd PM | 1st M | 2nd M | 3rd M |
| M    D | M    D | M    D | M    D | M    D | M    D | M    D | M    D |
| Both at incisal 3rd near incisal ridge | Incisal 3rd | | Cervical to the junction of occlusal and middle 3rd | | Center of middle 3rd of the crown | | |

**Contact Areas as Viewed Occlusally**
*Anteriors*: Contact areas are nearly centered labiolingually, and are small.
*Posteriors*:
Contact areas are broader than those of the anteriors.
The contacts areas on maxillary posterior teeth are placed buccal to the center of the crown buccolingually and at center in mandibular posteriors.

(CI: central incisor; LI: lateral incisor; C: canines)

## EMBRASURES (SPILLWAYS)

When two adjacent teeth of the same dental arch come in contact, their curvatures adjacent to the contact areas form "V"-shaped spaces called the *embrasures or spillway spaces*. An embrasure is a "V"-shaped space adjacent to the contact area of two adjacent teeth. Narrowest part of V-shaped space is at the contact area. From here the space widens facially to form the *labial or buccal embrasure,* lingually to form the *lingual embrasure,* and occlusally to form the *incisal or occlusal embrasure* **(Fig. 4.13)**.

The fourth triangular space that is cervical to the contact area is filled by interdental or gingival papilla and is appropriately called as the *interproximal space* though it is sometimes referred to as *gingival or cervical embrasure.*

The incisal or occlusal embrasures are observed when teeth are viewed from the facial aspect **(Fig. 4.14A)**. They are bounded by the marginal ridges as they join cusps and incisal ridges. The facial and lingual embrasures are seen from incisal or occlusal view **(Fig. 4.14B)**. The facial, lingual, and occlusal embrasures are continuous as they surround the area of contact.

### Characteristics of an Ideal Embrasure

- The embrasure should be symmetrical, thus the proximal surfaces of adjacent teeth should be mirror images of each other.
- Adjacent marginal ridges and cementoenamel junctions (cervical lines) should be of same height.
- The teeth should have tight proximal contacts.

*Form of embrasures in general, in all teeth:*
- Occlusal embrasure tends to be widened as one moves from incisors toward molars.
- Crowns of most teeth show lingual convergence. Therefore, usually the lingual embrasures are wider than the facial (labial or buccal) embrasures.

*In anterior teeth:*
- Incisal embrasures get widened from mesial of central incisor to distal of the canine.
- Incisal embrasure is very minimal in mandibular incisors as their contact areas are more incisally located (nearer to the incisal edge).
- Lingual embrasures in anteriors are much wider than the labial embrasures. This is due to marked lingual convergences seen in anterior teeth.

*In posterior teeth:*
- Embrasures are more regular and uniform in posteriors
- Occlusal embrasures are wider than those seen in anteriors (incisal embrasures).
- Facial and lingual embrasures tend to be similar in form, though lingual embrasure may be slightly bigger.

### Functions of Embrasures

The embrasures serve the following purposes:
- The embrasures provide a spillway for the escape of food during mastication.

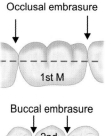
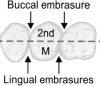
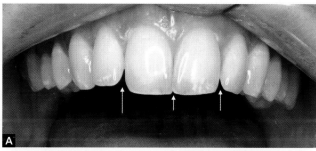

**Fig. 4.13:** Embrasures or spillway spaces.

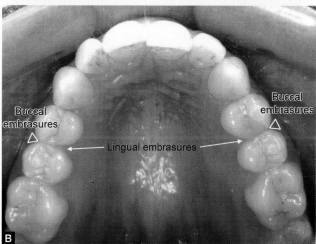

**Figs. 4.14A and B:** (A) Incisal or occlusal embrasures are seen from facial view; (B) Buccal and lingual embrasures are seen from occlusal view.

- They reduce forces imparted on teeth during reduction of any hard food material.
- They prevent food from being forced through the contact area. When the occlusal embrasure is lost due to attrition (e.g. in incisors), food is pushed into contact area between the teeth.
- They make the tooth self-cleansing as the rounded smooth surfaces of the crown are exposed to the cleaning action of fibrous foods and friction of cheeks and lips.
- Embrasures and contact areas protect the gingiva from undue trauma.

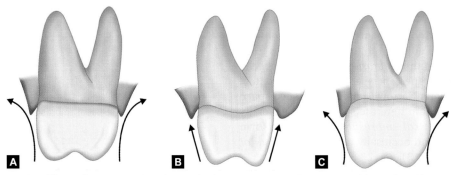

**Figs. 4.15A to C:** Facial and lingual contours of teeth: (A) Ideal contours; (B) Undercontoured buccal and lingual surfaces may cause food impaction; (C) Overcontoured buccal and lingual surfaces—no gingival stimulation.

### Clinical Significance

- During proximal restoration of teeth or when crown prosthesis is given, over- or undercontouring of proximal surface should be avoided.
- Overcontouring of the proximal surface at the expense of embrasure space results in food impaction.

## FACIAL AND LINGUAL PHYSIOLOGIC CONTOURS OF TEETH (FIGS. 4.15A TO C)

- When teeth are viewed from proximal aspects, the facial (labial or buccal) and lingual surfaces of the crowns show some bulge above the cervical line.
- The crests of curvature of buccal and lingual surfaces are at the cervical or middle third of their crowns. Such a form protects and stimulates gingiva by deflecting the food away from gingival tissue during mastication.
- These contours deflect food away from the gingival sulcus and prevent accumulation of food debris.
- If buccal and lingual surfaces are undercontoured, there is possibility of food impaction.

### *In anterior teeth (Fig. 4.16A):*
- The crests of curvatures or heights of contours labially and lingually are at cervical third of the crown.
- The crests of curvatures are at the same level and are opposite to each other labiolingually.
- The curvatures extend up to 0.5 mm beyond the cervical line.
- Lingually, the crest of curvature is on the cingulum.

### *In posterior teeth (Figs. 4.16B and C):*
- Buccal crest of curvature in both maxillary and mandibular posteriors is at the cervical third.
- Lingual crest of curvature in both maxillary and mandibular posteriors is at the middle third.
- Buccal and lingual curvatures in maxillary posteriors and buccal curvatures in mandibular posteriors extend about 0.5 mm beyond the cervical line.
- Extent of lingual curvature in mandibular posteriors is accentuated by lingual inclination of their crowns and the root base, which is about 1.0 mm from the cervical line.

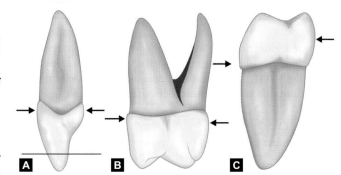

**Figs. 4.16A to C:** (A) Crest of labial and lingual contours in anterior teeth at cervical third, facing each other; (B and C) Crest of curvature of buccal and lingual contours in maxillary and mandibular posteriors: Crest of buccal curvature—cervical third; Crest of lingual curvature—middle third.

## CURVATURES OF CERVICAL LINE (CEMENTOENAMEL JUNCTION): MESIALLY AND DISTALLY

The curvature of cervical line on teeth signifies the location of cementoenamel junction. The epithelial attachment (soft tissue attachment at the neck of the tooth) and contour of alveolar crest follow the curvature of cementoenamel junction of the tooth.

Epithelial attachment is vulnerable to physical injuries. Thus, it is important to know the level of epithelial attachment proximally, so as to prevent injury during dental procedures like scaling, restorations, impression making, crown preparation, etc. Inadvertent probing should be avoided.

The following observations can be made regarding the curvature of cervical line:
- The curvature of cervical line on proximal surfaces of adjoining teeth is nearly at the same level **(Fig. 4.17)**. This produces symmetrical interproximal space which is ideal.
- In all teeth, the extent of the curvature is greater mesially than distally.
- In both the arches, the anterior teeth exhibit greater curvature than the posteriors.
- In general, the curvature of cervical line on distal surface is 1 mm less than that of the mesial surface of the tooth. For instance, the extent of cervical line curvature on mesial

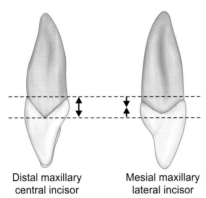

**Fig. 4.17:** Extent of cervical line curvature on proximal surface of adjoining teeth is at same level. Distal surface of maxillary central incisor and mesial surface of maxillary lateral incisor.

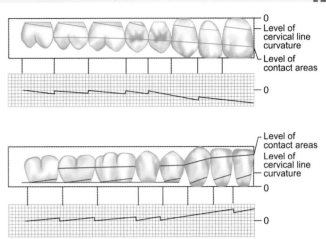

**Fig. 4.18:** The cervical line curvature is maximum at midline on mesial surface of central incisor (3.5 mm) and decreases gradually and becomes flat (0.0 mm) at the molars.

surface of central incisor is 3.5 mm and while it is 2.5 mm on the distal surface.

The extent of cervical line curvature dictates the level of contact areas.

The height of tooth crowns decreases as one moves away from midline toward distal of arch and the contact areas shift more cervically.

Incisors have long crowns with incisally placed contact areas. Therefore, the cervical line curvature is greater in incisors and tends to decrease toward the molars.

- The cervical line curvature is maximum at mesial surface of central incisor, i.e. 3.5 mm, from here it diminishes gradually to 0.0 mm at the molars, where there is no curvature at all **(Fig. 4.18)**.

## IMAGINARY OCCLUSAL PLANES AND CURVES

### Curve of Spee (Anteroposterior Curve or the Curve of Occlusal Plane) (Fig. 4.19A)

Curve of Spee is a naturally occurring phenomenon in the human dentition. It is defined as the anteroposterior curvature of the mandibular occlusal plane beginning at the tip of mandibular canine and following the buccal cusps of mandibular posterior teeth, continuing as an arc through the condyle. If the curve is extended, it would form a circle of about 4-inch radius.

This geometric arrangement is believed to provide most efficient pattern for maintaining maximum tooth contacts during chewing. Normal occlusal curvature of Spee is required for an efficient masticatory system. Exaggerated curve of Spee is frequently observed in dental malocclusions.

### Curve of Wilson (Side-to-Side Curve) (Fig. 4.19B)

Curve of Wilson is the mediolateral curve that contacts the buccal and lingual cusp tips of the mandibular posterior teeth. It results from the lingual inclination of the mandibular posterior teeth. Curve of Wilson provides optimum resistance to masticatory forces.

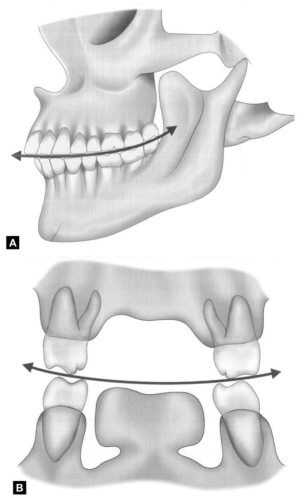

**Figs. 4.19A and B:** (A) Curve of Spee; (B) Curve of Wilson.

## GEOMETRIES OF CROWN OUTLINES

Although outlines of tooth crowns are curved, they can be generally included within geometric figures. All the aspects of tooth crowns except the incisal or occlusal aspects can be outlined schematically within three geometric figures, i.e. a triangle, trapezoid, and rhomboid.

Geometric shape or form of tooth crowns appears to conform to a general plan. Correct anatomy of tooth crowns can be understood better through the medium of schematic drawings.

### Facial and Lingual Aspects of all Teeth—Trapezoid with Narrow Cervical Area (Fig. 4.20, 4.21B to D)

When viewed from facial and lingual aspects, the crown outlines of all the teeth may be represented as trapezoids of various dimensions by disregarding the cuspal forms of cusped teeth, i.e. canines and posteriors.

A trapezium has two even sides (of equal length) and two uneven sides. The shortest uneven side of the trapezoid represents the cervical area of the crown while the longest uneven side represents the working (incisal or occlusal) surface.

The schematic diagram drawn by disregarding the overlap of anterior teeth and cuspal forms helps in visualizing the fundamental plan in form and arrangement of the teeth from facial aspect. The occlusal line that is drawn along the longest uneven side of each of the trapezoid represents the approximate line of occlusion of opposing teeth when the jaws are closed.

The trapezoid form of crowns and the arrangement portray the following fundamentals of form:
- Trapezoid crown form with narrow cervix creates interproximal spaces that can accommodate interproximal gingival tissue.
- Spacing between the roots of adjacent teeth allows sufficient bulk of investing and supporting tissues (alveolar bone, periodontal ligament) for proper investment and maintenance of nutrition and function of adjacent teeth.
- Each tooth crown in the dental arches makes contact with adjoining tooth or teeth. This arrangement provides mutual support and occlusal stability. It also helps protect the interproximal gingival tissue from trauma during mastication.

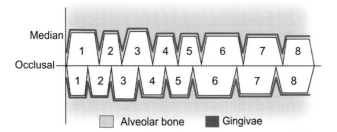

**Fig. 4.20:** The general form of all crowns from facial and lingual aspect is trapezoid with narrow cervical area. This arrangement creates interproximal spaces than can accommodate interproximal gingival tissue.

- Each tooth in a dental arch occludes with two teeth of the opposing arch when in occlusion. In other words, each tooth has two antagonists in the opposing arch except for the mandibular central incisor and maxillary third molar. When a tooth is lost, this arrangement helps to prevent extrusion of the antagonistic teeth and stabilizes the remaining teeth.

### Proximal Aspects of Anterior Teeth—Triangular (Fig. 4.21A)

The proximal aspects of all anterior teeth (both maxillary and mandibular) can be included within triangles. The base of the triangle is formed by the cervical portion of crown while the apex is represented by the incisal ridge.

Triangular proximal form of the anterior teeth portrays the following fundamentals of form:
- Base of the crown is wide providing strength
- Tapering labial and lingual outlines converge into a thin incisal ridge. This gives a wedge-shaped cutting edge to the anteriors that facilitates the penetration of food material.

### Proximal Aspects of Maxillary Posterior Teeth—Trapezoid with Narrow Occlusal Surface (Figs. 4.21E and F)

The proximal aspects of maxillary posterior teeth also appear trapezoidal like their facial and lingual aspects. The difference however is that, the longest uneven side of the trapezoidal figure is toward the base of the crown, i.e. cervical portion, rather than toward the occlusal surface. It must be noted that the tooth crowns are not always narrow at the cervix from all the aspects as it is often perceived to be.

The proximal aspects of maxillary posteriors bring about the following fundamentals of form:
- Since the crown is narrow occlusally, the tooth can be forced into food material more easily during mastication.
- If the occlusal surfaces were as wide as the base of the crown, the additional chewing surface would have increased the forces of mastication by many folds.

### Proximal Aspects of Mandibular Posterior Teeth—Rhomboidal (Figs. 4.21E and F)

Contrary to maxillary posteriors, the outline of proximal aspects of mandibular posterior teeth is rhomboidal. However, their occlusal surfaces are constricted in comparison to the bases, similar to the maxillary posteriors.
- The rhomboidal outline obtained is due to the fact that the tooth crowns are inclined lingual to the root bases in case of mandibular posteriors.
- This ensures proper intercuspation of mandibular teeth with their maxillary antagonists.
- If mandibular posterior crowns were upright on their root bases, upper and lower cusps would clash and proper intercuspation would not be possible.
- The maxillary posterior teeth have a slight buccal inclination while the mandibular posterior teeth have a slight lingual inclination.

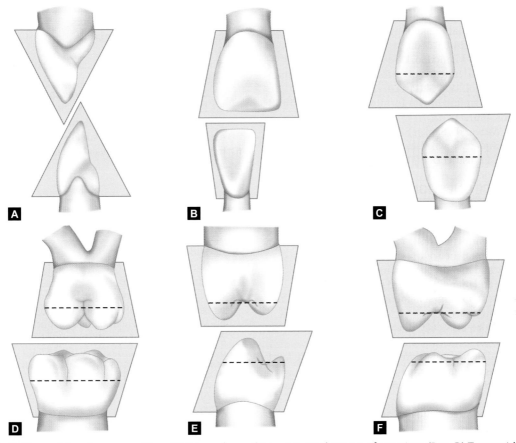

**Figs. 4.21A to F:** Geometrics of crown outline: (A) Triangular outline—proximal aspect of anteriors; (B to D) Trapezoidal outline with narrow cervix—facial and lingual aspect of all teeth; (E and F) Trapezoidal outline with narrow occlusal surface—proximal surface of all maxillary posteriors; Rhomboidal outline—proximal aspect of mandibular posteriors.

- Lingual inclination of mandibular teeth also ensures that the axes of maxillary and mandibular teeth are kept parallel in the jaws **(Fig. 4.22)**.
  **Box 4.2** summarizes the geometries of crown outlines.

**Box 4.2: Geometric crown outlines of teeth.**

*Triangular outline*: All maxillary and mandibular anterior teeth:
- Mesial aspect
- Distal aspect

*Trapezoidal outline*:
- Trapezoid with longest uneven side toward incisal or occlusal surface
  - Facial and lingual aspects of all the teeth (anteriors and posteriors of both the jaws)
- Trapezoid with shortest uneven side towards incisal or occlusal surface
  - Proximal (mesial and distal) aspects of maxillary posterior teeth

*Rhomboidal outline*: Proximal (mesial and distal) aspects of mandibular posterior teeth

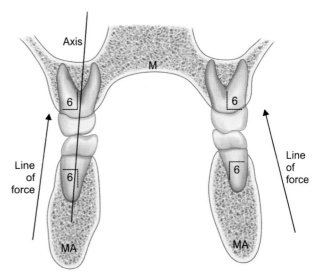

**Fig. 4.22:** Lingual inclination of mandibular teeth and slight buccal inclination of maxillary teeth ensure that the axes of maxillary and mandibular teeth are kept parallel in the jaws. This will be parallel to the line of force.

## BIBLIOGRAPHY

1. Perel ML. Periodontal consideration of crown contour. J Prosthet Dent. 1971;26-6:627-30.
2. Russell ES. Form and Function. Dutton: New York; 1917.
3. Shaw DM. Form and function of teeth: A theory of maximum shear. J Anat Physiol. 1917;52(Pt 1):97-106.
4. Wheeler RC. Complete crown form and periodontium. J Prosthet Dent. 1961;11:722.
5. Youdelis RA, Weaver JD, Sapkos S. Facial and lingual contours of artificial complete crown restoration and their effect on the periodontium. J Prosthet Dent. 1973;29(1):61-6.

## MULTIPLE CHOICE QUESTIONS

1. Each tooth in permanent dentition is in contact with two adjacent teeth, except:
   a. Maxillary central incisors
   b. Maxillary lateral incisors
   c. Maxillary and mandibular first molars
   d. Maxillary and mandibular third molars
2. Which of the following statement is false regarding the location of contact areas?
   a. Contact more cervically placed on posterior than in anteriors
   b. Mesial and distal contact areas are nearly at same level in posterior than in anteriors
   c. The contact areas are broader in posteriors than that of anteriors
   d. Mesial contact area is already cervically located than the distal contact area
3. The distal contact area is more cervically placed than the mesial contact area in all teeth, except in:
   a. Maxillary canine
   b. Mandibular first premolar
   c. Mandibular first molar
   d. Mandibular canine
4. Among anteriors, both mesial and distal contact areas are at the same level in:
   a. Maxillary central incisors
   b. Mandibular central incisors
   c. Mandibular lateral incisors
   d. Mandibular canine
5. Which of the following statements is false about the embrasures?
   a. Lingual embrasures are wider than facial embrasures
   b. They are "V"-shaped spaces between adjacent teeth
   c. Embrasures are more uniform in anteriors than posteriors
   d. Embrasures should be ideally symmetrical
6. In posterior teeth, the buccal crest of curvature is at:
   a. Occlusal third
   b. Middle third
   c. Cervical third
   d. None of the above
7. In posterior teeth, the lingual crest of curvature is at:
   a. Occlusal third
   b. Middle third
   c. Cervical third
   d. None of the above
8. The curvature of cervical line is maximum on:
   a. Mesial surface of maxillary central incisor
   b. Mesial surfaces of maxillary second molar
   c. Distal surface of mandibular third molar
   d. Distal surface of maxillary third molar
9. The geometric form of proximal aspect of anterior is:
   a. Triangular
   b. Rhomboid
   c. Trapezoid
   d. Quadrilateral
10. The proximal geometric form of mandibular molars is:
    a. Trapezoid
    b. Rhomboid
    c. Quadrilateral
    d. Circular

**Answers**

1. d    2. d    3. b    4. b    5. c    6. c    7. b    8. a
9. a    10. b

# Evolution of Teeth, Comparative Dental Anatomy and Forensic Odontology

**5**

**CHAPTER**

## INTRODUCTION

Teeth are highly mineralized appendages found in the entrance and the alimentary canal of both invertebrates and vertebrates. The teeth are mainly associated with prehension and processing of food. However, they frequently serve other functions such as defense, display of dominance, and phonetics as in humans.

This chapter gives an overview and evolution of teeth, comparative dental anatomy, and forensic application of dental anatomy.

## EVOLUTION OF TEETH

A huge amount of literature is devoted to the origin, evolution, and organogenesis of teeth, knowledge of which help to better understand the regulation of tooth development and associated pathogenesis.

Teeth can be classified into three types, based on where they are formed: jaw, mouth, and pharyngeal. The close relationship between past and present teeth can be demonstrated by a phylogenetic analysis. Using this type of analysis, amelogenesis appears to have been duplicated from SPARC (SPARC—secreted protein, acidic, rich in cysteine), some 630,000,000 years ago.

There is substantial evidence to suggest that teeth evolved from scale-like epidermal structures, the *odontodes* which "migrated" into the month after enough mutations. This process is visible in modern sharks, which have *placoid scales* on the skin that grade into the teeth on the jaws.

Teeth with the basic microscopic anatomy similar to that of recent vertebrates first appeared at ordovicium, approximately 460 million years ago. Some jawless fishes developed superficial dermal structures known as *odontodes* **(Fig. 5.1)**. These small tooth-like structures were located outside the mouth and served various functions, including protection,

sensation, and hydrodynamic advantage. Over the evolution, encroachment of odontodes into the oropharyngeal cavity created the buccal teeth, which covered the entire surface and later were localized to the jaw margins.

To begin with, teeth were of uniform conical shape *(homodont).*

Over the period, dietary habits and ecological adaptations have driven the teeth of higher vertebrates to acquire numerous anatomical forms and shapes, as represented by incisors, canines, premolars, and molars *(heterodont).*

It is interesting to note that there is close similarities in structure and development between the *dermal denticles or placoid scales* and the teeth of higher vertebrates.

Each placoid scale when seen in vertical section consists of a base of bone-like substance which is embedded in the dermis and the spine projects through the epidermis beyond the surface **(Figs. 5.2A and B)**. Each spine is covered on the outside with a hard transparent, shiny layer—*the enamel or enameloid* within which is the dentin. Numerous fine canals (canaliculi) ramify through the dentin. The center of the spine is occupied by a cavity—*the pulp cavity,* in which lie blood vessels, nerves,

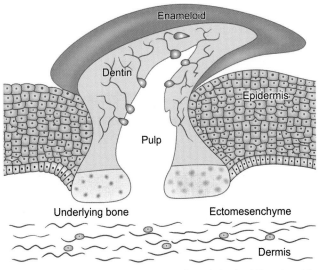

**Fig. 5.1:** Odontodes, the ancestors of teeth, looked like placoid scales of recent sharks.

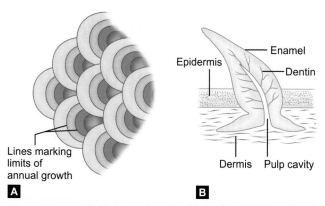

**Figs. 5.2A and B:** (A) Dermal scales of bony fish; (B) Placoid scale of a cartilaginous fish (e.g. Dogfish in section).

and the dentin forming cells *(odontoblasts)*, the protoplasmic extensions of which are continued into the fine canals of the dentin. The pulp cavity is continued into the base and had small aperture to admit the blood vessels and nerves.

The development of placoid scale is much similar to that of teeth **(Fig. 5.3)**.

The first sign of a developing scale is a condensation of mesenchymal cells in the dermis to form *dental or dermal papilla*. This becomes capped by a cone-like down growth of the epidermis. The layer next to the papilla forms a single layer of columnar cells called the *enamel organ*. The outermost cells of the papilla form collagen fibers are the organic basis of the scale.

Then the organic matter between the enamel organ and the outermost layers of the dental papilla get calcified to form the *enamel or enameloid.*

The scale is then thickened by further calcification on the outside of the cone to form the *dentin;* the cells secreting it are called *odontoblasts.* But the central cavity, the *pulp cavity,* is left within the scale which communicates with the dermis through a small opening.

As the scale grows in size, its spine pushes through the epidermis. As the scales get constantly worn away the new scales form, so that in a vertical section of the skin, denticles on various stages of development can be seen.

## Important Changes in the Course of Evolution of Teeth

The evolutionary pathway from fish to reptiles to mammals is characterized by:

- Reduction in number of teeth (from polydonty to oligodonty)
- Reduction on generations of teeth (from polyphyodonty to di- and/or monophyodonty)
- Increase in morphological complexity of the teeth (from homodonty to heterodonty).

## Evolution Favored an Increase in Teeth Complexity

Diet and mastication are regarded as central factors in teeth evolution. There is a strong correlation between teeth form and feeding habits.

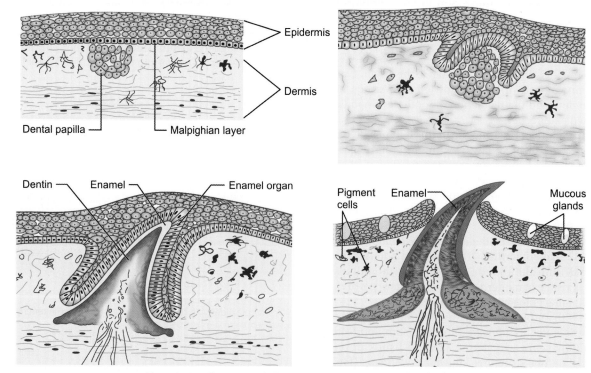

**Fig. 5.3:** Development of placoid scales is similar to that of teeth.

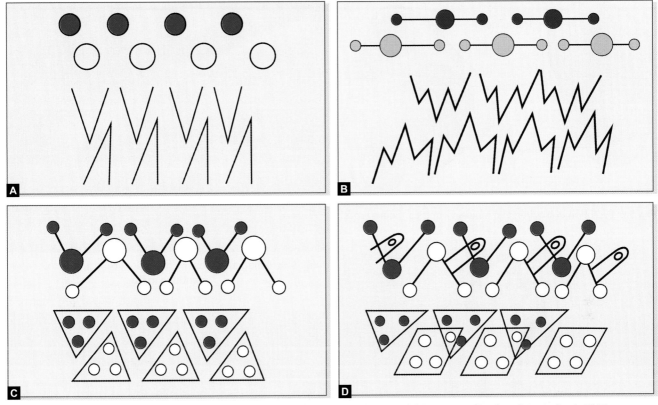

**Figs. 5.4A to D:** Phylogenetic classes of tooth forms: (A) Single cone *(haplodont)*; (B) Three cusps in a line *(triconodont)*; (C) Three cusps in a triangle *(tritubercular molar)*; (D) Four cusps in a quadrangle *(quadritubercular molar)*.

The most important anatomic and functional feature of the masticatory surface of an erupted tooth is the cusps. Cusp number, morphology, topology, and orientation are species specific; these features also differ between teeth of the same mammal. The evolution of the mammalian jaw and teeth created occlusal surfaces that are adequate for a great variety of food.

**Figures 5.4A to D** give four phylogenetic classes of tooth forms:

1. Single cone *(haplodont)*
2. Three cusps in line *(triconodont)*
3. Three cusps in a triangle *(tritubercular molar)*
4. Four cusps in a quadrangle *(quadritubercular molar)*.

The *haplodont class* has simplest form of tooth, single cone **(Fig. 5.4A)**. In haplodont animals (e.g. crocodiles, alligator), the jaws have many teeth and jaw movements are limited to simple open and close (hinge) movements. No occlusion of teeth occurs and teeth are mainly used for prehension of prey and defense **(Fig. 5.5)**.

The *triconodont class* has three cusps in line in posterior teeth **(Fig. 5.4B)**. The largest cusp is in center with smaller cusps located anteriorly and posteriorly. Purely triconodont dentitions are not seen, but the design can be appreciated in some teeth of carnivores.

The *tritubercular molar* evolved from the triconodont. The central cusp was separated from the other two outer cusps so that a triangle was formed on the occlusal surface of upper

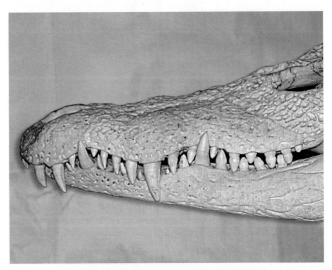

**Fig. 5.5:** Haplodont dentition in crocodile.
*Courtesy:* Crocodile park, La Vanille, Mauritius.

molars **(Fig. 5.6)**. The carnivores, like dogs, are considered to be in tritubercular class **(Fig. 5.7)**.

The *quadritubercular class* reflects an occlusal contact relationship between the teeth of the upper and lower jaw. There is dramatic increase in the masticatory efficiency of the molars. The humans have quadritubercular molars.

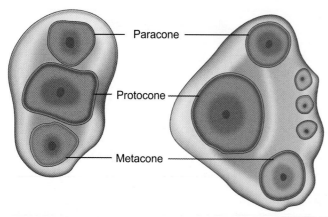

**Fig. 5.6:** Evolution of trituberular molars from triconodont tooth.

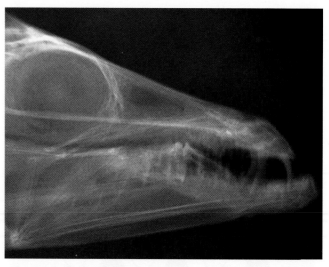

**Fig. 5.8:** Radiograph showing homodont (similar form of teeth) dentition in fish.

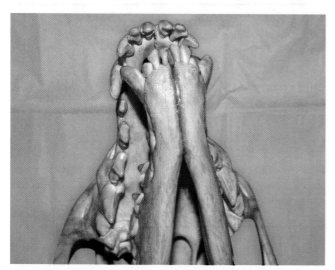

**Fig. 5.7:** Transition from triconodont to tritubercular molar in carnivores, like dog.

## COMPARATIVE DENTAL ANATOMY

To understand the human dentition, it is helpful to compare the dentitions and other vertebrates. Although human dentition is different in form and function from the dentitions of other vertebrates, it becomes obvious that overall plan is common to all.

The fishes, amphibians, reptiles, birds, and mammals together make up the vertebrate group of animals. They are similar to one another in that they all possess a vertebral column and teeth, unless the teeth have been lost as a secondary process of degeneration or specialization.

### Fishes

Most fishes have teeth, but in few teeth are absent. The primary function of teeth in them is to hold their prey. Teeth of the fishes usually exhibit continuous succession *(Polyphyodonty)*. The fishes are of two types—bony fishes and cartilaginous fishes.

Examples of *bony fishes* include herring and tront. Bony fishes have a wide variety of teeth. Some even appear on the

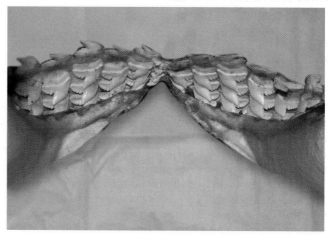

**Fig. 5.9:** Successional teeth in the jaw of a shark with cutting margins turned downward to avoid soft tissue injury.

tongue, palate, and in extreme cases—the throat. Most fishes have homodont (of similar form) dentitions **(Fig. 5.8)** but few exhibit heterodont teeth (teeth of different classes). In bony fishes teeth are attached to jaws by ankylosis.

Examples of *cartilaginous fishes* include sharks, rays, and dogfish. They have many successions of similar shaped teeth. The successional teeth are developed from a persistent dental lamina on the lingual side of the upper and lower jaws. The succeeding teeth lie behind and beneath each functional tooth in rows, with the cutting margins turned upward or downward so that the soft tissue is not damaged **(Fig. 5.9)**. Sharks have haplodont teeth (single cone), but the shape of teeth varies in different types of sharks **(Figs. 5.10A and B)**.

### Amphibians

Teeth are absent in some amphibians (e.g. toad). In others, they are present in one jaw only. In these, the teeth are usually

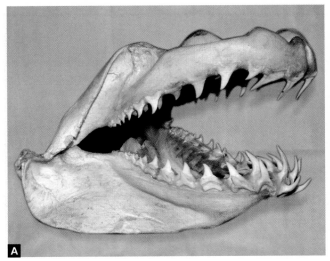

**Figs. 5.10A and B:** Sharks have haplodont (single coned) teeth, but shape vary in different types of sharks.

small conical structures attached by bony ankylosis and undergo continuous replacement.

The frog has a row of small teeth along the edges of the upper jaw only, and two small patches of teeth—vomer teeth on the roof of the mouth.

## Reptiles

The typical reptilian dentition consists of a row of conical teeth of varying sizes in each jaw, attached by bony ankylosis and undergoing a process of continuous succession. In some reptiles, like crocodiles, the teeth are attached by a periodontal membrane to bony sockets.

Crocodiles and alligators have conical shaped teeth of varying sizes that interlock when jaws are closed **(Fig. 5.11)**. Only opening and closing jaw movements are possible in them and the upper jaw is movable. All teeth have single roots.

Teeth are absent in turtles and are replaced by horny plates **(Fig. 5.12)**.

In some snakes **(Fig. 5.13)**, certain teeth are modified to form poison fangs. These contain a canal or a groove which conducts the venom from the base of the tooth to just below the tip in a manner similar to a hypodermic needle.

## MODERN MAMMALS

The characteristic dentition of modern mammals is heterodont, i.e. the teeth vary in form in different parts of the mouth. The typical mammalian dentition is generally considered to have the following dental formula:

$$I\frac{3}{3}, C\frac{1}{1}, P\frac{4}{4}, M\frac{3}{3}$$

There are however a great number of variations from this formula. The teeth are attached by a periodontal membrane to the walls of a bony socket in the jaws. There are usually two dentitions: the deciduous and the permanent.

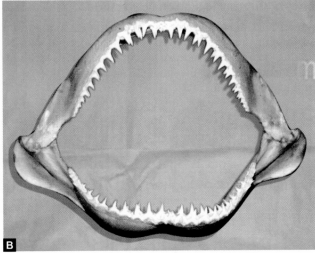

**Fig. 5.11:** Alligator has interlocking conical shaped teeth.
*Courtesy:* Crocodile Park, La Vanille, Mauritius.

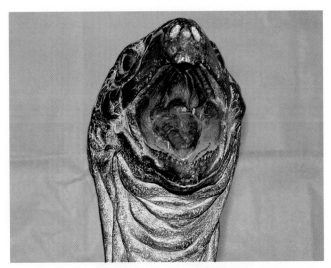

**Fig. 5.12:** In turtles, teeth are replaced by horny plates.
*Courtesy:* Crocodile Park, La Vanille, Mauritius.

### Rodents (Guinea Pig, Rat, and Hamster)

Rodents have most constant type of dentitions. At the front of the mouth are the specialized chisel shaped, continuously erupting, incisor teeth. At the back of the mouth is a series of cheek teeth that are usually similar in form **(Fig. 5.14)**. The dental formula for rat is:

$$I\frac{1}{1}, C\frac{0}{0}, P\frac{0}{0}, M\frac{3}{3}$$

There is only one dentition.

### Herbivorous Mammals (Sheep, Cow, and Horse)

The herbivorous animals have back teeth adapted for grinding up vegetation. The jaws move from side to side while chewing. Dental formula for horse is:

$$I\frac{3}{3}, C\frac{1}{1}, P\frac{4}{4}, M\frac{3}{3}$$

Dental formula for sheep and cow:

$$I\frac{0}{3}, C\frac{0}{1}, P\frac{3}{3}, M\frac{3}{3}$$

Interestingly, the herbivores like sheep and cow do not have upper anteriors. Instead, they have a horny pad against which the front teeth of lower jaw bite **(Figs. 5.15A and B)**.

### Carnivorous Mammals (Dog, Cat, and Seal)

Teeth in carnivores are adapted for catching and killing their prey. They have powerful blade-like cheek teeth called *carnassials*.

### Dog

The dental formula for dog is:

$$I\frac{3}{3}, C\frac{1}{1}, P\frac{4}{4}, M\frac{2}{3}$$

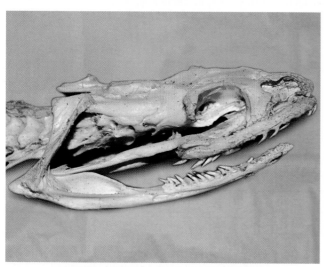

**Fig. 5.13:** Small conical teeth in a snake.
*Courtesy:* Dr DC Master, Professor and Head, Department of Anatomy, Medical Hospital, Vadodara, Gujarat, India.

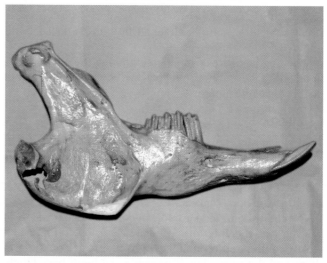

**Fig. 5.14:** Mandibular jaw of a rodent with continuously erupting incisors.

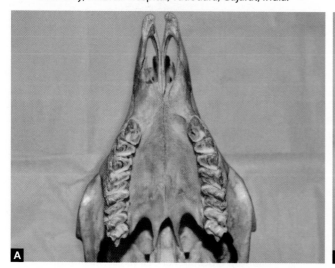

A

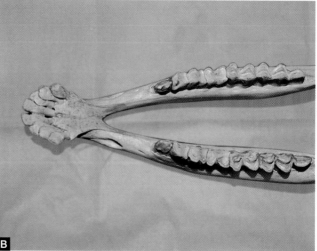

B

**Figs. 5.15A and B:** Dentition in a cattle does not have upper anteriors.

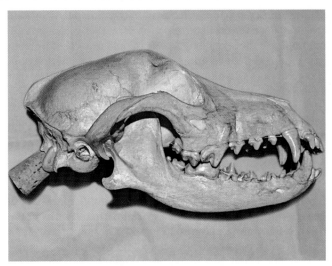

**Fig. 5.16:** Dentition of a dog.
*Courtesy:* Dr DC Master, Professor and Head, Department of
Anatomy, Medical Hospital, Vadodara, Gujarat, India.

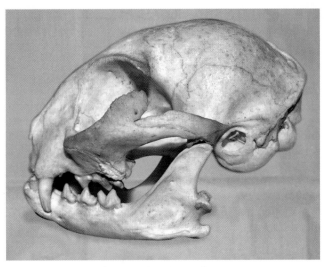

**Fig. 5.17:** Dentition of a cat.
*Courtesy:* Dr DC Master, Professor and Head, Department of
Anatomy, Medical Hospital, Vadodara, Gujarat, India.

They have three incisors and four premolars. The canines are the strongest and the longest teeth in the jaws **(Fig. 5.16)**.

## Cat

The dental formula for cat is:

$$I\frac{3}{3}, C\frac{1}{1}, P\frac{3}{2}, M\frac{1}{1}$$

Cat has three incisors lined in a straight line but has only one molar. Canine is large and sharp tooth **(Fig. 5.17)**.

## New World Monkey

Monkey's dentition is most similar to that of man; only difference being is an extra set of premolars. They have larger primate spaces **(Fig. 5.18)**.
The dental formula is:

$$I\frac{2}{2}, C\frac{1}{1}, P\frac{3}{3}, M\frac{3}{3}$$

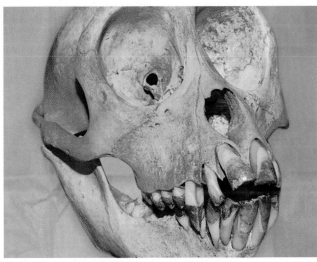

**Fig. 5.18:** Dentition of a monkey.

## FORENSIC ODONTOLOGY

Forensic odontology or forensic dentistry is a branch of forensic medicine that, in the interest of justice, deals with the proper examination, handling, and presentation of dental evidence in a court of law. The dental anatomy is the basis for any forensic dentistry investigation. The main responsibilities of a forensic dentist include the following:

- Identification of human remains, and identification in mass disasters
- Age estimation
- Gender determination
- Bite mark registration and analysis
- Assessment of cases of abuse (child, spousal, elder).

### Identification of Human Remains

Dentistry has much to offer in identification as the teeth are the most durable parts of human body and dentitions are unique due to custom dental restorations and developmental characteristics. The most common role of a forensic dentist is to identify the deceased individuals in whom other means of identification (e.g. finger prints, facial features) are not available. This is true in situations involving burns, decomposition such as air crashes, incineration, floods, and other similar disasters.

The *postmortem* (after death) teeth, jaw, prostheses, and appliances can yield a positive identification, when compared with the *antemortem* (before death) records. Even when

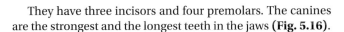

antemortem records are not available, useful information can be drawn by *postmortem dental profiling* which provides information on deceased individual's age, ancestry, sex, and socioeconomic status.

Postmortem and antemortem dental charts are prepared by carefully recording various features such as—number and identity of teeth, tooth rotation, spacing and malposition, anomalies, restorations, prosthesis or appliances, caries, endodontic treatment, implants and surgical repairs, pathology, bone patterns, occlusion, erosion and attrition.

The postmortem and antemortem dental charts are then compared to arrive at conclusion. Presence of unique and rare anatomical variations such as bifurcated mandibular canine, peg-shaped maxillary laterals, etc. may aid early positive identification.

## Age Estimation

Estimation of chronological age is an important aspect of forming the dental profile of an unknown individual both dead and alive. Age estimation by dental means is by far the most accurate method as tooth development is not much affected by nutritional and hormonal changes.

Tooth formation occurs in a programmed and sequential manner with a set sequence of events—from first evidence of calcification to crown formation, root growth, tooth eruption, and root apex closure—that can be accurately assessed on dental radiographs. Thus, age of young children can be accurately determined by the analysis of tooth development and subsequent comparison with standard developmental charts to the accuracy of ±1.5 years. The standard developmental charts given by Dimirjian et al., Moorrees et al., Schour and Massler are routinely used for this purpose. Age estimation after 14 years when most of the teeth are completely formed is difficult although third molars offer a unique advantage over other teeth as their root formation tends to continue over a longer period.

However, adult age estimation is less accurate although a number of methods are employed. Gustafson in 1950 for the first time gave a histological method to estimate adult age. He used six regressive alterations of teeth such as attrition, secondary dentin formation, root dentin translucency, cementum thickness, periodontal attachment, and root resorption to determine adult age to the accuracy of ±10 to 12 years. There have been numerous modifications of Gustafson's technique applied over the years. Certain biochemical methods such as aspartic acid racemization may give better accuracy. Adult age can also be estimated using nondestructive radiographic methods such as tooth:pulp ratio.

## Gender Determination

Determination of sex is of immense importance in forensic investigations. Prediction of gender makes the task simpler since the missing person of only one gender is to be evaluated. Although DNA (deoxyribonucleic acid) analysis is the most precise technique to determine the sex, sometimes lack of facilities and the cost factor may be a hindrance. Measurement of long bones particularly humerus and femur, pelvis, or skull are often used for sex determination. However, odontometric methods are more reliable in case of pediatric cases as teeth complete their development before skeletal maturation. Hence, dentist's opinion is often sought to answer queries that arise during a postmortem investigation.

Various odontometric parameters have been used for gender determination such as mandibular and maxillary and mandibular canine indices, maxillary first molar dimensions, and cumulative dimension of all teeth.

## Bite Marks

Human and animal teeth both leave conspicuous marks. Teeth leave behind noticeable bruises or punctuate marks in the flesh and the marks may also be left on other substances such as food stuffs (apple, cheese, chocolate, and chewing gum), leather, and wood. Bite marks are frequently seen on victims of attack and in cases of child abuse. The distinctiveness of the bite mark, where sufficient detail is available, may lead to identification of the person who caused the mark or exclusion of other suspects.

The physical characteristics of both the bite mark wound and the suspect's teeth that can be compared include— canine to canine distance, shape of dental arch, tooth out of alignment, teeth width, spacing between teeth, missing teeth, curves of biting edges and wear patterns such as chipping of teeth or grinding. Any unique anatomy, i.e. developmental anomalies or variations such as peg shaped laterals make positive identification using bite marks easier **(Figs. 5.19 A and B)**.

The bite marks are recorded and documented using photographs with measurement scales. Positive replicas can be poured using dental impression material. Corresponding morphological features found on the bite mark pattern and the suspect's teeth on a dental cast are then compared to arrive at a conclusion whether the bite mark is caused by the suspect or not.

## Role of DNA in Dental Identification

The oral cavity is a useful source of DNA. The DNA material can be obtained from saliva, the oral mucosal cells, and the teeth. Teeth represent an excellent source of DNA material since they are resistant to most environmental assaults. In teeth, DNA is found in the pulp tissue, dentin, cementum, and periodontal ligament. Due to the resistance of the hard tissues of the teeth to environmental actions such as incineration, immersion, trauma or decomposition, pulp tissue is an excellent source of DNA.

The DNA extracted from dental tissues can provide identity when conventional dental identification methods fail. DNA from dental tissues can be both genomic and mitochondrial DNA. Comparison of DNA from the teeth of an unknown individual can be matched to a known antemortem sample (stored blood, hair brush, biopsy, etc.) or to a parent or sibling.

Sex determination can also be done by targeting *AMEL* gene locus, i.e. *AMELX* and *AMELY* (coding for amelogenin protein of enamel), present in X and Y chromosomes, respectively.

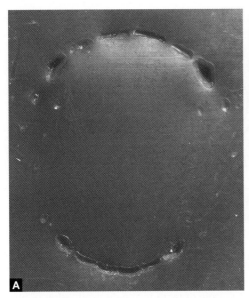
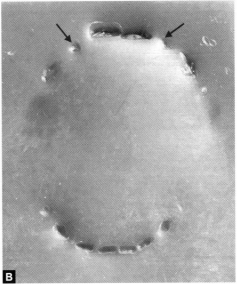

**Figs. 5.19A and B:** Human bite mark exemplars of two individuals. (A) Bite mark shows well aligned normal teeth; (B) Note the indentations left by peg-shaped laterals in this bite mark.

Sufficient DNA material can be extracted from pulp, dentin, and upon amplification using polymerized chain reaction; the length variation in the X and Y homologues of the amelogenin gene gives the basis of sex determination.

## Cheiloscopy/Lip Prints (Fig 5.20)

**Cheiloscopy** (*chelios* in Greek means lips) is a forensic investigation technique that deals with identification of humans based on lips traces. Fisher was the first to describe it in 1902. Studies have shown that it is possible to identify lip patterns as early as the sixth week of intrauterine life and the patterns rarely change thereafter. Lip prints bring valuable added evidence especially in cases lacking other evidence, like fingerprints. Lip prints can be found on tape when a person has been bound or gagged, prints on a drinking glass, cigarette butt and on a glass/window if they were pressed up against it.

Classification given by Suzuki and Tsuchihashi is commonly used to record lip prints which is as follows:
1. Type I: A clear cut groove running vertically across the lip
2. Type I': Partial length groove of Type I
3. Type II: A Branched groove
4. Type III: An intersected groove
5. Type IV: A reticular pattern
6. Type V: Other patterns.

## Palatal Rugoscopy (Fig 5.21)

Palatal rugae are irregular, asymmetric ridges of the mucous membrane extending laterally from the incisive papilla and the anterior part of the palatal raphe. Palatine rugae are unique and are reasonably stable during the lifetime of an individual. Rugoscopy can be of special interest in edentulous cases and also in certain conditions where peripheral body

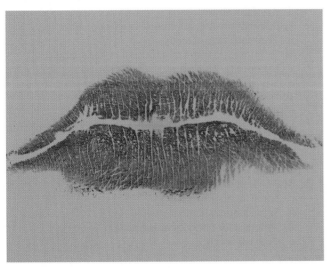

**Fig. 5.20:** Lip print.

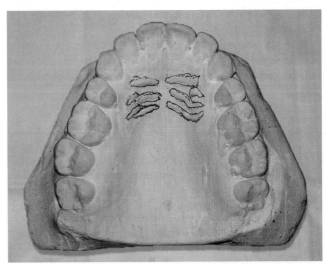

**Fig. 5.21:** Rugoscopy: Rugae patterns marked on a cast.

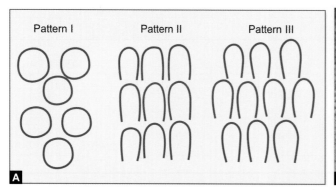 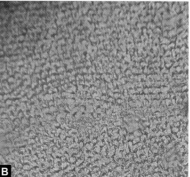

**Figs. 5.22A and B:** (A) Patterns of enamel prisms; (B) Keyhole pattern seen on enamel surface.

parts are burned or decomposed. The shapes of individual rugae are classified into 4 major types: curved, wavy, straight, and circular.

## AMELOGLYPHICS (FIGS. 5.22A AND B)

The term *ameloglyphics* means the study of enamel rod end patterns (amelo: enamel, glyphics: carvings). Enamel does not remodel once it is formed and the ameloblasts retract away from the enamel surface after enamel completion. They leave behind the prism morphology, which is evident on the surface enamel. The basic structural unit of enamel is the enamel prism consisting of several million hydroxyapatite crystals packed into a long thin rod 5–6 mm in diameter and up to 2.5 mm in length. These prisms run from the dentino-enamel junction to the surface. The adjacent enamel rods form a unique pattern due to undulating course of ameloblasts during formative stages.

The shape of the enamel prisms approximates to one of the three main patterns:
1. Pattern I: Prisms are circular.
2. Pattern II: Prisms are aligned in parallel rows.
3. Pattern III: Prisms are arranged in staggered rows such that the tail of prism lies between two heads in the next row, giving a keyhole appearance.

Biometric analysis reveals that the enamel rod end pattern is unique for each tooth in an individual. Studies are being carried out to examine the usefulness of ameloglyphics in forensic investigations.

## BIBLIOGRAPHY

1. Acharya AB, Sivapathasundharam B. Forensics odontology. In: Rajendran R, Sivapathasundharam B (Eds). Shafer's Textbook of Oral Pathology, 6th edition. Elsevier; 2009.
2. Anderson BL, Thompson GW, Popovich F. Evolutionary dental changes. Am J Phys Anthropol. 1975;43(1):95-102.
3. Ferreira da Silva R, Machado do Prado M, de Lucena Botelho T, et al. Anatomical variations in the permanent mandibular canine: forensic importance RSBO. 2012;9(4):468-73.
4. Grove AJ, Newell GE, Carthy JD. Animal Biology, 6th edition. University Tutorial Press Ltd; 1961.
5. Koussoulakou DS, Margaritis LH, Koussoulakos SL. Curriculum Vitae of Teeth: Evolution, Generation, Regeneration. Int J Biol Sci. 2009;5:226-43.
6. Pretty IA, Sweet D. A look at forensic dentistry. Part 1: The role of teeth in the determination of human identity. BDJ. 2001;190(7):359-66.
7. Phulari RG, Rathore RS, Patel AI. Evaluation of third molar development in a Gujarati population using modified Dimirjian method. Ind J Forensic Odontol. 2016;9(1):11-16.
8. Phulari RG, Rathore R, Talegaon T, et al. Comparative assessment of maxillary canine index and maxillary first molar dimensions for sex determination in forensic odontology. J Forensic Dent Sci. 2017;9(2):110.

## MULTIPLE CHOICE QUESTIONS

1. Forensic odontology deals with:
   a. Victim identification
   b. Bite mark analysis
   c. Age estimation
   d. All of the above
2. Up to adolescence, age estimation can be done by:
   a. Eruption stage of teeth
   b. Examining stage of root formation, radiographically
   c. Examining stage of crown formation, radiographically
   d. All of the above
3. Age estimation after adulthood can be done by:
   a. Eruption stage of teeth
   b. Examining stage of root formation, radiographically
   c. Examining stage of crown formation, radiographically
   d. Studying the regressive changes of teeth
4. The regressive changes of teeth include:
   a. Attrition
   b. Secondary dentin formation and apical cementum deposition
   c. Transparency and resorption of roots
   d. All of the above
5. DNA in humans is:
   a. Same for all the individuals
   b. Same for only identical twins
   c. Different for different individuals
   d. Both (b) and (c)

**Answers**

1. d     2. d     3. d     4. d     5. d

# 6

# Dental Anthropology

## INTRODUCTION

Anthropology is the study of humans in all places and at all times. The term anthropology comes from Greek, anthropos = man, logos = the study. The study of anthropology is an investigation into what we are now, from whence we came and how we got to be the way we are today. Anthropologists study modern humans and their direct ancestors generally referred to as hominids.

Anthropology is a recent discipline originating a little more than 100 years ago. The first course in the field was offered in 1879 at University of Rochester (New York). Dental anthropology has evolved more recently as a distinct subfield of physical anthropology, one of the major branches of anthropology.

## BRANCHES/SUBFIELDS OF ANTHROPOLOGY

There are four distinct branches of anthropology in current literature.

### Physical Anthropology

It is the study of people from a biological perspective. It utilizes both biological and physical sciences for the study of humans.

The following are some of the area of interest to physical anthropologists.

### Evolution

*Paleontology* is the study of fossils. It is especially useful in study of evolution and human origins. The study of the fossils of modern humans and human ancestors is called paleoanthropology.

The term *Hominids* refers to modern humans (Homo sapiens), the *Neanderthals,* Homo erectus and the many Australopithecines. The term *Hominids* is a more inclusive term for all the hominids and their closest primate relations, i.e. apes *(Gorilla,* Chimpanzee, Orangutan, and Gibbon).

### Human Variation

How and why physical traits vary around the world is studied. *Anthropometry* is the measuring of human physical characteristics; variations in skeletal shape and bone structure provide useful clues on the search for the origins of human species.

*Primatology* is the study of primates. Primates are our closest relations and are studied for their implications in evolutions and the insights they provide into human behavior.

*Forensic anthropology* is a specialized area of physical anthropology, which deals with identification of human remains for legal purposes.

*Dental anthropology* is the study of teeth as recorded in casts of living mouths or as seen in the skulls of archeological and fossil collections.

### Archeology

It is the study of human cultures and behavior through material remains such as caves, temples, mummies, etc. It mainly focuses on prehistoric cultures.

### Linguistics

It is the discipline that studies speech and language. According to anthropologists, language is conservative. When people move to new areas, they adapt new foods, and lifestyles, but their language is retained. Linguistics has been valuable in tracing the migrations of prehistoric human populations/communities such as that of Native American Indians.

### Ethnology

Ethnology is the study of the cultures of the present. Ethnography is the intensive study of a single culture. Ethnography studies human behavior as it can be experienced—about a particular culture and compares it with that of many cultures of today.

## DENTAL ANTHROPOLOGY

### Terms used in Dental Anthropology

Many of the terms used in anthropology are derived from Greek or Latin and are explained for ease in learning.

## Categories of Teeth by Shape

### *"Homodont" Dentition (Homo = Similar)*

Dentition in which all the teeth are uniformly of similar shape, e.g. teeth in reptiles such as crocodiles and in shark—all teeth are conical in shape **(Fig. 6.1)**.

### *"Heterodont" Dentition (Hetero = Different)*

Dentition in which teeth are regionally specialized into classes, e.g. majority of mammals have heterodont dentitions including humans and higher vertebrates such as dog, cat, sheep, etc.

In heterodont dentition, generally there are four classes of teeth, i.e.—(1) incisors, (2) canines, (3) premolars, and (4) molars **(Figs. 6.2A and B)**.

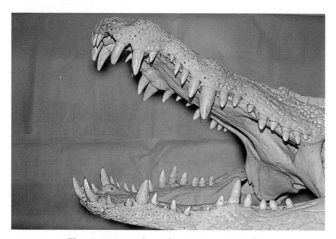

**Fig. 6.1:** Homodont dentition in crocodile.

## Categories of Teeth by Generation

### *Monophyodont Dentition (Mono = Single)*

A monophyodont dentition has a single generation of teeth in lifetime, e.g. dolphin and narwhal.

### *Diphyodont Dentition (Di = Double)*

If the condition of having two generations of teeth in lifetime, e.g. humans are diphyodont with two generations of teeth, i.e. deciduous and permanent dentitions.

### *Polyphyodont Dentition (Poly = Many)*

It refers to many generations of teeth in a lifetime, e.g. many reptiles including crocodiles are polyphyodont. Fishes such as sharks are also polyphyodont.

## Crown

### *Bunodont (Gr = Mound or Hell)*

Teeth have cone-shaped tubercles or cones. They are low crowned with well-developed roots, e.g. posterior teeth in pig.

### *Selenodont (Gr = The Moon)*

Selenodont teeth have cusps transformed into half-moon shapes, e.g. posterior teeth of sheep.

### *Secodont/Sectorial Teeth (L = Secare/To Cut)*

Sectorial teeth are blade-like teeth adapted to cutting the diet into pieces and swallowing them whole. A specialized variant in carnivores are the carnassials teeth, which consist of the last premolar in the upper jaw and the first molar of the lower jaw.

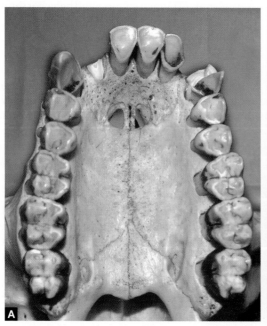
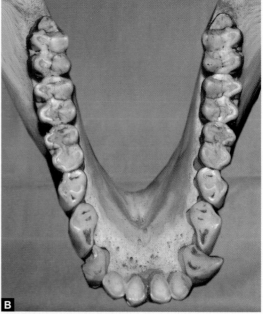

**Figs. 6.2A and B:** Heterodont dentition in monkey.

### Lophodont (Gr = Crest)

Lophodont molars are ridged teeth that have transverse ridges as in the tapir. Lophs are sharp crests that join the cusps in multicusped teeth, i.e. transverse ridges.

Bilophodont molars have two sets of transverse ridges. Polyphodont molars have many ridges, e.g. molar teeth of elephants.

### Brachydont (Gr = Short)

Brachydont teeth have low crowns and well-developed roots, e.g. humans have brachydont teeth.

### Hypsodont (Gr = Height)

Hypsodont teeth have long crown and short roots, e.g. this condition is seen in horse. It is a functional adaptation in these animals for continuous wear sustained by chewing grass with high abrasive silica content.

### Haplodont (Gr = Simple)

Haplodont teeth have simple conical crowns and roots, e.g. teeth in dolphin and crocodiles.

### Tusks

Tusks are incisors or canines of continuous growth that protrude beyond the lips when mouth is closed.

The following are some of the examples of tusks:
- The incisors of the elephant and hippopotamus
- The left incisors of narwhal
- Canines of the wild boar, warthog, and the walrus.

## TEETH IN THE STUDY OF HUMAN VARIATION

Physical traits of humans vary around the world, e.g. skin color, body size, eye color, and size and shape of teeth. Human variation is the combined result of genetic influences, as well as environmental factors such as climate and geographic location.

Teeth provide unique advantage in the study of human variations since tooth crowns are fully formed in childhood before eruption into oral cavity. This permits study of tooth morphology in mixed samples of teeth from ranging ages. This is not possible with skeletal material since only full grown adults show developed skeletons. Furthermore, tooth morphology can also be studied in living subjects by simply taking dental impressions. Scott and Turner II have divided humans into several population groups based on their geographic origin feature, e.g. presence/absence of Carabelli's cusp.

Dental features used to describe population differences are broadly classified as metric (tooth size) and nonmetric (tooth shapes).

### Metric Variation in Teeth

Metric variations are features that are directly measured. Generally, the maximum dimensions of the teeth are considered. Three basic dimensions are usually used:
1. Mesiodistal diameter of the crown
2. Buccolingual diameter of the crown
3. Crown height.

### Nonmetric Variations in Teeth

Several nonmetric variations in crown and root form have been used to study migration patterns of human populations. Some of the commonly recorded features are discussed below.

### Carabelli Trait (Cusp of Carabelli)

The Carabelli trait was first described in 1811 by George Carabelli, who was Court dentist to the Austrian Emperor Franz. The trait when present is located on the mesiolingual corner of upper first permanent molar and second deciduous molar. The trait shows varied expression. It can express itself as a pit, a groove, ridge, and tubercle or as a well-formed cusp **(Figs. 6.3A to C)**. When present as a cusp version, it can be larger than the main cusp.

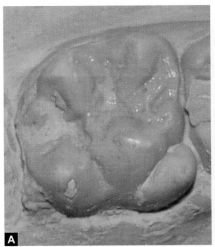 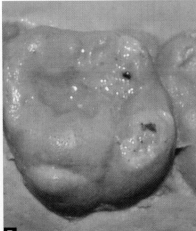 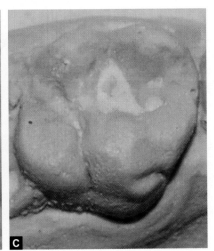

**Figs. 6.3A to C:** Varied expression of cusp of Carabelli.

The Carabelli trait is most frequently seen in Caucasoid populations and has a low incidence of expression in Mongoloid population. Sometimes, the trait expresses as a lingual cingulum; a similar feature is found amongst primates—gibbon, chimpanzee, gorilla, and orangutan.

### Shovel-shaped Incisors

Shoveling is a feature seen in incisors, where the marginal ridges are especially prominent and enclose a deep fossa in the lingual surface **(Fig. 6.4)**.

Shoveling is commonly seen on permanent and deciduous upper incisors but can sometimes appear in lower incisors also shoveling can also create a pit on the lingual surface of central incisors.

Shovel-shaped incisors show highest frequency of occurrence in Asians and Native Americans and lowest occurrence in Europeans.

Shovel-shaped incisors are found in Homo erectus, suggesting that this is a very ancient trait.

### Winged Incisors

Winging is an indirect crown trait. In this condition, distal margins of both the upper central incisors are rotated labially creating a "V"-shaped pattern of incisal edges when view occlusally **(Fig. 6.5)**.

### Protostylid of Molars

The protostylid is a feature on the buccal side of the lower molar crown characterized by a tubercle on the mesiobuccal cusp, ranging from a spot in the buccal groove, through a furrow to a prominent cusp **(Fig. 6.6)**.

The feature is seen especially on first or third permanent lower molars or in deciduous lower second molar population identification is based on protostylid on lower first molar.

### Lower Molar Groove Pattern

Occlusal groove configuration (X, Y, and "+") on the lower first and second molars is also used for population identification **(Fig. 6.7)**.

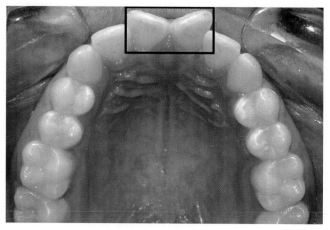

**Fig. 6.5:** Winged incisors.

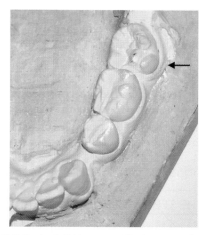

**Fig. 6.6:** Protostylid in a mandibular second molar.

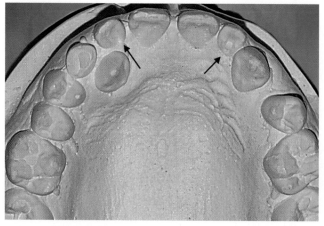

**Fig. 6.4:** Shoveling in maxillary lateral incisors.

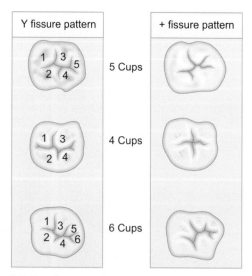

**Fig. 6.7:** Developmental grooves pattern in lower molars.

### Sixth Cusp on Lower Molar

Lower first molar may have a supernumerary cusp on the distal aspect between the distolingual and the distal cusp **(Fig. 6.8)**.

### Taurodontism (Taurus = Bull)

The term taurodontism is used to describe the bull-like condition on the multirooted posterior teeth in which the teeth have long root trunks with wide pulp chamber. Some consider this feature to be an atavistic tendency. Taurodontism is found prominently on Krapina Neanderthal specimens.

### Variation in Root Morphology

**Single-rooted upper first premolar:** Upper first premolar with single root is used for population identification **(Fig. 6.9A)**.

**Two-rooted lower canine:** Presence of double-rooted lower canine is rare in humans, but is a typical feature in primate dentition **(Fig. 6.9B)**.

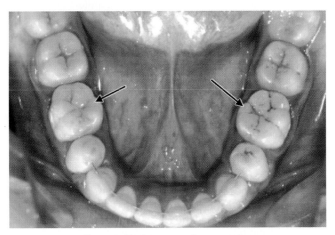

**Fig. 6.8:** Sixth cusp on lower molar.

**Three-rooted lower molars:** Presence of a third root on lower molars also helps in population identification **(Fig. 6.9C)**.

## SEXUAL DIMORPHISM AND TEETH

The sexual dimorphism of teeth is a well-known feature of higher animals and primates where size and shapes of teeth, especially those of canine teeth, are differ significantly among males and females. In many animals, large canines are considered to be a visual sexual sign of dominance and rank. Due to evolutionary changes, there has been a reduction in sexual dimorphism of teeth in humans.

However, studies have shown significant differences in males and females on metric and certain nonmetric features of teeth. In general, mesiodistal and buccolingual diameters of crowns are greater in males than in females.

### Metric Features

Various odontometric parameters have been used for gender determination such as mandibular and maxillary canine indices, mandibular canine dimensions, maxillary canine dimension, maxillary first molar dimensions, and cumulative dimension of all teeth. Human dental dimorphism is centered on canines, with lower canines showing the greatest dimorphism followed by the upper canines.

$$\text{Canine index} = \frac{\text{Mesiodistal crown width of canine}}{\text{Intercanine distance}}$$

### Nonmetric Features

*Sexual differences*: Females have a higher frequency of missing teeth and a lesser frequency of supernumerary teeth than in males.

A nonmetric feature of canine "distal accessory ridge" is the most sexually dimorphic (feature) trait in human dentition, with males showing higher frequencies than females.

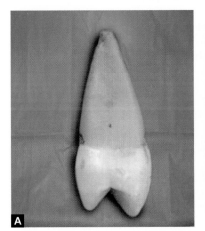 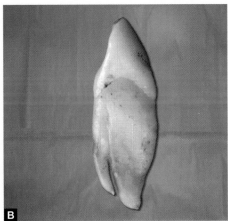 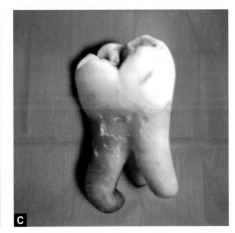

**Figs. 6.9A to C:** (A) Single-rooted upper first premolar; (B) Two-rooted lower canine; (C) Three-rooted lower first molar.

Presence of only four cusps in mandibular first molar (absence of 5th cusp) is more commonly seen in females than in males. In addition to tooth size, certain tooth proportions show sexual dimorphism.

## BIBLIOGRAPHY

1. Hillsons. Dental Anthropology. New York: Cambridge University Press; 1996.
2. Hrdlicka A. Shovel-shaped teeth. Am J Phy Anthro. 1920;3:429-65.
3. Khraisat A, Taha ST, Jung RE, et al. Prevalence, association, and sexual dimorphism of Carabelli's molar and shovel incisor traits amongst Jordanian population. Odontostomatol Trop. 2007;30(119):17-21.
4. Krogman WM. The role of genetic factors in the human face, jaws and teeth: a review. Eugen Rev. 1967;59(3):165-92.
5. Phulari RG, Rathore R, takvani MD, et al. Evaluation of occlusal groove patterns of mandibular first and second molars in an Indian population: A forensic anthropological study. Indian J Dent Res. 2017;28:252-5.
6. Phulari RG, Rathore R, Talegaon T, et al. Comparative assessment of maxillary canine index and maxillary first molar dimensions for sex determination in forensic odontology. J Forensic Dent Sci.2017;9(2):110.
7. Portin P, Alvesalo L. The inheritance of shovel shape in maxillary central incisors. Am J Phy Anthro. 1974;41:59-62.

## MULTIPLE CHOICE QUESTIONS

1. Homodont dentition refers to:
   a. Dentition in which all the teeth are uniformly of similar shape
   b. Dentition in which teeth are regionally specialized into classes
   c. Dentition has a single generation of teeth in lifetime
   d. Dentition having two generations of teeth in lifetime
2. Heterodont dentition refers to:
   a. Dentition in which all the teeth are uniformly of similar shape
   b. Dentition in which teeth are regionally specialized into classes
   c. Dentition has a single generation of teeth in lifetime
   d. Dentition having two generation of teeth in lifetime
3. The term monophyodont dentition refers to:
   a. Dentition in which all the teeth are uniformly of similar shape
   b. Dentition in which teeth are regionally specialized into classes
   c. Dentition has a single generation of teeth in lifetime
   d. Dentition having two generations of teeth in lifetime
4. The term diphyodont dentition refers to:
   a. Dentition in which all the teeth are uniformly of similar shape
   b. Dentition in which teeth are regionally specialized into classes
   c. Dentition has a single generation of teeth in lifetime
   d. Dentition having two generation of teeth in lifetime
5. An example of homodont dentition is:
   a. Reptiles
   b. Humans
   c. Fish
   d. Sheep
6. An example of heterodont dentition is:
   a. Reptiles
   b. Humans
   c. Fish
   d. Sheep
7. The term polyphyodont dentition refers to:
   a. Dentition in which all the teeth are uniformly of similar shape
   b. Dentition in which teeth are regionally specialized into classes
   c. Dentition has a single generation of teeth in lifetime
   d. Many generations of teeth
8. Which of the following is true regarding the selenodont teeth?
   a. Selenodont teeth have cusps transformed into half moon shaped
   b. Posterior teeth of sheep
   c. Both of the above
   d. None of the above
9. Which of the following is false statement?
   a. Sectorial teeth—blade like teeth
   b. Selenodont—half moon-shaped teeth
   c. Lophodont—confined to molars
   d. Bilophodont incisors—incisors having ridges
10. Bilophodont molars are seen in:
    a. Molars teeth of humans
    b. Molars teeth of elephant
    c. Molars teeth of fish
    d. Molars teeth of sheep

**Answers**

1. a    2. b    3. c    4. d    5. a    6. b    7. d    8. c
9. d    10. b

# 4

## SECTION

# Deciduous Dentition

### Section Outline

# 7

# Primary (Deciduous) Dentition

## INTRODUCTION

Humans are diphyodonts having two sets of dentitions in their life time. The first set of teeth is termed as the "*primary dentition*" or "*deciduous dentition*". The term "*deciduous*" comes from Latin word meaning "to fall off". The deciduous teeth are called so since they fall off or shed naturally similar to the leaves of deciduous trees. Both the terms are accepted and are used interchangeably to describe the first set of dentition in this book.

Sometimes, the deciduous teeth are also referred to as "*temporary teeth*", "*milk teeth*", "*baby teeth*" or "*lacteal teeth*".

However, these terms are improper and should be discouraged since they erroneously imply that these teeth are only useful for a short period and thus denote a lack of importance.

## DENTAL FORMULA FOR PRIMARY DENTITION

There are a total of 20 teeth in the primary dentition, 10 in each jaw **(Fig. 7.1A)**. Each jaw has four incisors, two canines, and four molars. Each quadrant has five teeth namely—central incisor, lateral incisor, canine, first molar, and second molar, beginning from the midline. *There are no premolars in primary dentition*. It is also important to note that, *there are no third molars either in primary dentition*. Thus, the premolars and the third molars are the teeth which are present only in the permanent dentition.

In mixed dentition period, when the permanent teeth (succedaneous teeth) replace their predecessors (primary teeth)—*the primary incisors are replaced by the permanent*

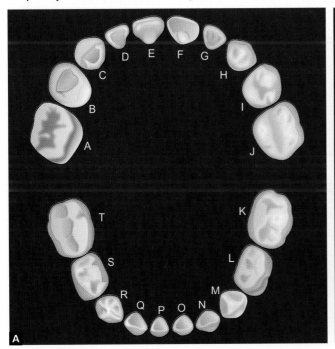

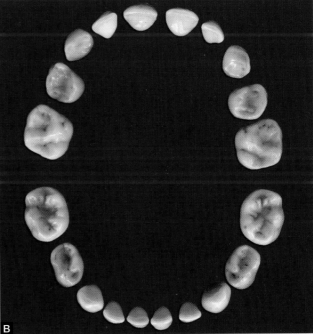

**Figs. 7.1A and B:** (A) Primary dentition has 20 teeth, 10 in each jaw (4 incisors, 2 canines, 4 molars); and no premolars (tooth notation in universal system); (B) A complete set of primary teeth specimen arranged here are from a single child preserved by her mother.

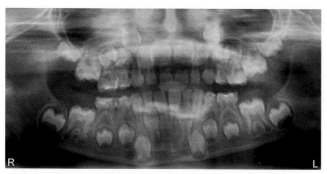

**Fig. 7.2:** Orthopantomogram (OPG) of a 6-year-old boy showing replacement of primary teeth by their respective successors—primary incisors by permanent incisors, primary canines by permanent canines, and primary molars by the permanent premolars. Note that the permanent molars are not succedaneous teeth and do not replace any primary teeth. (Note that 31 and 41 have already erupted, permanent first and second molars are developing distal to the primary molars. The third molar germs are not yet seen).

incisors; *the primary canines are replaced by the permanent canines.* However, *the primary molars are replaced by the permanent premolars.*

The permanent molars do not replace any teeth but erupt distal to the primary molars. In other words, *the permanent molars are not succedaneous teeth as they do not have predecessors in primary dentition* **(Fig. 7.2).** Thus permanent molars are sometimes referred to as *accessional teeth.*

Primary anteriors resemble their respective permanent anteriors. The primary first molars have unique crown form.

The primary maxillary first molars resemble the permanent premolars in crown form. However, they have three roots like permanent maxillary molars. *Primary mandibular first molars have unique occlusal anatomy and do not resemble any teeth in either of the dentitions.*

*The primary second molars closely resemble and appear like miniature permanent first molars of the respective dental arches* **(Fig. 7.1B).**

The dental formula (representing each half of mouth) for primary dentition in humans is as follows:

$$I\frac{2}{2}, C\frac{1}{1}, M\frac{2}{2} \text{ (10 per one side of mouth)}$$

On the other hand, the dental formula for human permanent dentition is:

$$I\frac{2}{2}, C\frac{1}{1}, P\frac{2}{3}, M\frac{3}{3} \text{ (16 per one side of mouth)}$$

## Life Cycle

*Development of the primary teeth occurs both prenatally and postnatally.* Primary teeth begin to develop prenatally about 14 weeks *in utero,* with the appearance of first evidence of calcification of primary central incisors. Development of all the primary teeth is completed postnatally at about 3 years of age. **Figure 7.3** illustrates the development of primary teeth.

Crown formation of all primary teeth is completed at about 12 months of age. Eruption of primary teeth into oral cavity usually begins with the emergence of mandibular central incisors at around 6 months **(Fig. 7.4)** and is completed with the eruption of maxillary second molars around 2.5 years

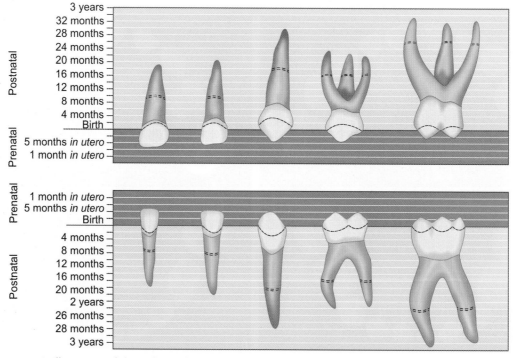

**Fig. 7.3:** Diagrammatic illustration of chronology of primary teeth. Eruption is completed at the time indicated by the dotted area on the root of teeth. Dotted line on crowns of teeth indicates the portion formed prenatally.

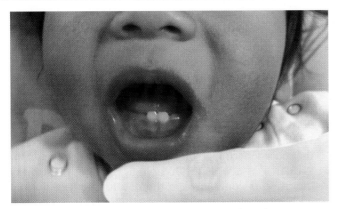

**Fig. 7.4:** Eruption of primary teeth usually begins with emergence of mandibular central incisors at around 6 months of age.

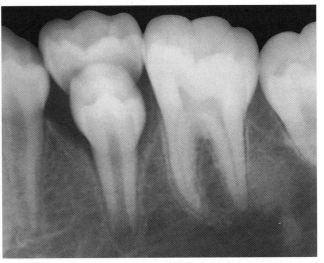

**Fig. 7.5:** A permanent successor tooth replaces its predecessor when most part of latter's root is resorbed and is shed naturally.

(24 ± 4 months). The roots of primary teeth are completely formed in just 1 year after eruption of the crowns into oral cavity; root formation of all the primary teeth is completed by 3 years of age. The complete set of primary dentition is functional in the mouth from 2 years to 6 years of age, after which the primary teeth are gradually replaced by the permanent teeth. Thus, primary dentition period lasts from 6 months to 6 years of age.

The roots of deciduous teeth begin to resorb just 2–3 years after their completion. Resorption begins at the apices of roots and continues gradually toward the crown. When most of the root is resorbed, the crown is shed naturally making way for eruption of the permanent successor tooth **(Fig. 7.5)**. The deciduous teeth are exfoliated between 7 years and 12 years of age.

*Transitional or mixed dentition period* begins with the emergence of permanent first molars. The permanent first molars erupt distal to deciduous second molars before any of the deciduous teeth are lost. The transitional period lasts from 6 years to 12 years of age, or ends when all the deciduous teeth have been shed. Permanent dentition stage begins at that time. Chronology of deciduous teeth is given in **Table 7.1**.

## SIGNIFICANCE OF DECIDUOUS DENTITION

A person with average life expectancy of 70 years would spend only 6% of his or her life masticating solely with primary teeth. Despite this small proportion of time they serve, care of deciduous dentition is very much essential for the normal growth and development of the jaws and establishment of normal occlusion of permanent dentition. Well-cared primary teeth ensure proper alignment of the permanent teeth by "preserving" space for the latter until they erupt. Malocclusion with severe crowding can occur when primary teeth are lost prematurely due to loss of space in the arch.

**Table 7.1:** Chronology of primary teeth.*

| Tooth | First evidence of calcification (weeks *in utero*) | Amount of enamel formed at birth | Crown completed | Eruption | Root completed |
|---|---|---|---|---|---|
| *Maxillary teeth:* | | | | | |
| Central incisor | 14 | Five-sixths | 1½ months | 10 months | 1½ years |
| Lateral incisor | 16 | Two-thirds | 2½ months | 11 months | 2 years |
| Cuspid | 17 | One-third | 9 months | 19 months | 3¼ years |
| First molar | 15½ | Cusps united | 6 months | 16 months | 2½ years |
| Second molar | 19 | Cusp tips still isolated | 11 months | 29 months | 3 years |
| *Mandibular teeth:* | | | | | |
| Central incisor | 14 | Three-fifths | 2½ months | 8 months | 1½ years |
| Lateral incisor | 16 | Three-fifths | 3 months | 13 months | 1½ years |
| Cuspid | 17 | One-third | 9 months | 20 months | 3¼ years |
| First molar | 15½ | Cusps united | 5½ months | 16 months | 2¼ years |
| Second molar | 18 | Cusp tips still isolated | 10 months | 27 months | 3 years |

*Chronology of teeth. Schour and Massler (1940); Logan and Kronfeld slightly modified by McCall and Schour (1933).

Importance of primary teeth can be listed as follows:

*Efficient mastication of food:*
- With the establishment of primary occlusion, child learns to masticate the food efficiently.
- Neuromuscular coordination required for masticatory process is established at primary dentition stage itself.

*Maintenance of a proper diet and good nutrition:*
- Primary teeth are the only teeth present until 6 years of age and thus it is important to provide the child with a comfortable functional occlusion of primary teeth.
- A child with missing or grossly decayed primary teeth may reject food that is difficult to chew.

*Maintenance of normal facial appearance:* A well-cared set of deciduous dentition contributes to establishment and maintenance of the normal facial appearance during the tender age of childhood **(Fig. 7.6A)**.
- It contributes to normal psychological and cognitive development of the child. Prematurely lost or rampantly carious front teeth may hamper a child's self-confidence due to mocking from their peers **(Fig. 7.6B)**.

*Development of clear speech:*
- Teeth, especially the anteriors, are essential for normal pronunciation of consonants.
- Speech is developed in early childhood and congenital absence or premature loss of anterior primary teeth can hamper the development of clear speech.

*Avoidance of infection and possible sequelae:*
- It is important to prevent and treat dental caries of primary teeth so as to prevent abscess formation and pain.
- Spread of infection from periapical abscess (especially in primary molars) may reach the underlying permanent tooth germs and can cause brown spots of their crowns (Turner's hypoplasia).

*Maintenance of normal eruption schedule of permanent successors:*
- A primary tooth is shed when its successor permanent tooth is ready to erupt.

- Generally, successor tooth erupts within 3 months of exfoliation of its predecessor tooth.
- However, this normal eruption schedule of permanent teeth is disturbed when primary teeth are lost prematurely due to caries or trauma. As a consequence malocclusion may develop.

*Maintenance of space for eruption of permanent successor teeth:*
- Primary teeth serve a very important function of "preserving" the space for eruption of their permanent successor teeth.
- Presence of adequate physiologic spacing in primary dentition is conductive to the development of normal occlusal relations in permanent dentition **(Fig. 7.7)**.
- Maintenance of space is especially important in canine and molar regions since their successors, the permanent canines and premolars, erupt relatively late in life.
- When primary teeth are lost prematurely, the adjacent teeth migrate into the available space leading to a decrease in the arch length. This causes a lack of space in the arch for the erupting permanent successors and results in the development of malocclusion. A lack of space associated with premature loss of primary teeth

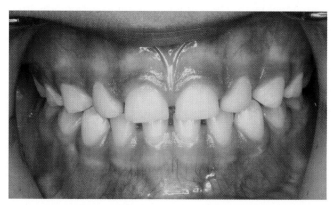

**Fig. 7.7:** Adequate physiologic spacing between the primary teeth in a 5-year-old child.

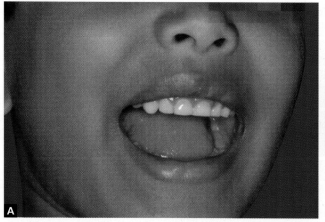
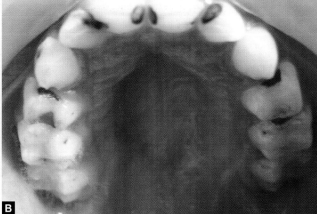

**Figs. 7.6A and B:** (A) Well-cared deciduous dentition contributes to normal facial appearance and boosts psychological and cognitive development of the child; (B) Carious or prematurely lost front teeth may hamper child's self-confidence.

is a common cause of malocclusion development **(Fig. 7.8)**.

- When a primary tooth is lost prematurely due to trauma, caries, etc. the space occupied by the lost tooth should be maintained using appliances known as "space maintainers" until the permanent successor erupts **(Fig. 7.9)**.

## DETAILED DESCRIPTION OF EACH PRIMARY TOOTH

### Deciduous Incisors

Deciduous incisors are the first teeth to erupt into oral cavity. The mandibular central incisors erupt at around

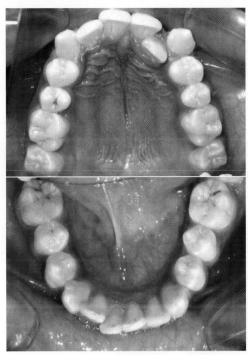

**Fig. 7.8:** Crowding in maxillary anterior region due to premature loss of primary molars and resultant anterior shifting of premolars, leaving inadequate space for canine eruption.

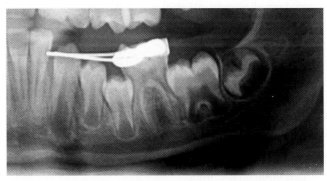

**Fig. 7.9:** A portion of orthopantomogram (OPG) showing band and loop type of space maintainer given on mandibular first molar to preserve the space for eruption of canine and premolars.

6–8 months of age, followed by mandibular lateral, maxillary central, and maxillary lateral incisors. Deciduous incisors are morphologically similar to permanent incisors. However, *primary teeth do not exhibit mamelons on their incisal ridges.* All deciduous incisors have single conical roots.

### Deciduous Maxillary Central Incisor (Figs. 7.10 and 7.11)

#### *Crown*

##### *Labial aspect (Figs. 7.10A and 7.11A)*

- *Geometric shape:* Trapezoidal with narrow cervix.
- Deciduous maxillary central incisors are the only incisors (in both deciduous and permanent dentition) in which mesiodistal width of the crown is greater than the cervicoincisal length.
- Labial surface is slightly convex in all planes. It is smooth and devoid of developmental grooves, depressions, and lobes.
- Unlike permanent incisors, the deciduous incisors do not show mamelons on their incisal ridge.
- More often than not, the incisal ridge is attrited to form a straight incisal edge.
- The mesioincisal angle is sharp and acute while the distoincisal angle is obtuse and rounded.

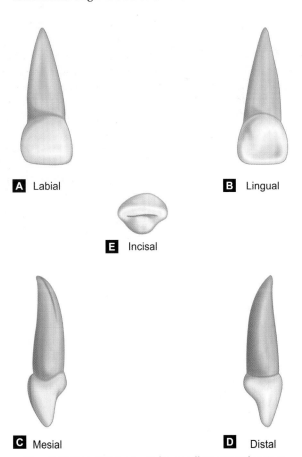

**A** Labial  **B** Lingual

**E** Incisal

**C** Mesial  **D** Distal

**Figs. 7.10A to E:** Primary right maxillary central incisor.

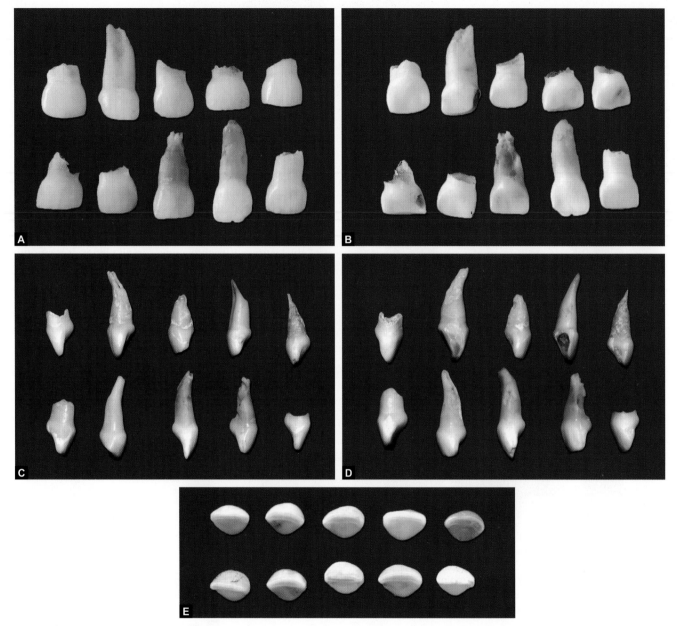

**Figs. 7.11A to E:** Primary maxillary central incisor—typical specimen from all aspects: (A) Labial aspect; (B) Lingual aspect; (C) Mesial aspect; (D) Distal aspect; (E) Incisal aspect.

***Lingual aspect:***

- *Geometric shape:* Trapezoidal.
- The cingulum is very well developed, proportionally larger than seen on permanent maxillary central incisors.
- It extends far more toward the incisal ridge than that of permanent maxillary central incisors, occupying major part of lingual surface.
- The lingual fossa is smaller and shallower.
- The marginal ridges are well developed and distinct.

- As with permanent incisors, the proximal walls of the crown taper toward lingual aspect, making lingual surface narrower than the labial surface.

***Mesial aspect:***

- *Geometric shape:* Triangular or wedge-shaped.
- The crown appears bulkier labiolingually at cervical area due to bulges of cervical enamel ridge on one side and cingulum on the other.
- The mesial surface is smooth and convex.

- Incisal ridge is located labial to the root axis line. In permanent maxillary central incisor, the incisal ridge is on line with its root axis line.

### Distal aspect:
- Distal aspect is similar to that of mesial aspect in terms of shape and crown outline.
- As with permanent incisors, the cervical line curvature is less in extent on the distal surface than on the mesial surface.

### Incisal aspect:
- *Geometric shape:* Diamond-shaped.
- The mesiodistal diameter is greater than the labiolingual diameter.
- The incisal edge is straight and is centered over the crown.
- Labial surface is smooth and convex mesiodistally.
- The crown tapers lingually toward the cingulum.

### Root
- Single conical root
- The root is longer in proportion to the crown than in permanent central incisor. It is about twice the length of its crown.
- Similar to the crown, the roots also converge lingually forming a ridge for its full length.
- Often the roots exhibit physiologic resorption.
- Resorption occurs on lingual aspect of the roots since the permanent successors of deciduous anteriors are located apical and lingual to them in the jaws.
- Apical portion of the root may show a labial curvature. This arrangement is believed to provide room for the developing permanent teeth that is located in an apical and lingual portion in the jaw.

## Deciduous Maxillary Lateral Incisor (Figs. 7.12 and 7.13)

### Crown

The lateral incisor crown is smaller in all dimensions than the central incisor.

### Labial aspect:
- The crown is longer cervicoincisally than it is wide mesiodistally.
- The distoincisal angle is much more rounded than seen in the deciduous maxillary central incisor.
- The incisal ridge may form a semicircular arc rather than a straight line. There are no mamelons on the incisal margin.

### Lingual aspect:
- The cingulum is less pronounced than seen on the central incisor. It does not extend incisally as far as seen in the central incisor.
- Marginal ridges are well-marked and concavity of the lingual fossa is deeper than that of the central incisor.

### Mesial and distal aspects:
- The lateral incisor crown appears similar to the central incisor from proximal aspects.
- However, faciolingually, the crown looks less bulky due to less pronounced cingulum and cervical enamel ridge.
- Constriction of the neck of the tooth is visibly more apparent from proximal views.

### Incisal aspect:
- *Geometric shape:* Circular.
- Incisal ridge is more curved.
- Looking from this view, the labial surface is more convex than seen on the central incisor.
- Lingual surface tapers toward cingulum and the lingual fossa is distinct.

### Root
- Single, conical and slender root
- The deciduous lateral incisor root is much longer in proportion to its crown than in case of the central incisor. The root is more than twice the length of its crown.
- The root is often resorbed and the resorption pattern is typically on the lingual surface of the root.

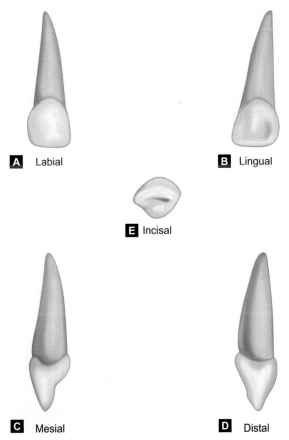

**A** Labial   **B** Lingual

**E** Incisal

**C** Mesial   **D** Distal

**Figs. 7.12A to E:** Primary right maxillary lateral incisor.

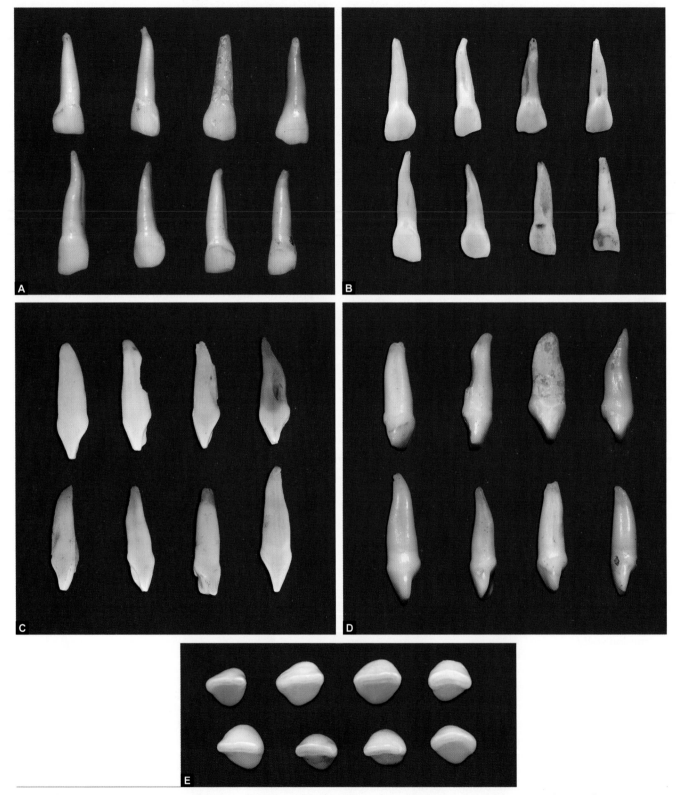

**Figs. 7.13A to E:** Primary maxillary lateral incisor—typical specimen from all aspects: (A) Labial aspect; (B) Lingual aspect; (C) Mesial aspect; (D) Distal aspect; (E) Incisal aspect.

## Deciduous Mandibular Central Incisor
(Figs. 7.14 and 7.15)

Deciduous mandibular central incisors are the smallest teeth in human dentitions.

### Crown

**Labial aspect:**
- *Geometric shape:* Trapezoidal narrow cervix.
- The tooth is bilaterally symmetrical like that of its permanent successor.
- The cervicoincisal length of the crown is slightly greater than the mesiodistal width.
- Both the mesioincisal and distoincisal angles are sharp and make right angles.
- The labial surface is smooth, slightly convex, and unmarked by developmental grooves and depressions.

**Lingual aspect:**
- *Geometrical shape:* Trapezoidal.
- *Crown outlines:* Similar but reversal to that seen on labial aspect.
- The lingual surface is narrower than the labial surface as the proximal walls converge toward lingual aspect.

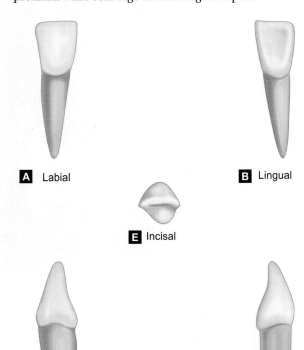

**A** Labial  **B** Lingual

**E** Incisal

**C** Mesial  **D** Distal

**Figs. 7.14A to E:** Primary right mandibular central incisor.

- The cingulum is not well developed although as prominent as seen on deciduous maxillary central incisor.
- The marginal ridges are not well developed.
- The lingual fossa is shallow and smooth.
- The cervical line is positioned more apically lingual than on labial surface.

**Mesial and distal aspects:**
- *Geometrical shape:* Triangular
- The incisal ridge is centered over the root axis line. In case of permanent central incisor, the incisal ridge is located lingual to the root axis line.
- The mesial and distal surfaces are smooth and convex.
- The crown appears robust from proximal as compared to its small size; although small, the tooth is bulkier in labiolingual dimension.

**Incisal aspect:**
- *Geometrical shape:* Circular.
- The incisal ridge is centered over the bulk of the crown.
- Major bulk of the crown is located at cervical third.
- Labial surface is convex and tapers lingually.
- The mesiodistal dimension is almost equal to labiolingual dimension of the crown.

### Root
- Single, conical root is twice the length of the crown.
- Similar to all incisors, the root also converges toward lingual aspect, making lingual surface narrower than the labial surface.
- The root shows physiologic resorption on lingual aspect the whole root may be gone.

## Deciduous Mandibular Lateral Incisor
(Figs. 7.16 and 7.17)

As in permanent dentition, morphology of the mandibular lateral incisor is similar to the central incisor but is larger than the latter. The mandibular lateral incisor is larger than the central incisor in all dimensions. However, both the incisors are of same bulk labiolingually.

### Crown

**Labial aspect:**
- The mandibular deciduous lateral incisor is slightly larger than the mandibular deciduous central incisor.
- Unlike the deciduous mandibular central incisor, the lateral incisor is asymmetrical and has sharp mesioincisal angle and the distoincisal angle is rounded.
- As the distoincisal angle is markedly rounded, the tooth mimics maxillary deciduous lateral incisor. Sometimes, it may be difficult to distinguish the two teeth.
- It is observed that, the incisal ridge or edge has a tendency to slope downward in a distal direction.

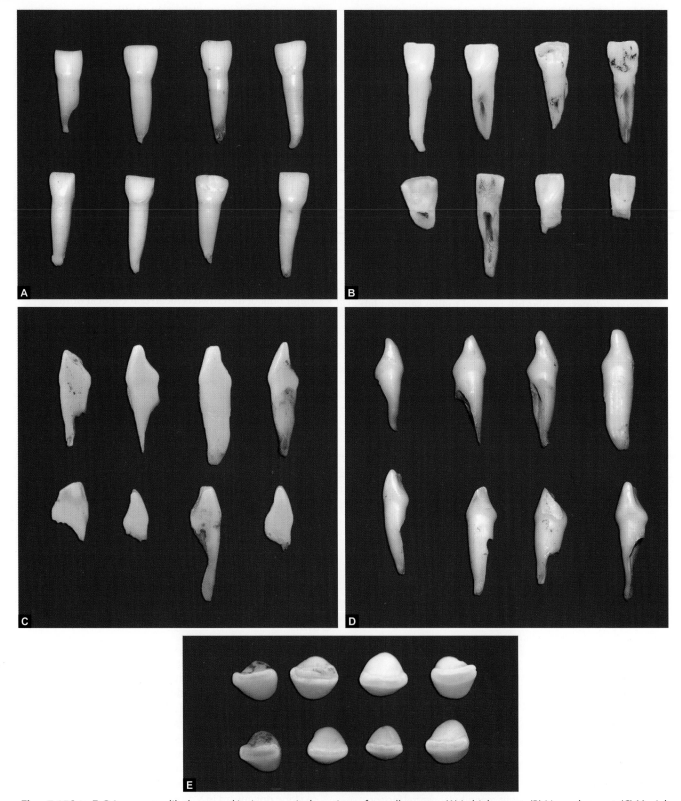

**Figs. 7.15A to E:** Primary mandibular central incisor—typical specimen from all aspects: (A) Labial aspect; (B) Lingual aspect; (C) Mesial aspect; (D) Distal aspect; (E) Incisal aspect.

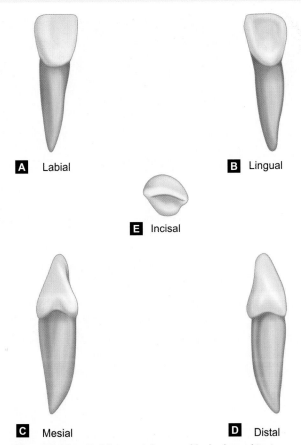

**A** Labial  
**B** Lingual  
**E** Incisal  
**C** Mesial  
**D** Distal

**Figs. 7.16A to E:** Primary right mandibular lateral incisor.

#### Lingual aspect:
- When compared to the deciduous mandibular central incisor, the cingulum may be well developed in deciduous mandibular lateral incisor.
- The lingual fossa of the deciduous mandibular lateral incisor may be deeper.

#### Mesial and distal aspects:
- The deciduous mandibular lateral incisor appears identical to the deciduous mandibular central incisor from proximal view.
- Labiolingual dimension is greater at the cervical third in both the teeth.

#### Incisal aspect:
- *Geometric shape:* Circular.
- The mesiodistal and labiolingual dimension of the crown is equal from this view.
- The convexity of the lingual surface is more generous than on the mandibular deciduous central incisor.

### Root
- Single, conical root.
- Longer than that of mandibular central incisor.
- Root apex when not resorbed may be sharp.
- The apical half of the root shows a labial tilt.

## DECIDUOUS CANINES

### Deciduous Maxillary Canine (Figs. 7.18 and 7.19)

Deciduous maxillary canines are the most common deciduous teeth to be over retained in the oral cavity. This is due to delayed eruption timing or schedule of permanent maxillary canine which erupts after the eruption of premolars in the arch. When the arch length is reduced, the permanent canine may erupt labially or lingually leading to malocclusion.

### Crown

#### Labial aspect:
- *Geometrical shape:* Diamond-shaped with broader sides, pointed tip, and constricted neck.
- In deciduous maxillary canine, the crown is more bulbous in proportion to its root than in its permanent successor. There is marked cervical constriction at the neck.
- The mesiodistal diameter of the crown is greater than its cervicoincisal length. This along with the marked cervical constriction makes the crown look bulbous.
- When not worn, the cusp is much longer, shaper, and more pointed compared with that of the permanent maxillary canine.
- The two cusp ridges meet at an acute angle.
- Mesial cusp ridge is longer.
- In general, *the distal cusp ridge is longer than the mesial in all teeth except in permanent maxillary first premolar and deciduous maxillary canine.*
- The labial surface is smooth and convex.
- There is cervical enamel ridge near the cervix. A labial ridge may be noted running from the cervical ridge to the cusp tip on labial surface.

#### Lingual aspect:
- *Geometric shape:* Diamond-shaped.
- The cingulum is pronounced that may cover more than half of the length of the crown.
- As in permanent maxillary canine, linear palatal or lingual ridges arise from cingulum to the cusp tip. It divides the lingual fossa into two small mesial and distal fossae.

#### Mesial and distal aspects:
- *Geometric shape:* Triangular.
- The crown is much more bulky at the cervical third when compared with primary incisors.
- The labial cervical ridge appears as prominently as the cingulum from proximal aspect.
- The incisal ridge or cusp tip is located labial to the root axis line.

#### Incisal aspect:
- *Geometric shape:* Diamond-shaped.
- The canine crown is bulkier in mesiodistal dimension than that of deciduous incisors.
- The crown appears somewhat angular.
- The labial outline is more convex and the crown tapers toward the cingulum.

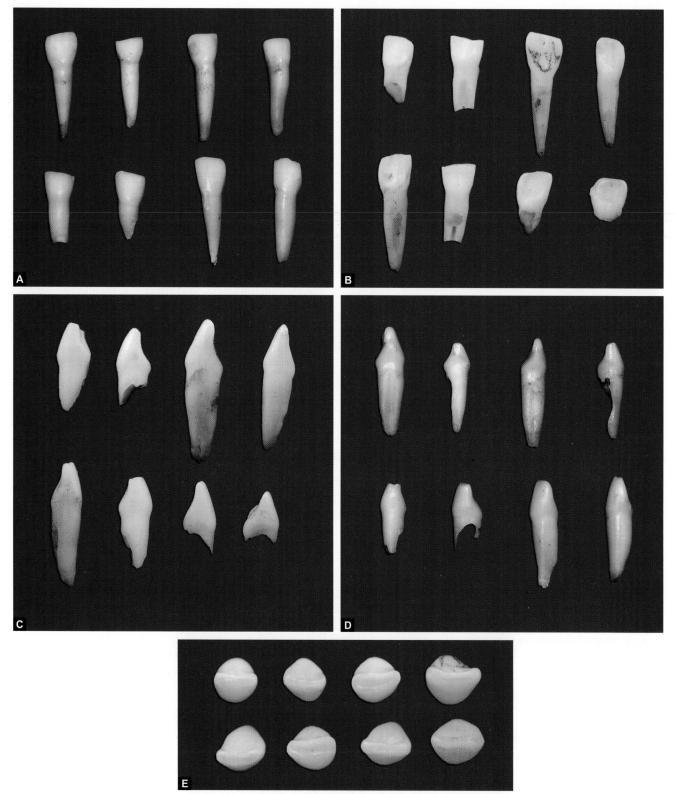

**Figs. 7.17A to E:** Primary mandibular lateral incisor—typical specimen from all aspects: (A) Labial aspect; (B) Lingual aspect; (C) Mesial aspect; (D) Distal aspect; (E) Incisal aspect.

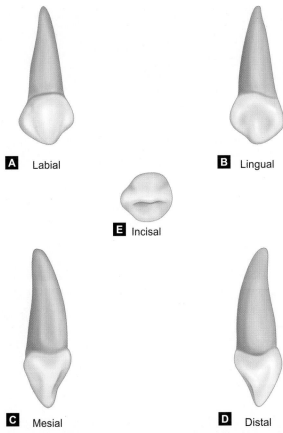

**Figs. 7.18A to E:** Primary right maxillary canine.

- The cusp tip is located distal to the center of the crown.
- The mesial half of the crown is thicker than the distal half. This is true for permanent maxillary canine as well.

### Root

- Single root, and is more than twice its crown length.
- The root is conical and appears slender in proportion to its wider crown.
- Like the crown, the root also tapers lingually.
- The root is wider labiolingually and gives good resistance against masticatory force.
- Roots are often resorbed. Resorption occurs on lingual and apical aspects.

## Deciduous Mandibular Canine (Figs. 7.20 and 7.21)

The deciduous mandibular canine is smaller than the deciduous maxillary canine in all dimensions. The crown is more asymmetrical and slender than the deciduous maxillary canine.

### Crown

#### Labial aspect:
- *Geometrical shape*: *Pentagonal* from labial and lingual aspects.

- The deciduous canine crown's length is greater than its mesiodistal width.
- Cervical constriction at the neck is not as marked as in the maxillary canine.
- Maximum mesiodistal dimension of the crown is comparable to the mesiodistal width of the root at cervix. Thus, the root appears thicker at the cervix.
- The mesial cusp ridge is shorter than the distal. The opposite is true for deciduous maxillary canine. This helps in proper intercuspation during mastication.
- Labial ridge is not prominent.
- *Contact areas*: Distal contact area is cervically placed than the mesial contact area.

#### Lingual aspect:
- *Geometric shape:* Pentagonal.
- The marginal ridges are less developed
- The cingulum is placed more cervically and is less pronounced than that of deciduous maxillary canine. The lingual ridges are distinct and there is a single lingual fossa.

#### Mesial and distal aspects:
- *Geometric shape:* Triangular.
- Proximal form of deciduous mandibular canine is comparable to that of the deciduous maxillary central incisors.
- The crown is noticeably less bulkier in labiolingual dimension at cervix portion than in deciduous maxillary canine.
- The mesial and distal surfaces are smooth and convex.
- The tip of the cusp is located lingual to the root axis line as seen in case of permanent lower canine.

#### Incisal aspect:
- *Geometric shape:* Diamond-shaped.
- The cusp tip is located mesial to the center of the crown.
- The crown seems to have slightly more bulk on the distal half.

### Root

- Single root is proportionally larger comparable to its slender crown.
- It is about 2 mm shorter than the deciduous maxillary root.
- The root is conical, appears bulky in cervical and middle thirds, and tapers more in the apical third.
- The root is usually resorbed, sometimes up to the cervix.

## Deciduous Molars

- There are only two molars in each quadrant in deciduous dentition.
- There are no third molars in deciduous dentition.
- Primary molars erupt immediately distal to the primary canines since premolars are absent in primary dentition.
- They are wider mesiodistally than their successors—first and second premolars. Thus, they save space in the arch for the permanent premolars.

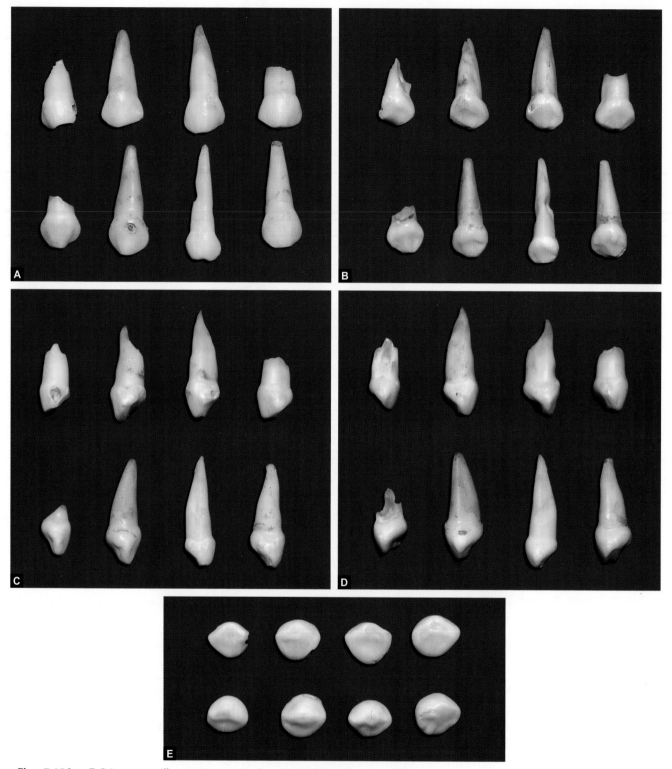

**Figs. 7.19A to E:** Primary maxillary canine—typical specimen from all aspects. (A) Labial aspect; (B) Lingual aspect; (C) Mesial aspect; (D) Distal aspect; (E) Incisal aspect.

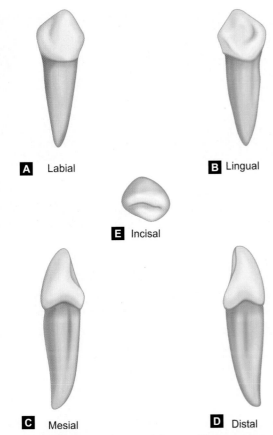

**A** Labial **B** Lingual

**E** Incisal

**C** Mesial **D** Distal

**Figs. 7.20A to E:** Primary right mandibular canine.

- The combined mesiodistal width of the primary canines, first and second molars is greater than the combined mesiodistal width of the permanent successors that is permanent canines, first and second premolars. This difference in their mesiodistal dimension is known as *Leeway space of Nance* and provides space for mesial migration of permanent first molar and subsequent establishment of normal occlusion.
- It is interesting to note that *the primary second molars are larger than primary first molars.* On the contrary, in permanent dentition, the first molars are generally the largest.
- Primary first molars are more unique in their morphology, while the primary second molars closely resemble the permanent first molars.
- *Primary maxillary first molar is regarded as the most atypical of all molars* (in both dentitions) by many authors. Some feel that they somewhat resemble the permanent premolars. Others postulate that their morphology appears to be an intermediate between a premolar and a molar.
- The primary mandibular first molar is very unique in its crown morphology.
- *It is generally agreed that the primary mandibular first molar does not resemble any tooth in either of the dentitions.*

- The roots of the primary molars are delicate, slender, and diverge widely to make room for developing permanent successor teeth.
- Care has to be taken while extracting deciduous molars. Extraction of deciduous molars before their roots have begun to resorb, may lead to inadvertent removal of the permanent successor tooth germs along with the primary molars.
- Inflammation from deciduous pulp can easily reach to the developing permanent tooth germ (Turner's hypoplasia). The primary molars provide chewing surface to the child in early growing years from 2½ to 6 years.
- After 6 years until they are shed, the primary molars are assisted in function by the permanent first molars that erupt distal to them in the dental arch before any of the deciduous teeth are shed.

## Deciduous Maxillary First Molar (Figs. 7.22 and 7.23)

Primary maxillary first molar is the smallest among all the molars in both the dentitions. The crown has unique form that is regarded as an intermediate between a premolar and a molar. Like permanent maxillary molars it has three roots. Primary maxillary first molar is much smaller than the maxillary second molar in all the dimensions.

### Crown

**Buccal aspect:**
- *Geometric shape:* Trapezoidal.
- The *cervical line* is quite distinct. It is sinuous, higher mesially than distally.
- The much smaller size of the primary first molar compared to the maxillary second molar is easily appreciated from this aspect.
- The tooth is wider mesiodistally than its cervico-occlusal height.
- It is noticeably constricted at the neck, with proximal walls diverging occlusally.
- The buccal surface is smooth, generally devoid of any developmental grooves.
- The mesiobuccal cusp is prominently visible from this view.
- The cervical ridge that runs mesiodistally is most prominent on primary first molar both maxillary and mandibular.
- It is more prominent on maxillary first molar than on mandibular first molar.
- The bulge is thicker mesially than distally.

**Lingual aspect:**
- *Geometric shape:* Trapezoidal.
- The crown noticeably tapers toward the lingual aspect, making the lingual surface narrower than the buccal aspect. From this aspect, the mesiolingual cusp, which is the longest and sharpest cusp of this tooth, is prominently visible. The smaller and shorter distolingual cusp may also be seen.
- The lingual surface is smooth. It is more convex mesiodistally and less convex cervico-occlusally.

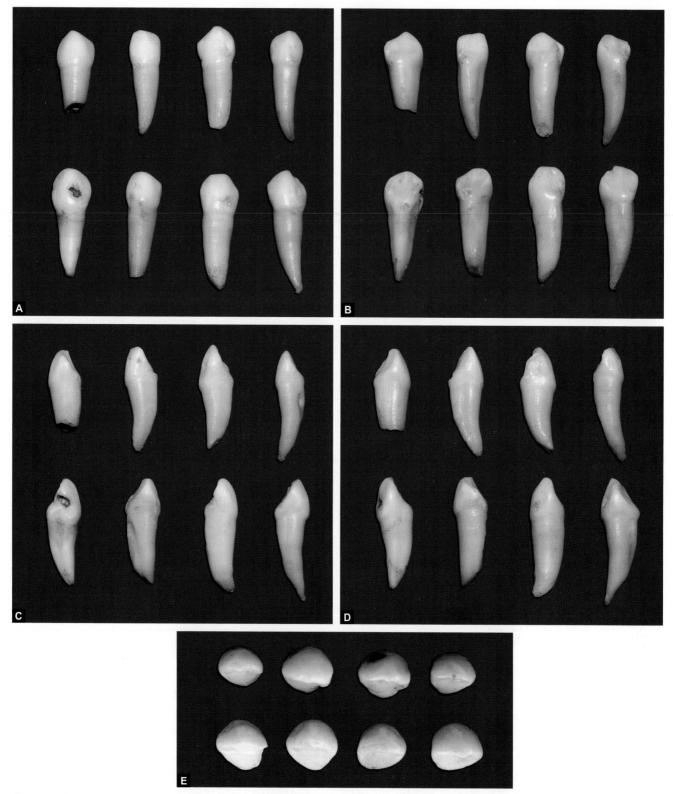

**Figs. 7.21A to E:** Primary mandibular canine—typical specimen from all aspects: (A) Labial aspect; (B) Lingual aspect; (C) Mesial aspect; (D) Distal aspect; (E) Incisal aspect.

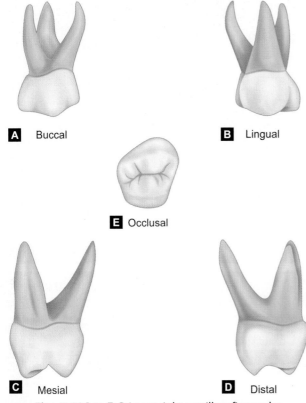

**Figs. 7.22A to E:** Primary right maxillary first molar.

### Mesial aspect:
- *Geometric shape:* Trapezoidal.
- The crown appears much wider cervically than occlusally in case of all primary molars.
- The crown tapers drastically toward the occlusal surface from their buccal and lingual convexities.
- The mesial surface is broader than distal surface.
- It is smoothly convex.

### Distal aspect:
- *Geometric shape:* Trapezoidal.
- The distal surface is narrower buccolingually than the mesial surface.
- This is because the buccal and the lingual surfaces of the crown converge from mesial to distal aspect.
- The distal surface is more convex than the mesial surface.

### Occlusal aspect:
*Geometric shape:* Quadrilateral.

*Crown form:*
- The primary maxillary first molar resembles a maxillary premolar and is regarded as the premolar section of primary dentition.
- The resemblance is nicely appreciated from occlusal view.
- However, the tooth is essentially a molar in junction with three roots giving good anchorage in the alveolar bone.

*Cusps:*
- The primary maxillary first molar generally has four cusps: two larger and two smaller.
- The two larger cusps namely, *mesiobuccal and mesiolingual cusps,* confer premolar like form to the tooth especially from an occlusal view.
- The two smaller cusps are the *distobuccal* and the often inconspicuous *distolingual cusp.*
- Not uncommonly, the distolingual cusp may be absent giving a triangular occlusal form to the tooth that resembles a maxillary premolar more closely. This is also referred to as a *three cusp molar.*

*Cusp ridges:*
- The mesial and distal marginal ridges form the two smaller sides or arms of the occlusal quadrilateral form.
- The distal marginal ridge is much smaller than the mesial since the crown converges distally.
- The mesiobuccal and mesiolingual cusps have well-defined triangular ridges.
- Sometimes, a well-developed triangular ridge connects the mesiolingual and distobuccal cusp and is called the oblique ridge.

*Fossae:*
- The primary maxillary first molar has three fossae—a central fossa, a mesial triangular fossa, and a distal triangular fossa.
- The mesial triangular fossa is larger than the distal triangular fossa.

*Grooves and pits:*
- The groove pattern is often described as an H-pattern.
- The *central developmental groove* runs mesiodistally across the center of the occlusal surface from the mesial pit in the mesial triangular fossae to the distal pit in the distal triangular fossae.
- The *buccal developmental groove* separates the mesiobuccal and distobuccal cusps and may extend onto buccal surface.
- It joins the central developmental groove in the central fossae to form a central pit.
- The *distal developmental groove* divides the smaller distolingual cusps. It may or may not extend onto the lingual surface.

### Root
- In line with maxillary arch traits, the primary maxillary 1st molar has three roots: mesiobuccal, distobuccal and palatal.
- The tooth has three long, slender and widely diverging roots.
- The palatal root is the longest and largest. The distobuccal root is shorter than the mesiobuccal root.
- The roots flare out widely to accommodate the developing permanent successor between the roots.
- The trifurcation begins nearly at the cervical line itself thus having a very small root trunk if it is present at all.
- This feature is true for all the primary molars, which is in contrast to permanent molars. In permanent molars, bifurcation and trifurcation begins at some distance

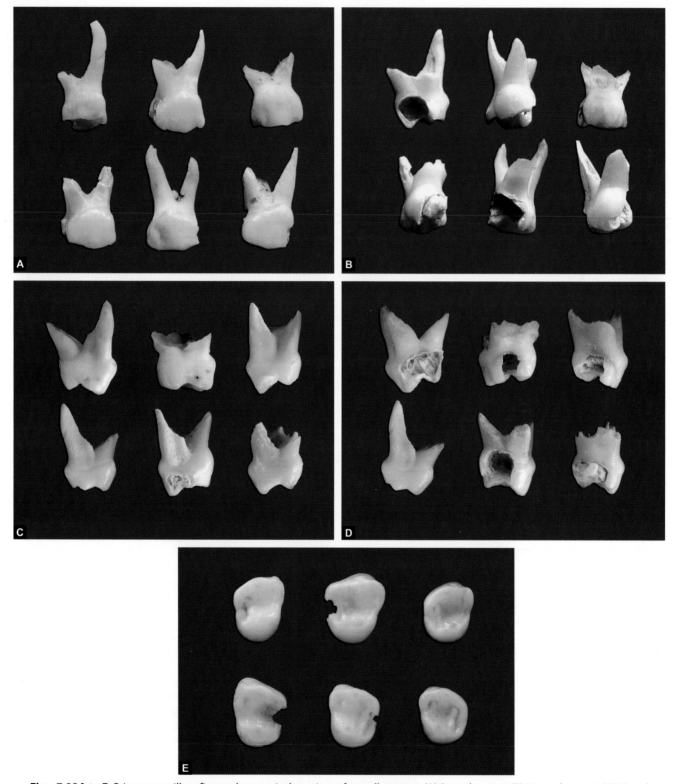

**Figs. 7.23A to E:** Primary maxillary first molar—typical specimen from all aspects: (A) Buccal aspect; (B) Lingual aspect; (C) Mesial aspect; (D) Distal aspect; (E) Occlusal aspect.

(4–5 mm) from the cervical line, thus they have a well-defined and strong root trunks.

## Deciduous Maxillary Second Molar
## (Figs. 7.24 and 7.25)

As discussed earlier, the primary second molars closely resemble the permanent first molars that erupt distal to the tooth. It is the replica of permanent molar in form, albeit smaller. However, the primary second molar can be easily distinguished from the permanent first molar by its smaller size, whitish color, prominent buccal cervical ridge, and widely diverging roots. Like the permanent maxillary first molars, it also has the major cusps namely the mesiobuccal, mesiolingual, distobuccal, distolingual, and a small accessory cusp referred to as cusp of Carabelli or the 5th cusp.

### Crown

**Buccal aspect:**
- *Geometric shape:* Trapezoidal.
- The primary maxillary second molar is considerably larger than the primary maxillary first molar.
- As with all primary molars, the crown has a much constricted cervix on comparison to its mesiodistal dimension at the contact areas.

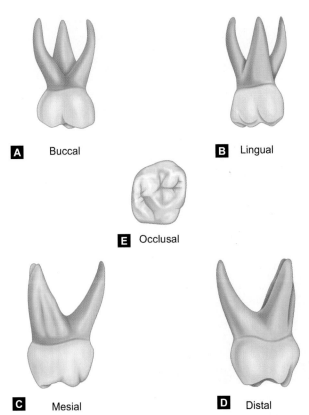

**Figs. 7.24A to E:** Primary right maxillary second molar.

- Two buccal cusps are nearly of same size and development.
- The crown is longer mesially than distally.
- The buccal surface is convex except for buccal developmental groove that separates the two buccal cusps.
- The bulge of buccal cervical ridge is prominent and runs mesiodistally at the cervical third of crown.

**Lingual aspect:**
*Geometric shape:* Trapezoidal.
Three cusps are seen from the lingual view:
1. *Mesiolingual cusp:* Larger and well-developed
2. *Distolingual cusp:* That is more well-developed than seen on primary maxillary first molar.
3. *Cusp of Carabelli or the 5th cusp:* Less prominent than seen in permanent maxillary first molar.

**Mesial aspect:**
- *Geometric shape:* Trapezoidal with shortest and uneven sides toward the occlusal surface.
- The crown form appears similar to permanent maxillary first molar from this aspect.
- The buccolingual dimension is narrower occlusally than cervically.
- The bulge of buccal cervical ridge is not as prominent as seen on the primary maxillary first molar.

**Distal aspect:**
- *Geometric shape:* Trapezoidal.
- The distal surface of crown is narrower than the mesial surface as the crown tapers distally. The distobuccal cusp is long and sharp while the distolingual cusp is poorly developed.
- It is from the occlusal aspect that the tooth appears as exact replica of the permanent maxillary first molar.

**Occlusal aspect:**
- *Geometric shape:* Rhomboidal as in case of permanent maxillary first molar.
- However, the crown somewhat tapers toward lingual (this is not true in case of maxillary first molar).
- The crown also tapers toward distal surface.
- The mesiolingual angle is much more obtuse than seen on permanent maxillary first molar.
- The mesiolingual corner of the crown appears to be flattened or compressed toward distal.
- This makes the mesiolingual cusp shift in a distal direction; and thus the oblique ridge has a more straighter and less oblique course buccolingually.

**Cusps and cusp ridges:** There are four major cusps—
1. Mesiolingual
2. Mesiobuccal
3. Distobuccal
4. Distolingual.
And one minor cusp—*the cusp of Carabelli.*

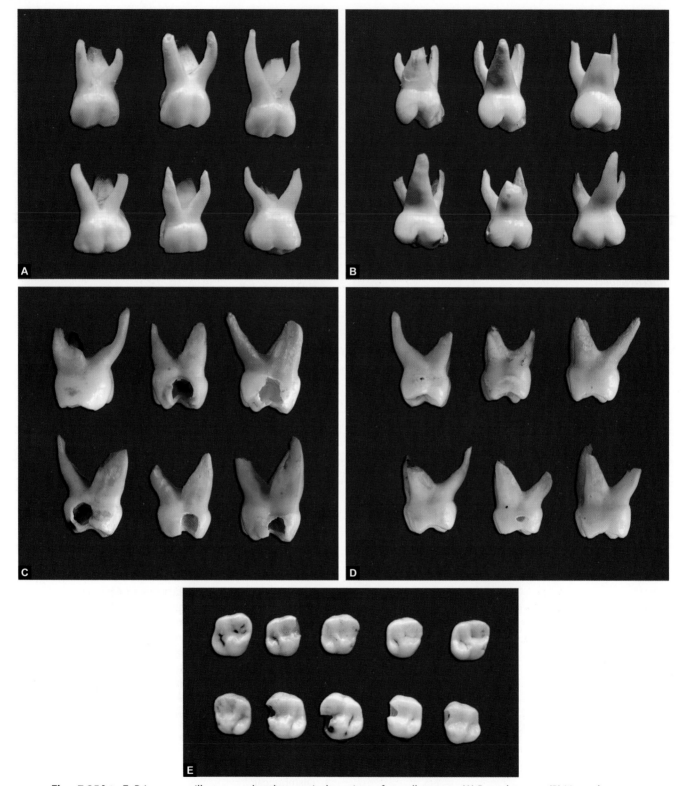

**Figs. 7.25A to E:** Primary maxillary second molar—typical specimen from all aspects: (A) Buccal aspect; (B) Lingual aspect; (C) Mesial aspect; (D) Distal aspect; (E) Occlusal aspect.

- The mesiolingual is the largest cusp.
- The prominent oblique ridge connects the mesiolingual and the distobuccal cusps.
- It is less oblique and more straighter in its course than that seen on permanent 1st maxillary molar.

***Fossae, grooves, and pits:***
- There is a *central fossa, mesial triangular* and smaller distal *triangular fossa.*
- The *central developmental groove* runs at the bottom of the sulcus that connects the mesial triangular fossa with the central fossa.
- The *buccal developmental groove* runs buccally from the central pit in the central fossa and separates the mesiobuccal and distobuccal cusps.
- The *distal fossa* is located distal to the oblique ridge.
- At the bottom of distal fossa, the *distal developmental groove* runs a short course.
- A less distinct distal triangular fossa is seen just mesial to the distal marginal ridge which shows supplementary groove.
- The distal developmental groove separates the mesiolingual and the distolingual cusps and continues onto the lingual surface as the lingual developmental groove.

## Root

- *Three roots:* mesiobuccal, distobuccal, and palatal.
- The roots are much longer and stronger than that of maxillary first primary molar.
- Palatal root is larger and heavier than the other roots.
- The roots are slender and longer in proportion to the crown.
- They diverge widely from their point of trifurcation. Trifurcation occurs immediately near the cervical line leaving no root trunk.

## Deciduous Mandibular First Molar (Figs. 7.26 and 7.27)

*The primary mandibular first molar does not resemble any other tooth in both primary and permanent dentitions.* It has a very unique morphology that is sometimes described as primitive in nature. Unlike primary maxillary first molar it is molariform. The tooth has four cusps and the two roots. The crown height varies from different aspects. The cervical line curvature is unique, different from all other teeth.

## Crown

***Buccal aspect:***
- *Geometric shape:* Trapezoidal
- Buccal aspect offers some unique features of primary mandibular first molar.
- The crown is much wider mesiodistally than it is cervicoincisally.
- The distal portion of the crown is noticeably shorter than the mesial portion. This is due to the cervical line design on buccal surface that dips apically on the mesial half of the crown.
- Two buccal cusps are visible from this view.

- The mesiobuccal cusp is larger than distobuccal cusp occupying two-thirds of the buccal surface. The two cusps are separated by a depression or fissure rather than a groove on the buccal surface.
- The linear cervical ridge is very prominent and is located on the mesial portion of crown.
- The apical slope of cervical line on buccal surface is accentuated by the mesiobuccal cervical ridge and appears to encircle the prominent bulge.
- The buccal surface is convex mesiodistally and is flat cervicoincisally above buccocervical ridge slanting in a lingual direction. This arrangement is true for all mandibular molars—primary and permanent.

***Lingual aspect:***
- *Geometric shape:* Trapezoidal.
- From lingual aspect, the crown length is nearly equal mesially and distally since cervical line is straighter.
- This makes the lingual surface as wide as buccal surface mesiodistally.
- The mesial wall of the crown and root converges noticeably in a lingual direction; however, the distal proximal wall converges buccally rather than lingually.
- The mesiolingual cusp is larger than distolingual cusp.
- The mesiolingual cusp is longer and sharper at the tip and is located nearly at the center lingually.
- *The prominent conical and sharp mesiolingual cusp is the outstanding feature of this tooth.*

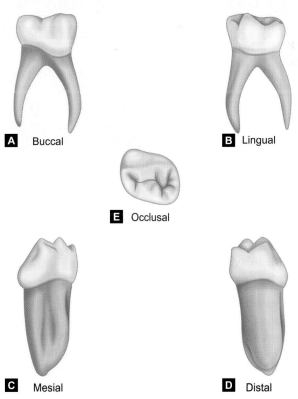

**A** Buccal     **B** Lingual

**E** Occlusal

**C** Mesial     **D** Distal

**Figs. 7.26A to E:** Primary right mandibular first molar.

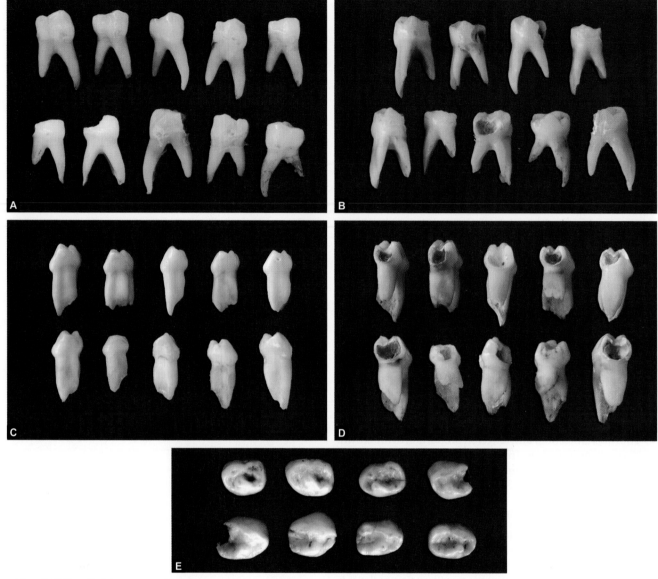

**Figs. 7.27A to E:** Primary mandibular first molar—typical specimen from all aspects: (A) Buccal aspect; (B) Lingual aspect; (C) Mesial aspect; (D) Distal aspect; (E) Occlusal aspect.

- The distolingual cusp is small and is more rounded.
- The mesial marginal ridge is extremely well developed in primary mandibular first molar and appears as a small cusp from this view.

***Mesial aspect:***
- *Geometric shape:* Rhomboidal.
- *Buccal outline* shows prominent convexity of the *buccal cervical ridge* at the cervical third of the crown.
- Primary maxillary and mandibular first molars exhibit extreme curvature of buccal cervical ridge on their buccal outlines when viewed from proximal aspects.

- Although the buccal cervical ridge is a common feature exhibited by all primary teeth. It is most dramatic in maxillary first molar followed by mandibular first molar.
- This prominent bulge on the buccal surface has to be considered while crowns are planned on these teeth.
- The tooth shows a typical proximal form of any mandibular molar with a lingual tilt of the crown at its root base.
- The crown appears to lean lingually on the root base. This feature is accentuated by prominent bulge of buccal cervical ridge.
- Like all mandibular molars, crest of curvature buccally is at cervical third and lingually is at middle third of the crown.

- The crown length is greater buccally than lingually when viewed from mesial aspect.
- Mesiobuccal and mesiolingual cusps are seen along with prominent mesial marginal ridge.
- The buccal cusps are centered over the root base. A line bisecting the root would pass through cusp tips of buccal cusps.
- The lingual cusp outline extends outward lingually beyond the confines of root base.
- The mesial surface of the crown is relatively flat cervicoincisally and converges in a lingual direction on the buccal aspect.

### Distal aspect:

- *Geometric shape:* Rhomboidal.
- The crown is of uniform height buccally and lingually when viewed from distal aspect.
- The distobuccal and distolingual cusps are not as long as mesial cusps.
- The distal marginal ridge is not as well developed as the mesial marginal ridge.
- The distal surface converges buccally rather than lingually. This feature is not seen in any other mandibular molar.

**Occlusal aspect:** Occlusal aspect offers most unique and characteristic feature of primary mandibular first molar.

**Geometric shape:** Occlusal outline of the tooth is *rhomboidal* and is elongated mesiodistally. It is to be noted that all other mandibular molars have rectangular occlusal outline that converge lingually. The mesiobuccal corner of the rhombus is extended due to the mesiobuccal cervical ridge. The mesiolingual angle and distobuccal angle is markedly obtuse and corner is flattened.

### Cusps and ridges:

- The primary mandibular first molar has four cusps: two buccal and two lingual.
- The mesial cusps are larger than the distal cusps with distolingual cusp as the smallest and poorly developed.
- The mesiolingual cusp is longest, sharpest, and very well developed. The sharper and prominent mesiolingual cusp as viewed occlusally is the outstanding feature of this tooth.
- The mesiobuccal cusp is larger than the distobuccal cusp occupying two-thirds of buccal half of the occlusal surface.
- The mesiobuccal cusp is well formed with long mesial and distal cusp ridges while in occlusion, with opposing during mastication. It is sort of compressed buccolingually.
- The distolingual cusp is smaller and shorter than mesiobuccal cusp, appears as a small protuberance.
- A *transverse ridge* may be noted which is formed by joining of triangular ridges of mesiobuccal and mesiolingual cusps.
- The mesial marginal ridge is prominent, longer buccolingually, and is so well developed that it appears as a small cusp lingually and occlusally.

- The distal marginal ridge is shorter and cervically placed than that of the mesial marginal ridge.
- The occlusal table between the cusp ridges and marginal ridges is rhomboidal and narrower buccolingually. It is wider, larger and distal to transverse ridge.

### Fossae, grooves, and pits:

- The occlusal table is divided buccolingually by *central developmental groove*. It runs mesiodistally from mesial pit in mesial triangular fossa to a central pit toward distal portion of the occlusal aspect. The central developmental groove separates mesiobuccal and mesiolingual cusps.
- A short *buccal developmental groove* divides two buccal cusps extending occlusally and joins the central developmental groove at the central pit. The buccal developmental groove does not extend onto buccal surface.
- Since both the lingual cusps are larger occupying two-fourths of the occlusal surface, the central pit is in large distal fossa. There is no central fossa. A distal pit may also be seen in the smaller distal triangular fossa just mesial to distal marginal ridge.
- A short *lingual developmental groove* extends from central pit toward distolingual line angle, separating the mesiolingual and distolingual cusps. It ends as a fissure.
- Two to three short supplementary grooves may be seen in mesial triangular fossa and distal triangular fossa.

## Root

- The primary mandibular first molar has two roots: mesial and distal. This is in line with the mandibular arch traits of the both dentition.
- Both the roots are flatter mesiodistally and wider buccolingually. The mesial root is much longer and wider than the distal root.
- As with all primary molars the bifurcation is immediately apical to the cervical line.
- The mesial and distal roots diverge from point of bifurcation, are slender, and long in comparison to the crown. The distal root is smaller and sharper.
- The mesial root form is unique and does not resemble any other root form. Buccal and lingual outlines of the mesial root drop down straight from the cervical line, running parallel to each other nearly up to the apex, where they converge to form a squarish root tip. There is a developmental depression at the center of the mesial root running to its full length.
- The distal root is smaller and shorter. The buccal and lingual outlines of the distal root converge steadily from middle third to its apex.
- Apex of mesial root is squarish and blunt. Apex of the distal root is sharp.
- Mesial root shows distal curvature at the apex. Distal root is straighter or curves mesially.

## Deciduous Mandibular Second Molar
## (Figs. 7.28 and 7.29)

Deciduous mandibular second molar is similar to permanent mandibular first molar in morphology although there are some differences. It has five cusps—mesiobuccal, distobuccal, mesiolingual, distolingual, and distal. There are two roots—mesial and distal.

### Crown

#### Buccal aspect:

- *Geometric shape:* Trapezoidal with shorter uneven side toward the cervix.
- From buccal aspect, the tooth exhibits marked cervical constriction, i.e. the crown is narrower cervically and broader occlusally.
- The buccal surface of the crown occlusally is divided into three cuspal portions by mesiobuccal and distobuccal developmental grooves.
- Thus, the primary mandibular second molar has a straight buccal surface with three equal buccal cusps: mesiobuccal, distobuccal, and distal cusps. This arrangement differs from permanent first mandibular molar in which buccal surface is uneven with two buccal cusps and one small distal cusp.

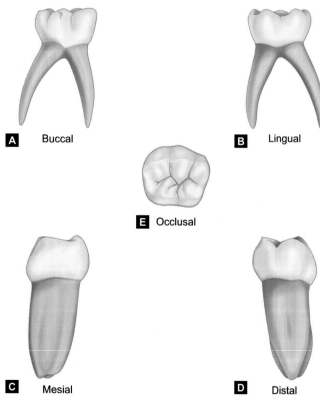

A    Buccal        B    Lingual

E    Occlusal

C    Mesial        D    Distal

**Figs. 7.28A to E:** Primary right mandibular second molar.

#### Lingual aspect:

- *Geometric shape:* Trapezoidal like buccal aspect.
- Two lingual cusps of equal size are seen from this view, which are separated by the lingual development groove.
- The lingual surface is narrower than the buccal surface as the crown tapers lingually.

#### Mesial aspect:

- *Geometric shape:* Rhomboidal.
- The crown shows lingual inclination over the root base, which is true for all mandibular posteriors.
- The mesiobuccal and mesiolingual cusps are seen from this view.
- Mesiolingual cusp is higher than the mesiobuccal cusp.
- Buccal cervical ridge is very prominent, which is not so in mandibular permanent second molar.
- Crown is constricted occlusally due to flattened buccal surface above the cervical ridge.

#### Distal aspect:

- *Geometric shape:* Rhomboidal
- The distal surface is narrower and shorter than that of the mesial surface.
- Distal marginal ridge is shorter and at a lower level than the mesial marginal ridge. Thus a portion of occlusal surface can be seen from distal view.

#### Occlusal aspect:

- *Geometric shape:* It is roughly *rectangular.*
- Mesiodistal width of the crown is greater than the buccolingual dimension. Crown shows slight lingual convergence, i.e. crown is narrower lingually.

#### Cusps and cusp ridges:

- There are five cusps as seen in permanent mandibular first molar. Three buccal cusps of nearly equal size:
  1. Mesiobuccal cusp
  2. Distobuccal cusp
  3. Distal cusp.
- Two lingual cusps of equal size:
  1. Mesiolingual
  2. Distolingual.
- In the deciduous mandibular second molar, the three buccal cusps are of nearly equal size and development. Whereas, in the permanent mandibular first molar, the distal cusp is much smaller than the other buccal cusps.
- Well-defined triangular ridges extend occlusally from each other of these cusp tips.
- Mesial marginal ridge is well developed than the distal marginal ridge, which is shorter and at a lower level.

#### Fossae, grooves and pits:
#### Fossae:

- There are two fossae—mesial triangular fossa and distal triangular fossa.

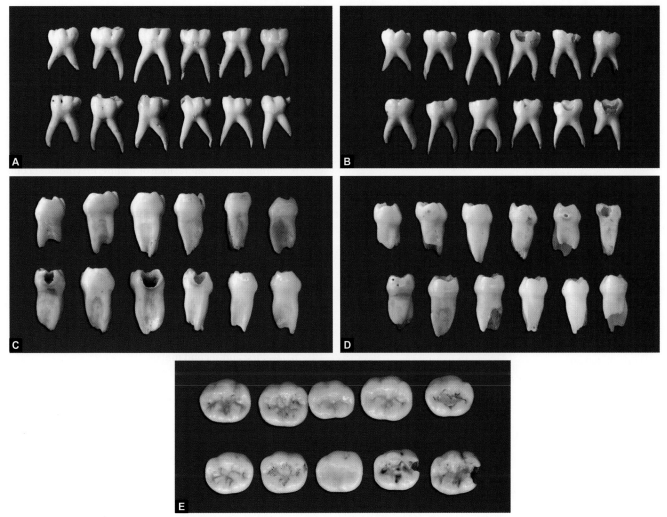

**Figs. 7.29A to E:** Primary mandibular second molar—typical specimen from all aspects: (A) Buccal aspect; (B) Lingual aspect; (C) Mesial aspect; (D) Distal aspect; (E) Occlusal aspect.

- Mesial and distal marginal ridges form the base of the triangle while mesial and distal pits form the apex for the respective triangular fossae.

*Grooves:* There are four grooves:

1. *Central developmental groove* has a zigzag course in across the center of the occlusal surface running from mesial pit to distal pit dividing the buccal and lingual cusps.
2. Mesiobuccal developmental groove
3. *Distobuccal developmental groove* originates from central pit and runs in a buccal direction extending onto the buccal surface to separate the three buccal cusps.
4. *Lingual developmental groove* originates from the central pit and runs lingually onto the lingual surface, separating the two lingual cusps.

*Pits:*

- *Central pit* in the center.
- *Mesial and distal pits* in mesial and distal triangular fossae.

*Root*

- There are two roots—mesial and distal.
- The roots are slender and twice as long as the crown and both roots are of equal length.
- The point of bifurcation of roots starts immediately below the cementoenamel junction without much root trunk left.
- The roots characteristically flare out to accommodate permanent successor tooth germ in the alveolus.
- The roots are thin mesiodistally and broad and flattened buccolingually.
- The apical third and roots may curve toward center to face each other.

## BIBLIOGRAPHY

1. Barker BC, Parsons KC, Williams GL, et al. Anatomy of root canals: IV. Deciduous teeth. Aust Dent J. 1975;20(2):101-6.
2. Fanning EA. Effect of extraction of deciduous molars on the formation and eruption of their successors. Angle Orthod. 1962;32:44.

3. Morrees CFA, Chadha M. Crown diameters of corresponding tooth groups in the deciduous and permanent dentition. J Dent Res. 1962;41:466.
4. Richardson AS, Castaldi CR. Dental development during the first two years of life. J Canad Dent Assoc. 1967;33:418.
5. Woo RK, Miller J. Accessory canals in the deciduous molars. J Int Assoc Dent Child. 1981;12(2):51-7.

## MULTIPLE CHOICE QUESTIONS

1. Primary or deciduous dentition consists of:
   a. 30 teeth, 15 in each jaw
   b. 32 teeth, 16 in each jaw
   c. 20 teeth, 10 in each jaw
   d. 12 teeth, 6 in each jaw
2. Each quadrant in deciduous dentition consists of:
   a. 4 teeth
   b. 5 teeth
   c. 6 teeth
   d. 8 teeth
3. The term "deciduous" comes from Latin meaning:
   a. The first set
   b. The important
   c. The small
   d. To fall off
4. The following terms are also used to describe primary teeth, except:
   a. Milk teeth
   b. Lacteal teeth
   c. Succedaneous teeth
   d. Baby teeth
5. The following classes of teeth are present in primary dentition:
   a. Incisors, canines, premolars, molars
   b. Incisors, canines, molars
   c. Incisors, premolars, molars
   d. Canines, premolars, molars
6. Teeth that are not present in primary dentition are:
   a. Premolars
   b. Canines, premolars
   c. Premolars, molars
   d. Premolars, third molar
7. Each quadrant in primary dentition contains the following teeth:
   a. Central incisor, lateral incisor, canine, first premolar, first molar
   b. Central incisor, lateral incisor, canine, first molar, second molar
   c. Central incisor, lateral incisor, first molar, second molar
   d. Central incisor, lateral incisor, canine, first premolar, second premolar, first molar, second molar, third molar
8. In mixed dentition period, the primary molars are replaced by:
   a. Permanent molars
   b. Permanent canines
   c. Permanent premolars
   d. None of the above
9. How many molars are there in primary dentition?
   a. 3—First, second, and third molars
   b. 2—First and second molars
   c. 4—First, second, third, and fourth molars
   d. 1—First molar
10. How many premolars are there in primary dentition?
   a. 2
   b. 1
   c. 3
   d. There are no premolars in primary dentition

**Answers**

1. c   2. b   3. d   4. c   5. b   6. d   7. b   8. c
9. b   10. d

# 8 CHAPTER

# Differences between Primary and Permanent Dentitions

## INTRODUCTION

In general, primary teeth pretty much resemble their corresponding permanent teeth in morphology **(Figs. 8.1A and B)**. One major exception is that the deciduous mandibular first molar does not resemble any tooth in the permanent dentition **(Fig. 8.2A)**. In addition, deciduous maxillary first molar resembles a permanent maxillary premolar rather than a permanent molar in crown anatomy; however, it has three roots, a trait common to all the maxillary molars **(Fig. 8.2B)**. The deciduous second molars closely resemble the permanent

first molars in both the arches and appear as their miniature replicas **(Figs. 8.3A to C)**.

Smaller sized jaws of the child functionally require and can accommodate fewer and smaller teeth. Thus, there are only 20 teeth in deciduous dentition as against 32 in the permanent dentition. *There are no premolars in the deciduous dentition.* Furthermore, there are only two molars (first and second deciduous molars) in the deciduous dentition. In other words, *there are no third molars in deciduous dentition.*

Furthermore, there are some important differences between primary and permanent teeth in terms of external morphology, structure, mineral density, etc. that have to be borne in mind while rendering dental treatment. Many of the routine dental procedures for instance, restorative cavity cutting, crown preparation, extractions, etc. have to be modified while treating primary teeth so as to accommodate these differences.

The differences between primary and permanent teeth are listed in **Table 8.1**.

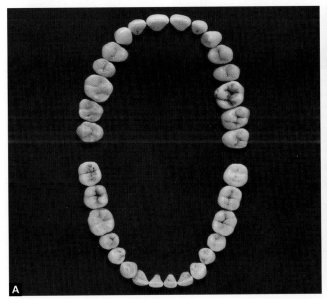
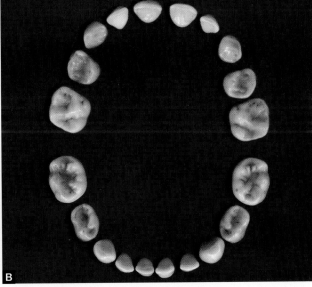

**Figs. 8.1A and B:** Primary anteriors resemble their corresponding permanent anteriors.

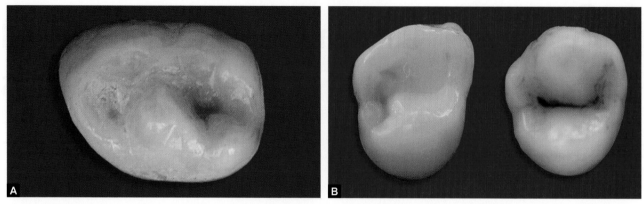

**Figs. 8.2A and B:** (A) Primary mandibular first molar has unique crown morphology and do not resemble any tooth in either of the dentitions; (B) Primary maxillary first molar crown resembles a permanent premolar.

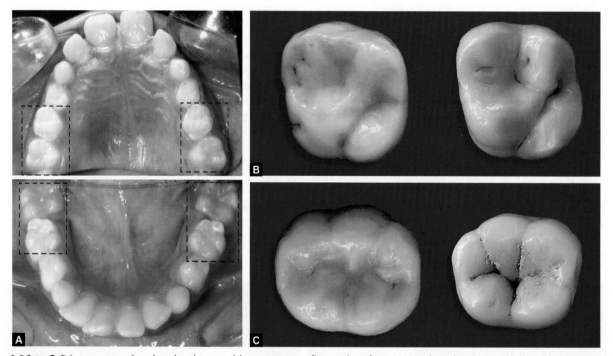

**Figs. 8.3A to C:** Primary second molar, closely resembles permanent first molar of respective dental arches—(A) Clinical photograph; (B) Teeth specimen of primary maxillary second molar and permanent first molar; (C) Teeth specimen of primary mandibular second molar and permanent first molar.

**Table 8.1:** Differences between primary and permanent teeth.

| | Primary dentition | Permanent dentition |
|---|---|---|
| | **General features** | |
| Number **(Fig. 8.1)** | A total of 20 teeth 10 in each jaw, 5 in each quadrant | A total of 32 teeth 16 in each jaw, 8 in each quadrant |
| Classes of teeth present | There are 2 incisors, 1 canine, 2 molars in each quadrant (*premolars* and *third molars* are not there in deciduous dentition) | There are 2 incisors, 1 canine, 2 premolars and 3 molars in each quadrant |
| Dental formula | $I\frac{2}{2}$, $C\frac{1}{1}$, $M\frac{2}{2}$ (on each side) | $I\frac{2}{2}$, $C\frac{1}{1}$, $P\frac{2}{2}$, $M\frac{3}{3}$ (on each side) |

*Contd...*

*Contd...*

| | Primary dentition | Permanent dentition |
|---|---|---|
| Duration of dentition | 6 months to 6 years | 12 years and beyond |
| Eruption | Primary teeth begin to erupt at 6 months. By 2½ to 3 years of age, a child would have his/her complete set of deciduous teeth | Eruption begins at 6 years and completes at 12–13 years except for 3rd molars |
| Eruption sequence | $\dfrac{AB \quad D \quad C \quad E}{A \quad B \quad D \quad CE}$  (ABDCE) | *Maxillary teeth:* 6 1 2 4 3 5 7 or 6 1 2 4 5 3 7 <br> *Mandibular teeth:* 6 1 2 3 4 5 7 |

| *Macroscopic features* | | |
|---|---|---|
| **Crown** | | |
| Size | Smaller in overall size and crown dimensions when compared to their permanent counterparts | Larger in overall dimension |
| Color* <br> *Thus for primary resin restorations, lighter shades should be selected.* | Primary teeth are lighter in color. They appear bluish-white (milky white) and are also called as milk teeth. Their refractive index is comparable to that of milk | Darker in color. Appear yellowish, white or grayish, white |
| Shape | Crowns of primary teeth are wider mesiodistally in comparison to their crown height <br> This gives a cup-shaped appearance to anterior teeth and "squat" shaped appearance to deciduous molars **(Fig. 8.4A)** | The crowns appear longer as their cervicoincisal height is greater than mesiodistal width **(Fig. 8.4B)** |
| Cervical constriction **(Figs. 8.4A and B)** | Marked cervical constriction present | No cervical constriction |
| Cervical ridge **(Figs. 8.5A and B)** | Cervical ridges on buccal aspect of deciduous crown are more prominent, especially on 1st molars | Cervical ridges on permanent crowns are flatter |
| ***Incisors:*** | | |
| Mamelons **(Figs. 8.6A and B)** | *Primary incisors do not exhibit mamelons* | Newly erupted permanent incisors exhibit mamelons |
| Crown width | Primary incisors are noticeably wider mesiodistally than they are longer cervicoincisally | Permanent incisors are *longer cervicoincisally* than they are wider mesiodistally |
| ***Canines*** | Primary canines tend to be more conical in shape and cusp tip is more pointed and sharp | Permanent canines are less conical; their cusps tips are less pointed |
| ***Molars:*** | | |
| Number | There are only 2 molars in each quadrant. No third molars in deciduous dentition | There are 3 molars in each quadrant—First, second and third molars |
| Size | Crown of second molar is larger than the crown of first molar | First permanent molar is larger than second and third molars. Size of crown gradually decreases from first to third molars |
| Shape* | Deciduous molars are more bulbous, bell-shaped and with marked cervical constriction <br> Cervical ridges are more pronounced especially on buccal aspect of 1st primary molars <br> *These cervical bulges have to be reproduced during restoration/ crown prosthesis* <br> *Sharp cervical constriction has to be kept in mind and special care should be taken while forming gingival floor during class II cavity preparation* | Permanent molars have less constriction of neck |
| Occlusal table **(Figs. 8.7A and B)** | Buccal and lingual surfaces of primary molars, especially that of 1st molars converge sharply occlusally, thus forming narrow occlusal table in buccolingual dimension | There is less convergence of buccal and lingual surfaces of molars towards occlusal surface |

*Contd...*

*Contd...*

| | Primary dentition | Permanent dentition |
|---|---|---|
| | *Deciduous molars are functionally adapted to withstand less occlusal load*<br>*Occlusal cavity preparations should be kept narrow in buccolingual plane* | Thus have broader occlusal table |
| Grooves **(Figs. 8.8A and B)** | Supplemental grooves are more<br>*Primary molars are more caries prone due to easy food lodgment*<br>*Pit and fissure sealants are advisable to prevent caries* | Supplemental grooves are less |
| Contact areas | Contact areas between primary molars are broader, flatter and situated gingivally | Contact areas between permanent molars are narrower and situated occlusally |
| Upper first molar | Has 3 cusps (resembles a premolar) | Has 4 cusps + 1 accessory cusp |
| Upper second molar | 4 cusps + one accessory cusp (resembles permanent upper first molar) | Has 4 cusps |
| Lower first molar | 4 cusps (does not resemble any permanent tooth) | Has 5 cusps |
| Lower second molar | 5 cusps (resembles permanent lower 1st molar) | Has 4 cusps |
| **Root (Figs. 8.9A and B)** | | |
| Size | Primary roots are more delicate<br>Roots are proportionately longer and more slender in comparison to crown size | Permanent roots are stronger and provide good anchorage in jaw bone<br>They are shorter and bulkier in comparison to their crown |
| Width | Roots are narrower mesiodistally | Roots are broader mesiodistally |
| Trunk | Root trunk is much shorter/absent | Root trunk is longer |
| Flaring | Roots of primary molars are flared out to accommodate permanent tooth buds between their roots | Marked flaring of roots is absent |
| Resorption | Primary roots undergo physiologic resorption and the primary teeth are shed naturally | Physiologic resorption is absent. |
| **Pulp (Figs. 8.10A and B)** | | |
| Pulp chamber | Pulp chambers of deciduous teeth are proportionately larger when compared to crown size | Pulp chamber is smaller in relation to crown size |
| Pulpal outline | Pulpal outline of primary tooth follows DEJ more closely than that of permanent tooth | Pulp outline follows DEJ less closely |
| Pulp horns | Pulp horns of deciduous molars (especially mesial horns) are higher and closer to outer surface than that of permanent molars. Primary pulp horns are more pointed and longer than cusps would indicate<br>*Depth of cavity preparation in primary teeth should be kept shallow. Care should be taken not to expose the pulp* | Pulp horns are comparatively lower and away from outer surface |
| Root canals | Root canals are more ribbon-like, follow a thin, tortuous and branching path<br>*Multiple ramification of primary pulp make complete debridement almost impossible!* | Root canals of permanent teeth are well-defined and less branching |
| Accessory canals | Floor of the pulp chamber is more porous. Accessory canals in pulp chambers of primary molars directly lead to inter-radicular furcation areas<br>*Inflammation/infection from pulp can easily reach periodontium and vice versa in case of primary molars*<br>*Enamel of underlying permanent successor teeth may become hypoplastic due to spread of inflammation. This can result in 'turner's hypoplasia' of permanent tooth* | Floor of the pulp chamber do not have many accessory canals |
| Apical foramen | Apical foramen is wider | Apical foramen is smaller/narrower |

*Contd...*

*Contd...*

| | Primary dentition | Permanent dentition |
|---|---|---|
| | **Microscopic/Histologic features** | |
| **Enamel** | | |
| Thickness **(Figs. 8.10A and B)** | Enamel is thinner and is about 1 mm thick but of uniform thickness<br>*Less pressure/force is required during cavity preparation of primary teeth. Depth of the cavity preparation is less* | Enamel is 2–3 mm thick and is not uniform in thickness |
| Direction of rods **(Figs. 8.11A and B)** | Enamel rods at the cervical third of primary crowns are directed occlusally instead of apically as seen in permanent teeth<br>*Due to this difference in the direction of enamel rods, gingival bevel is not given in class II cavity preparation* | Enamel rods at the cervix are directed apically<br>*In class II cavity preparation of permanent teeth, gingival bevel should be given to remove unsupported enamel* |
| Incremental lines | Incremental lines of Retzius are less common in enamel<br>*This may be partly responsible for bluish-white color of enamel. Primary enamel is less mineralized and more organic content is present* | Lines of Retzius are more common in enamel. Enamel is highly mineralized |
| Enamel prisms | Enamel is more prismatic<br>*Etching time in primary teeth is prolonged to 90–120 seconds* | *Less prismatic enamel*<br>*Usual etching time for permanent teeth is 30 seconds* |
| **Dentin** | | |
| Thickness **(Figs. 8.10A and B)** | Dentin thickness is half that of permanent teeth. (However, comparatively greater thickness of dentin is present over the pulpal wall at the occlusal fossa of primary molars)<br>*Depth of occlusal cavity preparation in primary molars should be kept shallow (There is less thickness of protective dentin over pulp)* | Greater thickness of dentin is present over pulpal roof |
| Dentinal tubules | Dentinal tubules are less regular | Dentinal tubules are more regular |
| Interglobular dentin | Interglobular dentin is absent | Interglobular dentin is present beneath the well-calcified mantle layer of dentin |
| **Pulp** | | |
| Blood supply | Primary roots have wide enlarged apical foramen. Thus primary teeth have abundant blood supply and exhibit a more typical inflammatory response<br>Thus, poor localization of infection and inflammation | Apical foramen is constricted. Reduced blood supply follows healing by calcific scarring<br>Thus, infection and inflammation are comparatively well-localized |
| Nerve supply | Primary pulp is less densely innervated<br>Nerve fibers terminate near odontoblastic zone as free nerve endings | Permanent pulp is densely innervated<br>Nerve fibers terminate among odontoblasts and even pass beyond predentin |
| Cementum | In primary teeth the cementum is thin and made-up of only primary cementum<br>*Anchorage of primary teeth is comparatively less firm and easily resorbed, and can be easily extracted* | Cementum is thick<br>Both primary and secondary cementum are present<br>*This shows that permanent teeth are firmly anchored in alveolar bone and are not easily resorbed* |
| Mineral content | Both enamel and dentin are less mineralized and less dense<br>*This difference can be easily appreciated clinically by the less resistance offered during cavity cutting. Primary teeth dentin is cut more easily* | Enamel and dentin are more mineralized |
| Neonatal line | Neonatal lines are present in all primary teeth both in enamel and dentin | Neonatal lines are seen only in first molars (since mineralization begins at birth) |

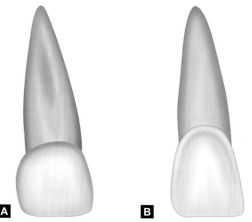

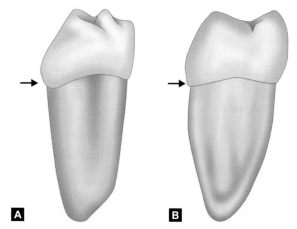

**Figs. 8.4A and B:** Comparison of mesiodistal dimensions of crown—(A) Primary teeth wider mesiodistally; (B) Permanent anteriors have greater length than width.

**Figs. 8.5A and B:** (A) Prominent cervical ridge; (B) Flatter cervical ridge.

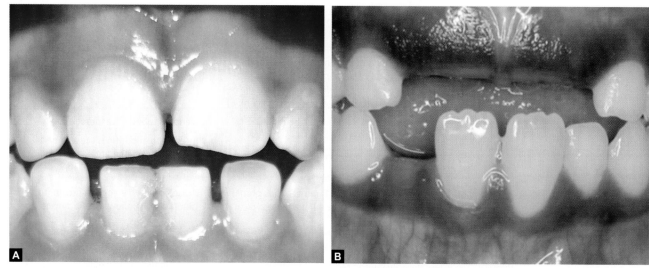

**Figs. 8.6A and B:** (A) Mamelons absent in primary incisor; (B) Mamelons present in permanent incisor.

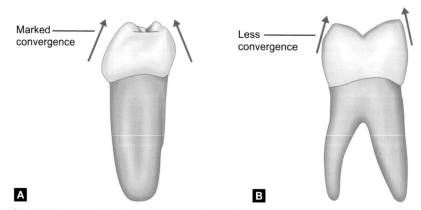

Marked convergence

Less convergence

**Figs. 8.7A and B:** (A) Primary molars have narrow occlusal table; (B) Permanent molars have wider occlusal table.

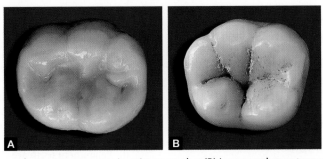

**Figs. 8.8A and B:** (A) More supplementary grooves in primary molar; (B) Less supplementary grooves in permanent molar.

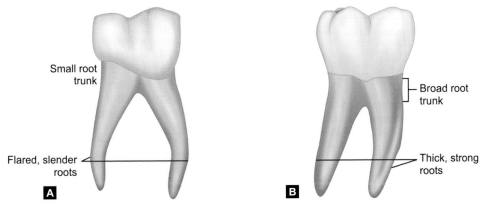

**Figs. 8.9A and B:** (A) Primary roots are slender, narrower, proportionately longer, and flare out markedly, root trunk is smaller; (B) Permanent roots are stronger, wider, do not flare much and have long root trunk.

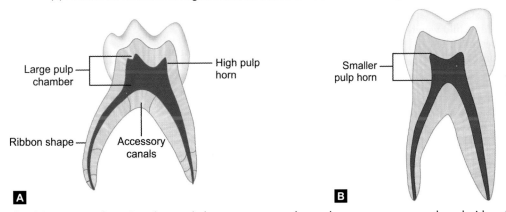

**Figs. 8.10A and B:** (A) Primary pulp cavity—long pulp horns, tortuous pulp canal, more accessory canals and wide apical foramen; (B) Permanent pulp cavity—shorter pulp horns, well-defined pulp canals, less accessory canals and constricted apical foramen.

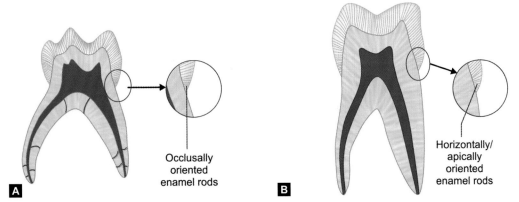

**Figs. 8.11A and B:** (A) Enamel rods are directed occlusally at the cervical third; (B) Enamel rods at cervical third are directed apically.

## BIBLIOGRAPHY

1. Barker BC. Anatomy of root canals. IV deciduous teeth. Aust Dent J. 1975;20:101-16.
2. Kraus B, Jordan R, Abrams L. Dental Anatomy and Occlusion. Baltimore: Williams and Wilkins; 1969.
3. Moorrees CFA, Chadha M. Crown Diameters of Corresponding Tooth Groups in the Deciduous and Permanent Dentition. J Dent Res. 1962; 41(2):466-70.
4. Woo RK, Miller J. Accessory canals in deciduous molars. J Int Assoc Dent Child. 1981;12(2):51-7.

## MULTIPLE CHOICE QUESTIONS

1. Total number of deciduous teeth in each quadrant are:
   a. 20
   b. 10
   c. 5
   d. 8
2. The differences between deciduous and permanent teeth with regards to classes of teeth are:
   a. 3 classes of teeth seen in deciduous dentition
   b. 4 classes of teeth seen in permanent dentition
   c. Both of the above
   d. None of the above
3. The dental formula for the permanent dentition is:
   a. I 2/2 C 1/1 M 2/2
   b. I 2/2 C 1/1 PM 2/2 M 3/3
   c. I 1/1 C 1/1 M 1/1
   d. I 2/2 C 2/2 M 2/2
4. By what age the child would have his/her complete set of deciduous dentition:
   a. 2½–3 years of age
   b. 1–2 years
   c. 0–1½ years
   d. 3½–6 years
5. The sequence of eruption of maxillary permanent teeth is:
   a. 6 1 2 4 5 3 7 8
   b. 6 1 2 3 4 5 7 8
   c. 6 1 2 4 3 5 7 8
   d. Both (a) and (c)
6. Which of the following statements is incorrect?
   a. Crown of deciduous teeth are more wider mesiodistally than cervicoincisally
   b. Crowns of permanent anterior are longer and more cervicoincisally and less mesiodistally
   c. Deciduous teeth are more constricted at the cervical portion of the crown
   d. Permanent teeth are constricted at their necks.
7. In deciduous dentition, the contact area between molars is:
   a. More broader and flatter
   b. Narrower
   c. Situated occlusally
   d. Both (b) and (c)
8. In comparison to crown size of permanent teeth, the roots of primary teeth are:
   a. Proportionately longer and more slender
   b. Proportionately smaller and less slender
   c. Proportionately smaller and more slender
   d. Proportionately longer and less slender
9. In permanent dentition, the dentinal tubules are:
   a. Less regular
   b. More regular
   c. Less irregular
   d. More irregular
10. Direction of enamel rods in the primary teeth at cervical thirds of crown is:
    a. Directed occlusally
    b. Directed apically
    c. Absent in deciduous teeth
    d. Absent in permanent teeth

**Answers**

1. c  2. c  3. b  4. a  5. d  6. d  7. a  8. a  9. b  10. a

# 5

## SECTION

# Permanent Dentition

### Section Outline

# 9

# The Permanent Maxillary Incisors

## INTRODUCTION

There are eight incisors; four in each arch and two in each quadrant. The central incisors are at the center of their respective arches, one on either side of the midline. The lateral incisors are distal to the central incisors. In the maxillary arch, the central incisor is larger than the lateral incisor, whereas in the mandibular arch the lateral incisor is larger. All the incisors have single roots.

## FUNCTIONS OF INCISORS

- Incisors are used for biting, cutting, and shearing the food during masticatory process.
- Maxillary and mandibular incisors act as cutting blades.
- They are of great importance in esthetics and phonation too.

## COMMON CHARACTERISTICS (CLASS TRAITS) OF INCISORS

- All incisors develop from four lobes; three labial lobes and one lingual lobe for cingulum. They have single, cone-shaped tapering roots.
- Their labial and lingual aspects are trapezoidal and the proximal aspects are triangular in shape. The incisal portions of the incisors are designed like the edges of blades.
- The newly erupted incisors have three rounded eminences on their incisal portion called the *mamelons,* which represent the three labial lobes.
- All incisors have cingulum at the cervical portion of their lingual aspects and concave lingual fossa at the center of lingual surfaces
- The contact areas are relatively smaller and are nearly at the same level, especially so in the mandibular incisors.
- Their labial surfaces are convex and lingual surfaces are concavoconvex.
- The crests of both labial and lingual contours are at the same level, in the cervical third of the crown, facing each other.

Positioned at the center of dental arches, the incisors are important for the esthetics and phonetics.

- The cervical lines on their proximal surfaces exhibit greater curvature than on other teeth.

## PERMANENT MAXILLARY CENTRAL INCISOR

The maxillary central incisors are esthetically the most prominent teeth in the mouth. An ideal smile should have incisal dominance, i.e. maxillary incisors should be the most prominent teeth visible when one smiles **(Fig. 9.1)**. Any defects in the form and alignment of these teeth are easily noticed, and adversely affect the normal facial appearance **(Fig. 9.2)**.

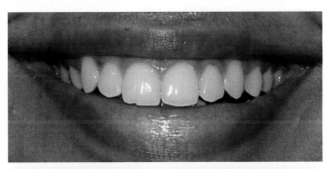

**Fig. 9.1:** An ideal smile has incisal dominance.

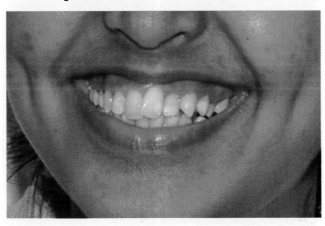

**Fig. 9.2:** Maxillary central incisors are esthetically the most prominent teeth and any defect is easily noticed. Overlapping of maxillary central incisors in this patient is adversely affecting the facial esthetics.

**Table 9.1:** Maxillary central incisor—chronology and dimensions.

| Chronology | |
|---|---|
| First evidence of calcification | 3–4 years |
| Enamel completed | 4–5 years |
| Eruption | 7–8 years |
| Root completed | 10 years |
| **Measurements** *Dimensions suggested for carving technique (in mm)* | |
| Cervicoincisal length of crown | 10.5 |
| Length of root | 13.0 |
| Mesiodistal diameter of crown | 8.5 |
| Mesiodistal diameter of crown at cervix | 7.0 |
| Labiolingual diameter of crown | 7.0 |
| Labiolingual diameter of crown at cervix | 6.0 |
| Curvature of cervical line—mesial | 3.5 |
| Curvature of cervical line—distal | 2.5 |

The mesiodistal dimension of maxillary central incisor is wider than that of any other anterior tooth. The chronology and measurement of the maxillary central incisor is given in **Table 9.1**.

Morphologically, there are two basic forms of maxillary central incisors **(Figs. 9.3A and B)**:
1. *Square form*: The tooth is relatively wider at cervix (neck of tooth) in comparison with the mesiodistal diameter of the crown at the contact areas.
2. *Tapering form*: With relatively narrow cervical width in comparison with the mesiodistal width at the contact areas.

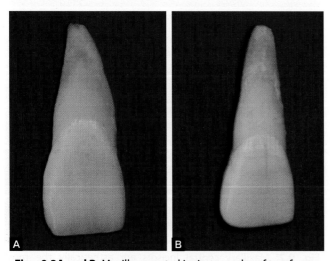

**Figs. 9.3A and B:** Maxillary central incisors can be of two forms: (A) Square form; (B) Tapering form.

## DETAILED DESCRIPTION OF MAXILLARY CENTRAL INCISOR FROM ALL ASPECTS (FIGS. 9.4 TO 9.6)

### Crown

*Labial Aspect (Fig. 9.7)*

***Geometric shape:*** Trapezoid with shortest of the uneven sides toward the cervix.

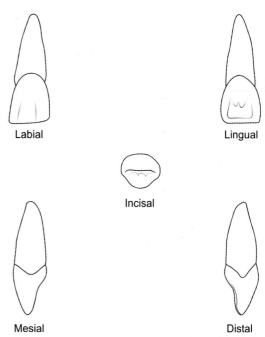

**Fig. 9.4:** Maxillary central incisor—line drawings.

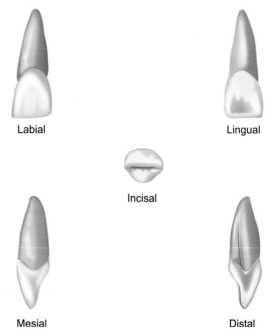

**Fig. 9.5:** Maxillary central incisor—graphic illustration.

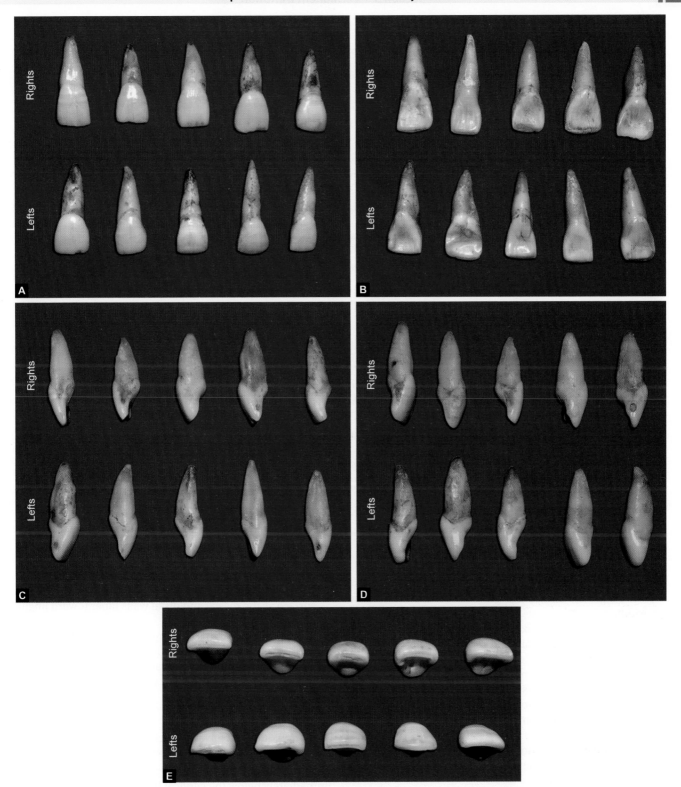

**Figs. 9.6A to E:** Maxillary central incisor—typical specimen from all aspects: (A) Labial aspect; (B) Lingual aspect; (C) Mesial aspect; (D) Distal aspect; (E) Incisal aspect.

← Distal            Mesial →

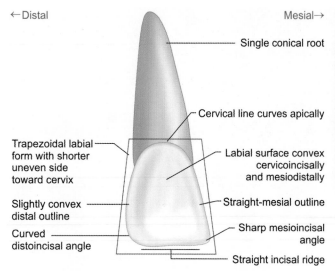

- Single conical root
- Cervical line curves apically
- Trapezoidal labial form with shorter uneven side toward cervix
- Labial surface convex cervicoincisally and mesiodistally
- Slightly convex distal outline
- Straight-mesial outline
- Curved distoincisal angle
- Sharp mesioincisal angle
- Straight incisal ridge

**Fig. 9.7:** Maxillary central incisor—labial aspect.

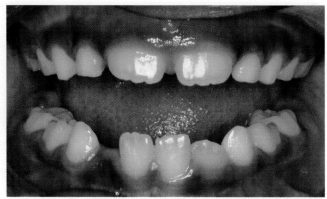

**Fig. 9.8:** Mamelons on erupting incisor teeth.

*Crown outlines:*

*Mesial outline:*
- It is relatively straight and meets incisal edge at a sharp angle.
- The crest of curvature of mesial outline *(mesial contact area)* is at incisal third of the crown near the mesioincisal angle.

*Distal outline:*
- It is more convex than the mesial outline. The distoincisal angle is more rounded.
- The crest of curvature of the distal outline *(distal contact area)* is higher toward the cervical line, at the junction of incisal and middle third of the crown.

*Incisal outline:* It is a straight line formed by the incisal ridge.

*Cervical outline:*
- It is formed by the cervical line.
- It is a semicircular curvature toward the root.

*Labial surface within the outlines:*
- The length of the crown is greater than the mesiodistal width.
- The labial surface of maxillary central incisor is smooth and convex both mesiodistally and cervicoincisally.
- Convexity is more near cervical third and becomes flattened toward the mesial and incisal third of the crown.
- Newly erupted incisors show three elevations at incisal portion called "mamelons" corresponding to three labial lobes **(Fig. 9.8)**. The mamelons disappear soon as the incisal surface of the tooth gets worn by mastication.

**Figures 9.4 to 9.6** show permanent maxillary central incisor from various aspects.

### Lingual Aspect (Fig. 9.9)

**Geometric shape:** Trapezoid

**Crown outlines:** Outlines are similar to that of labial aspect.

← Mesial            Distal →

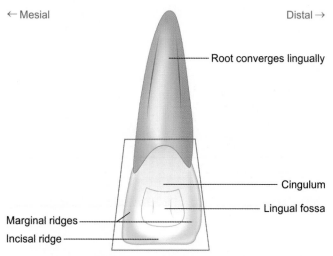

- Root converges lingually
- Cingulum
- Lingual fossa
- Marginal ridges
- Incisal ridge

**Fig. 9.9:** Maxillary central incisor—lingual aspect.

*Lingual surface within the outlines:*
- The lingual topography gives a scoop-like form to the crown.
- Lingual surface of crown and root is narrower than the labial surface as the mesial and distal walls taper toward lingual aspect (lingual convergence).
- Because of this lingual convergence, the labial line angles can be viewed from lingual aspect.
- The convexity found immediately below the cervical line is called the *"cingulum,"* and the central concavity is the *"lingual fossa".*

*Cingulum:*

*Definition:* It is the convexity encircling the lingual surface of anteriors at the cervical third like a girdle.

*Location:* It is found on lingual surfaces of all anteriors immediately below the cervical line. It occupies the cervical third of lingual surface.

*Development:* It develops from the lingual developmental lobe of the anterior teeth.

*Anatomy:*

- The cingulum is smooth and convex both mesiodistally and cervicoincisally. It makes up the bulk of cervical third of the lingual surface.
- There is a concavity next to the cingulum incisally, called the lingual fossa.
- Cingulum forms the cervical boundary of the lingual fossa.
- Usually two developmental grooves extend from cingulum into the lingual fossa, especially on canines and maxillary incisors.

*Lingual fossa:*

- There is a concavity in the center of lingual aspect of all anteriors called lingual fossa.
- Lingual fossa is bordered cervically by the cingulum, mesially by the mesial marginal ridge, distally by the distal marginal ridge, and incisally by the incisal ridge.
- Lingual grooves and pit may be present.

## Mesial Aspect (Fig. 9.10)

**Geometric shape:** Triangular. It is true for proximal aspects of all the anteriors. Base of the triangle is at the cervix and the apex of the triangle is toward the incisal ridge.

**Crown outlines:**

*Labial outline:*

- It is convex and curves smoothly from the cervical line to incisal ridge.
- Height of labial contour of the crown is at the cervical third.

*Lingual outline:*

- It is irregular with a convexity formed by cingulum in the cervical portion and a concavity formed by lingual fossa toward the incisal portion.
- Height of lingual contour is also at the cervical third.

*Incisal outline:* It is formed by a rounded *incisal ridge* in a newly erupted tooth and a flat *incisal edge* in a worn functional tooth.

*Cervical outline:*

- The cervical line on mesial and distal surfaces curves incisally.
- Curvature of the cervical line on mesial aspect of central incisor is greater than that of any other tooth, on any aspect—about 3.5 mm.

**Mesial surface within the outlines:**

Mesial surface is convex labiolingually and cervicoincisally with less convexity at the cervical area.

An imaginary line bisecting the tooth labiolingually passes through the incisal ridge, i.e. incisal ridge is in line with the root axis line.

Mesial contact area—at incisal third, immediately next to incisal edge.

## Distal Aspect (Fig. 9.11)

**Geometric shape:** Triangular

**Crown outlines:**

- *Labial, lingual, and incisal outlines* are similar to that of mesial aspect.
- *Curvature of cervical line* is less in extent on distal surface than on mesial surface. This feature is true for all other teeth.

**Distal surface within the outlines:**

- Distal surface is similar to mesial surface except that the crown appears thicker toward the incisal third.
- *Distal contact area* is at the junction of incisal and middle thirds of the crown cervicoincisally and at the center labiolingually.

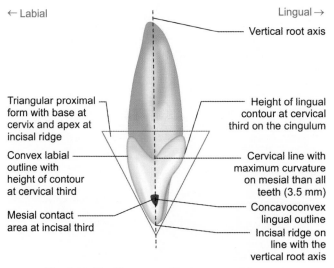

←Labial     Lingual→
—— Vertical root axis

Triangular proximal form with base at cervix and apex at incisal ridge

Convex labial outline with height of contour at cervical third

Mesial contact area at incisal third

Height of lingual contour at cervical third on the cingulum

Cervical line with maximum curvature on mesial than all teeth (3.5 mm)

Concavoconvex lingual outline

Incisal ridge on line with the vertical root axis

**Fig. 9.10:** Maxillary central incisor—mesial aspect.

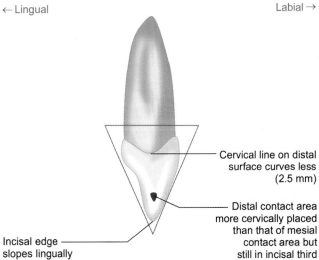

←Lingual     Labial→

Cervical line on distal surface curves less (2.5 mm)

Distal contact area more cervically placed than that of mesial contact area but still in incisal third

Incisal edge slopes lingually

**Fig. 9.11:** Maxillary central incisor—distal aspect.

### Incisal Aspect (Fig. 9.12)

**Geometric shape:** Triangular in shape with base of the triangle toward the labial surface and apex toward the cingulum.

### Relative dimensions:

- The mesiodistal dimension of the crown is only slightly greater than the buccolingual dimension. But the linear incisal ridge extending mesiodistally gives an illusion of much greater mesiodistal dimension.
- From this aspect, the crown appears bulkier than other aspects. Most of the labial surface is seen from this aspect, which is more convex cervically and flatter incisally.
- The cingulum forms a smaller convex arc and the crown tapers rapidly from the labial surface toward the cingulum.
- The mesiolabial and distolabial line angles are prominent from this aspect.
- The incisal ridge or edge is at right angle to a line bisecting the tooth buccolingually. The incisal edge in a worn tooth shows a lingual slope.

### Incisal ridge and incisal edge:

*Incisal ridge:*

- It is the rounded incisal portion of a newly erupted incisor, which merges with the mesioincisal and distoincisal angles and the labial and lingual surfaces.
- This linear elevation on incisal aspect of crown is called the *incisal ridge* (**Fig. 9.10**).

*Incisal edge:*

- In a functional tooth with occlusal wear, an incisal edge can be seen.
- The term "edge" means an angle formed by the merging of two flat surfaces. Incisal edge is not present in newly erupted incisor. In a functional incisor, a flattened surface is created linguoincisally due to occlusal wear (attrition). This linguoincisal surface forms an angle with the labial surface.
- This angle formed by incisal surface and labial surface is called *incisal edge.*

### Root

Morphology of the root can be described under the following headings:

| | |
|---|---|
| *Number:* | Single root |
| *Size:* | The root is about one and a half times as long as the crown |
| *Form:* | • It is cone-shaped, tapering gradually from cervical line to apex<br>• Root surface is narrower on lingual aspect due to lingual convergence. |
| *Curvature:* | Root is usually straight without any curvature |
| *Apex:* | Apex is usually blunt |
| *Cross-section:* | Triangular shaped with rounded border<br>Base of the triangle is formed by labial aspect and the apex by lingual aspect |

### Variations (Fig. 9.13)

- Short root
- Long root
- Shovel-shaped incisor (prominent marginal ridge seen in Mongoloid races).

### Developmental Anomalies (Figs. 9.14A to D)

- *Mesiodens* is a supernumerary tooth between the maxillary central incisors in midline (**Fig. 9.14A**)

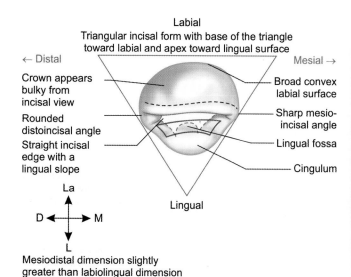

Labial
Triangular incisal form with base of the triangle toward labial and apex toward lingual surface

← Distal        Mesial →

Crown appears bulky from incisal view

Rounded distoincisal angle

Straight incisal edge with a lingual slope

Broad convex labial surface

Sharp mesio-incisal angle

Lingual fossa

Cingulum

La

D ←→ M

L

Lingual

Mesiodistal dimension slightly greater than labiolingual dimension

**Fig. 9.12:** Maxillary central incisor—incisal aspect.

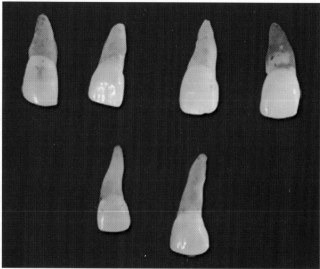

**Fig. 9.13:** Maxillary central incisor—variations.

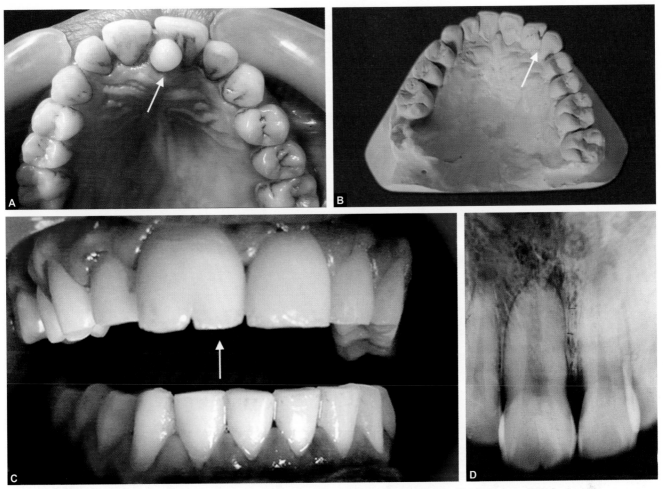

**Figs. 9.14A to D:** Developmental anomalies related to maxillary central incisors: (A) Mesiodens; (B) Talon's cusp; (C and D) Gemination of maxillary central incisor.

- Talon's cusp **(Fig. 9.14B)**
- Fusion
- Gemination **(Figs. 9.14C and D)**
- Dens invaginatus.

## Clinical Considerations

Maxillary central incisors ideally should be the most prominent teeth when one smiles. This is called incisal dominance. Maxillary central incisors are more prone to trauma especially in class II malocclusion (forwardly placed upper incisors).

A brief summary of maxillary central incisor anatomy is given in **Flowcharts 9.1 and 9.2**.

**Box 9.1** lists the identification points.

## PERMANENT MAXILLARY LATERAL INCISOR

The maxillary permanent lateral incisor has close resemblance to maxillary permanent central incisor and it supplements the latter in function. It is smaller than the central incisor in all dimensions except root length. The chronology and measurement of the maxillary lateral incisor is given in **Table 9.2**.

**Flowchart 9.1:** Maxillary central incisor—major anatomic landmarks.

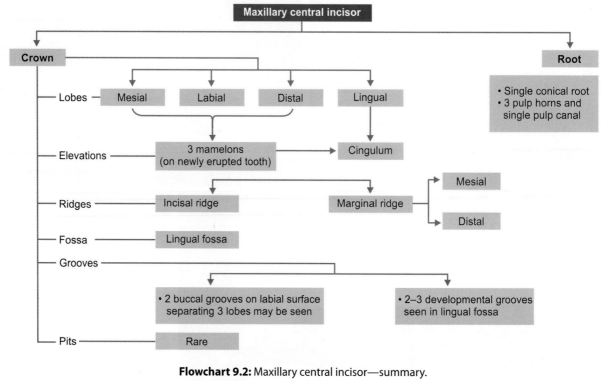

**Flowchart 9.2:** Maxillary central incisor—summary.

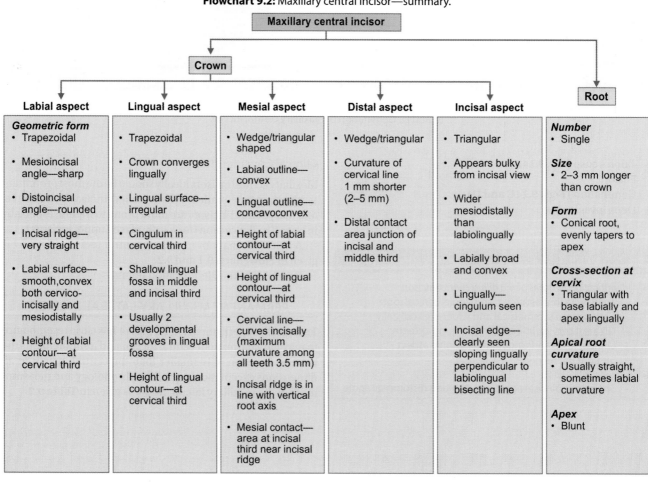

**Table 9.2:** Maxillary lateral incisor—chronology and dimension.

| Chronology | |
|---|---|
| First evidence of calcification | 1 year |
| Enamel completed | 4–5 years |
| Eruption | 8–9 years |
| Roots completed | 11 years |
| **Measurements** *Dimensions suggested for carving technique (in mm)* | |
| Cervicoincisal length of crown | 9.0 |
| Length of root | 13.0 |
| Mesiodistal diameter of crown | 6.5 |
| Mesiodistal diameter of crown at cervix | 5.0 |
| Labiolingual diameter of crown | 6.0 |
| Labiolingual diameter of crown at cervix | 5.0 |
| Curvature of cervical line—mesial | 3.0 |
| Curvature of cervical line—distal | 2.0 |

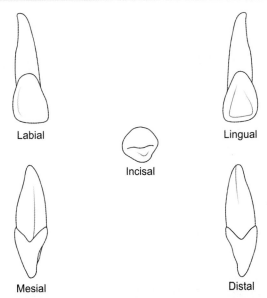

**Fig. 9.15:** Maxillary lateral incisor—line drawings.

*Maxillary lateral incisors show greater variation in morphology than any other teeth except third molars.* Variations in development and form are considered later.

## DETAILED DESCRIPTION OF MAXILLARY LATERAL INCISOR FROM ALL ASPECTS (FIGS. 9.15 TO 9.17)

### Crown

#### Labial Aspect (Fig. 9.18)

*Geometric shape:* Trapezoid, similar to labial aspect of maxillary permanent central incisor.

*Crown outlines:*

*Mesial outline:*
- It is slightly convex and the mesioincisal angle is rounded.
- *Height of mesial contour*—at the junction of middle and incisal thirds.

*Distal outline:*
- It is shorter than mesial outline.
- It is more convex than found in maxillary permanent central incisor with more rounded distoincisal angle.
- In some maxillary permanent lateral incisors, the distal outline may be a semicircle extending from cervix up to center of the incisal ridge.
- *The height of distal contour*—at the center of the middle third.

*Incisal outline:*
- It is formed by the incisal ridge.
- Mesial half of incisal outline is relatively straight and distal half is more rounded.

*Cervical outline:* The cervical line is more curved apically than that of maxillary permanent central incisor.

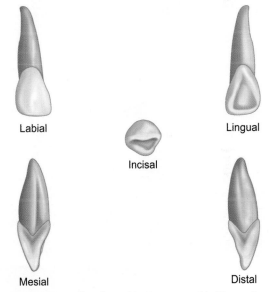

**Fig. 9.16:** Maxillary lateral incisor—graphic illustration.

*Labial surface within the outlines:*
- Labial surface is about 2 mm narrower and 2–3 mm shorter than the maxillary permanent central incisor.
- It is more convex than that of maxillary permanent central incisor.

#### Lingual Aspect (Fig. 9.19)

*Geometric shape:* Trapezoid similar to the labial aspect.

*Crown outlines:* Similar to labial aspect.

*Lingual surface within the outlines:*
- There is lingual convergence of proximal walls as seen in maxillary permanent central incisor.

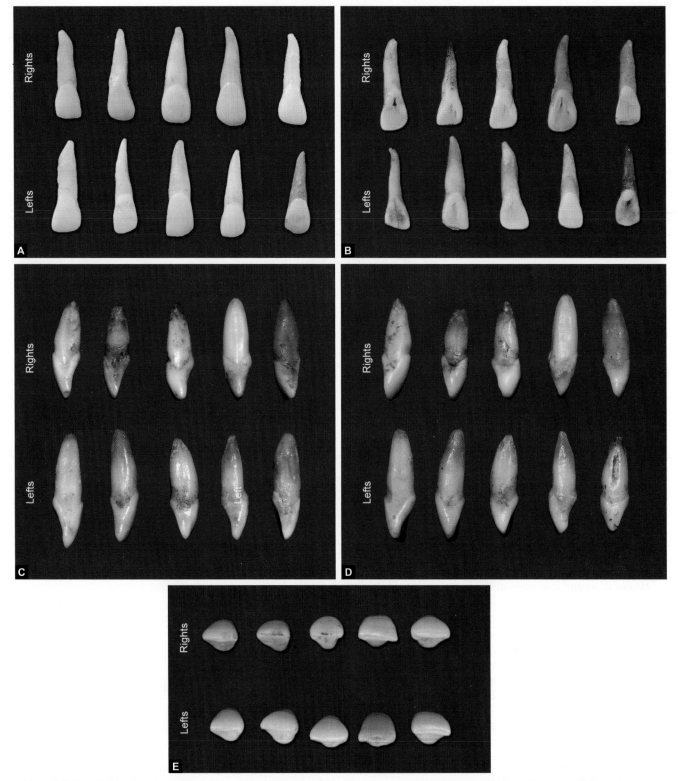

**Figs. 9.17A to E:** Maxillary lateral incisors—typical specimen from all aspects: (A) Labial aspect; (B) Lingual aspect; (C) Mesial aspect; (D) Distal aspect; (E) Incisal aspect.

← Distal                                    Mesial →

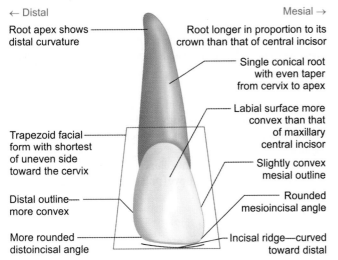

Root apex shows distal curvature

Root longer in proportion to its crown than that of central incisor

Single conical root with even taper from cervix to apex

Labial surface more convex than that of maxillary central incisor

Trapezoid facial form with shortest of uneven side toward the cervix

Slightly convex mesial outline

Distal outline—more convex

Rounded mesioincisal angle

More rounded distoincisal angle

Incisal ridge—curved toward distal

**Fig. 9.18:** Maxillary lateral incisor—labial aspect.

- Marginal ridges are more prominent and stronger than found on central incisor. Lingual fossa is deeper and well circumscribed.
- Cingulum is more prominent.
- There may be a deep developmental groove crossing the distal side of the cingulum extending on the root for a varying length—*palatogingival groove or palatoradicular groove.*

## Mesial Aspect (Fig. 9.20)

**Geometric shape:** Triangular or wedge-shaped.

**Crown outlines:**
- *Labial outline* of maxillary permanent lateral incisor is less convex than labial outline of maxillary permanent central incisor with crest of curvature at cervical third.
- *Lingual outline* is concavoconvex, similar to that of central incisor.

← Mesial                                    Distal →

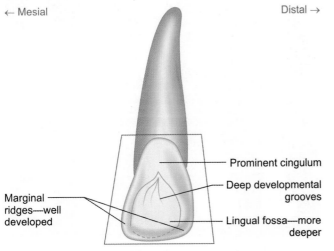

Marginal ridges—well developed

Prominent cingulum

Deep developmental grooves

Lingual fossa—more deeper

**Fig. 9.19:** Maxillary lateral incisor—lingual aspect.

← Labial                                    Lingual →

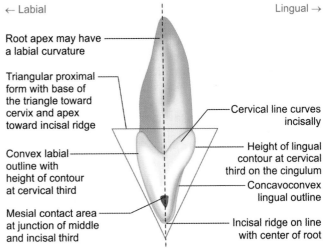

Root apex may have a labial curvature

Triangular proximal form with base of the triangle toward cervix and apex toward incisal ridge

Cervical line curves incisally

Convex labial outline with height of contour at cervical third

Height of lingual contour at cervical third on the cingulum

Concavoconvex lingual outline

Mesial contact area at junction of middle and incisal third

Incisal ridge on line with center of root

**Fig. 9.20:** Maxillary lateral incisor—mesial aspect.

- *Incisal outline* is formed by the incisal ridge which is more rounded.
- *Cervical line* shows marked curvature incisally.

**Mesial surface within the outlines:**
- From this aspect, incisal portion appears thicker than that of maxillary permanent central incisor as incisal ridge is heavily developed.
- The incisal ridge is in line with the central root axis.
- *Mesial contact area* is at the junction of incisal and middle thirds.

## Distal Aspect (Fig. 9.21)

**Geometric shape:** Triangle or wedge-shaped.

**Crown outlines:** Labial, lingual, and incisal outlines are similar to the mesial aspect.

← Lingual                                    Labial →

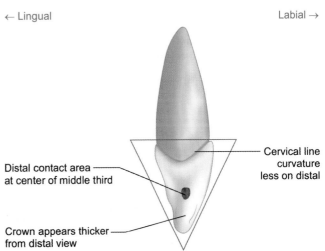

Distal contact area at center of middle third

Cervical line curvature less on distal

Crown appears thicker from distal view

**Fig. 9.21:** Maxillary lateral incisor—distal aspect.

*Cervical outline:* The curvature of cervical line on distal side is 1 mm less in extent than on mesial surface.

### Distal surface within the outlines:

- The crown appears thicker from distal aspect.
- Palatogingival or palatoradicular developmental groove may be seen on distal side of crown extending onto the root.
- *Distal contact area* is at the middle third.

### Incisal Aspect (Fig. 9.22)

### Geometric shape:

- Most maxillary permanent lateral incisors resemble maxillary permanent central incisors from this aspect, i.e. *triangular* outline.
- Some maxillary permanent lateral incisors resemble small maxillary permanent canines from incisal aspect, i.e. *oval* outline, due to their prominent large cingulum and occlusal ridges.
- *Relative dimensions*: Mesiodistal dimension is slightly greater than labiolingual dimension.
- *Labially*: Crown is more convex than that of maxillary permanent central incisors.
- *Lingually* crown at cervical third appears more convex than that of maxillary permanent central incisor.

### Root

Morphology of the root can be described under the following headings:

| | |
|---|---|
| *Number:* | Single root |
| *Size:* | • Root is long and slender |
| | • Root length is greater in proportion to the crown length when compared to central incisor |
| *Form:* | • The shape of maxillary permanent lateral incisor is flat labiolingually |
| | • Root tapers evenly from cervical line up to two-thirds of root length |
| | • May show developmental groove on mesial and distal surfaces |

| | |
|---|---|
| *Curvature:* | Apical third of root usually shows distal curvature |
| *Apex:* | Apex is usually pointed |
| *Cross-section:* | The cross-section of the root at cervix is oval. |

## Variations (Fig. 9.23)

Maxillary permanent lateral incisor shows great variation in development and morphology. This tooth exhibits greater variation in morphology than any other teeth except the third molars.

- Large size resembling a maxillary permanent central incisor.
- Deep developmental groove (palatoradicular groove) on the lingual aspect.
- Pit in the lingual fossa
- Twisted crown or root
- Lingual tubercle may be present.

## Developmental Anomalies (Figs. 9.24A to E)

- *Congenitally missing laterals* **(Fig. 9.24A)**: Most common tooth to be missing next to third molars.
- *Peg-shaped laterals* **(Fig. 9.24B)**: Small conical pointed crown
- *Talon's cusp* **(Fig. 9.24C)**
- Supplemental laterals or *supernumerary* lateral incisor **(Fig. 9.24D)**
- *Dens invaginatus* **(Fig. 9.24E)**: Most common tooth affected.

## Clinical Considerations

- Congenitally missing lateral incisors may need prosthetic replacement such as implants.

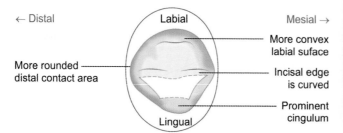

Fig. 9.22: Maxillary lateral incisor—incisal aspect.

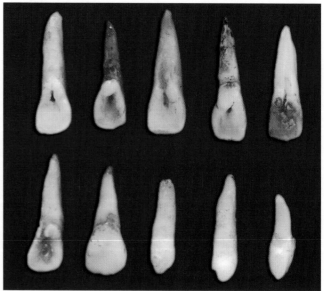

**Fig. 9.23:** Maxillary lateral incisor—variations.

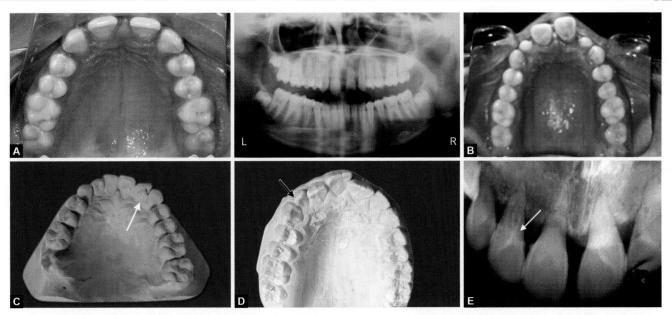

**Figs. 9.24A to E:** Developmental anomalies related to maxillary lateral incisors: (A) Congenitally missing laterals; (B) Peg-shaped laterals; (C) Talon's cusp; (D) Supplemental lateral; (E) Dens invaginatus.

- Microdontic or peg-shaped laterals may require crown or veneers for esthetic purpose.
- Deep palatogingival developmental groove may cause localized periodontal disease.

**Flowcharts 9.3 and 9.4** give the brief summary of maxillary lateral incisor morphology. **Box 9.2** shows the identification features of the tooth.

Type traits of maxillary central and lateral incisors are given in **Table 9.3**.

**Flowchart 9.3:** Maxillary lateral incisor—major anatomic landmarks.

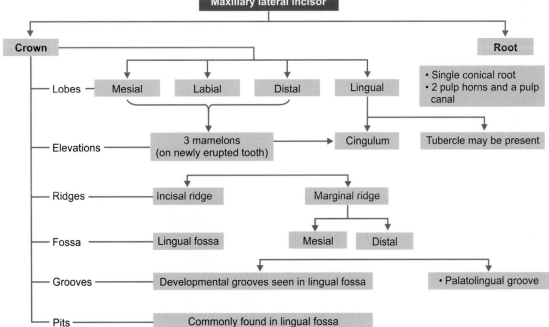

**Flowchart 9.4:** Maxillary lateral incisor—summary.

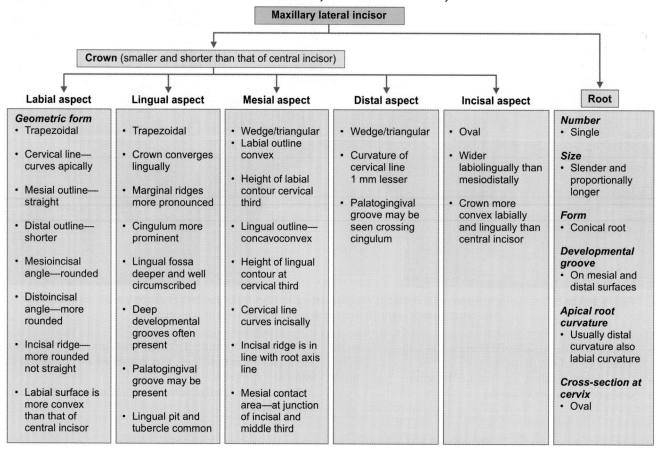

**Maxillary lateral incisor**

**Crown** (smaller and shorter than that of central incisor)

**Labial aspect**

*Geometric form*
- Trapezoidal

- Cervical line—curves apically

- Mesial outline—straight

- Distal outline—shorter

- Mesioincisal angle—rounded

- Distoincisal angle—more rounded

- Incisal ridge—more rounded not straight

- Labial surface is more convex than that of central incisor

**Lingual aspect**

- Trapezoidal

- Crown converges lingually

- Marginal ridges more pronounced

- Cingulum more prominent

- Lingual fossa deeper and well circumscribed

- Deep developmental grooves often present

- Palatogingival groove may be present

- Lingual pit and tubercle common

**Mesial aspect**

- Wedge/triangular
- Labial outline convex

- Height of labial contour cervical third

- Lingual outline—concavoconvex

- Height of lingual contour at cervical third

- Cervical line curves incisally

- Incisal ridge is in line with root axis line

- Mesial contact area—at junction of incisal and middle third

**Distal aspect**

- Wedge/triangular

- Curvature of cervical line 1 mm lesser

- Palatogingival groove may be seen crossing cingulum

**Incisal aspect**

- Oval

- Wider labiolingually than mesiodistally

- Crown more convex labially and lingually than central incisor

**Root**

*Number*
- Single

*Size*
- Slender and proportionally longer

*Form*
- Conical root

*Developmental groove*
- On mesial and distal surfaces

*Apical root curvature*
- Usually distal curvature also labial curvature

*Cross-section at cervix*
- Oval

**Box 9.2: Maxillary lateral incisor—identification features.**

- *Identification features of maxillary lateral incisor:*
  - Tooth with small asymmetrical crown
  - Slender and proportionately long root
  - Round mesioincisal and more rounded distoincisal angle
  - Rounded incisal ridge
  - Deep lingual fossa with grooves and pits
- *Side identification:*
  - More rounded distoincisal angle
  - Incisal ridge slants distally
  - Root shows distal curvature at apical third

**Table 9.3:** Differences between maxillary permanent central and lateral incisors (type traits).

| Characteristics | Maxillary permanent central incisor | Maxillary permanent lateral incisor |
|---|---|---|
| *Tooth nomenclature* | | |
| Universal system | Right 8; left 9 | Right 7; left 10 |
| Zsigmondy/Palmer system | 1⌋ Right, Left ⌊1 | 2⌋ Right, Left ⌊2 |
| FDI system | Right 11; left 21 | Right 12; left 22 |
| *Chronology* | | |
| Calcification begins | 3–4 months | 10–12 months |
| Eruption | 7–8 years | 8–9 years |

*Contd...*

*Contd...*

| Characteristics | Maxillary permanent central incisor | Maxillary permanent lateral incisor |
|---|---|---|
| Root completion | 10 years | 11 years |
| **General features** | | |
| Lobes | 4 lobes | 4 lobes |
| Dimension | Crown is larger, root is thicker | Smaller than central incisor in all dimension except root length. Crown smaller, root slender and comparatively longer |
| Variations | No much variations seen | Most common tooth to exhibit variation in form and development next to third molars, e.g. peg-shaped lateral and agenesis |
| **Crown** | | |
| *Labial aspect:* | | |
| Mesiodistal width | Comparatively wider | Comparatively narrow |
| Cervicoincisal length | Longest crown among incisors | Shorter crown |
| Incisal ridge | Makes straight line | Rounded incisal ridge, slopes cervically toward distal |
| Incisal angles | • Mesioincisal angle is sharp, right angled<br>• Distoincisal angle rounded | Both the incisal angles are rounded |
| Proximal contact areas | | |
| • Mesial contact area | At the incisal third | Junction of incisal and middle third |
| • Distal contact area | Junction of incisal and middle third | At the middle third |
| Labial surface | Slightly convex | More convex |
| *Lingual aspect:* | | |
| Cingulum | Moderately pronounced | Comparatively more prominent |
| Marginal ridge | Moderately developed | More prominent |
| Lingual fossa | Moderately deep | Deeper and well circumscribed |
| Grooves | Few grooves in lingual fossa | Deep palatogingival groove may be present |
| Lingual pits | Less common | More common |
| *Proximal aspects:* | | |
| Labial and lingual contours | More curved | Less curved |
| Height of labial and lingual contours | Both at cervical third | Both at cervical third |
| Incisal ridge | On line with vertical root axis | On line with vertical root axis |
| Curvature of cervical line | Shows the maximum curvature on mesially 3.5 mm, distally 2.5 mm | 1 mm less than that of central incisor |
| Contact areas | • Mesial—at incisal third<br>• Distal at—at incisal third | • Mesial—at junction of incisal and middle third<br>• Distal—at middle third |
| *Incisal aspect:* | | |
| Geometric form | Triangular | Ovoid or round |
| Relative dimension | Crown markedly wider mesiodistally | Mesiodistal and labiolingual dimensions of crown nearly same |
| Incisal ridge | straight | curved |
| **Root** | | |
| Number | Single | Single |
| Size | Thick conical root | Delicate and slender root, comparatively longer root |
| Developmental groove | Usually not present | May present on mesial and distal surfaces |
| Curvature | Usually straight | Distal and labial curvature of apical third is common |
| Cross-section of root at cervix | Triangular | Oval |
| Pulp horns | Three pulp horns from labial view | Usually two from labial view |
| Pulp canals | One canal | One canal, apical accessory canals are more frequent |

(FDI: Federation Dentaire Internationale)

## BIBLIOGRAPHY

1. Cecília MS, Lara VS, de Moraes IG. The palato-gingival groove: A cause of failure in root canal treatment. Oral Surg Oral Med Oral Pathol Oral Radiol Endod. 1998;85(1):94-8.
2. Garib DG, Alencar BM, Lauris JR, et al. Agenesis of maxillary lateral incisors and associated dental anomalies. Am J Orthod Dentofacial Orthop. 2010;137(6):732-3.
3. Kogon SL. The prevalence, location and conformation of palato-radicular grooves in maxillary incisors. J Periodontol. 1986;57:231-4.
4. Oliver RG, Mannion JE, Robinson JM. Morphology of the maxillary lateral incisor in cases of unilateral impaction of the maxillary canine. J Orthodont. 1989;16:9-16.
5. Shaju JP. Palatogingival developmental groove. Quintessence Int. 2001;32:349.

## MULTIPLE CHOICE QUESTIONS

1. Which of the following teeth show great variation in development and form?
   a. Permanent maxillary lateral incisor
   b. Permanent third molars
   c. Both (a) and (b)
   d. Permanent maxillary molars
2. The permanent maxillary lateral incisor is smaller than the maxillary permanent central incisor in all dimensions, *except*:
   a. Crown length
   b. Root length
   c. Both (a) and (b)
   d. None of the above
3. Distal outline of maxillary permanent lateral incisor is:
   a. Shorter than mesial outline
   b. Larger than mesial outline
   c. Similar to that of mesial
   d. None of the above
4. In comparison to maxillary permanent central incisor, the labial surface of maxillary permanent lateral incisor is:
   a. More convex
   b. Less convex
   c. More concave
   d. Less concave
5. When present, the developmental groove crossing the distal side of the cingulum extending on the root of maxillary permanent lateral incisor is called as:
   a. Palatogingival groove
   b. Palatoradicular groove
   c. Palatocervical groove
   d. Both (a) and (b)
6. The geometric shape of maxillary permanent lateral incisor from the mesial aspect is:
   a. Triangular
   b. Trapezoidal
   c. Cuboidal
   d. Rectangular
7. Mesial contact area of permanent maxillary lateral incisor is located at:
   a. Junction of middle and cervical third
   b. Center of middle third
   c. Junction of incisal and middle third
   d. Center of incisal third
8. Distal contact area of permanent maxillary lateral incisor is located at:
   a. At the middle third
   b. At the cervical third
   c. At the incisal third
   d. None of the above
9. Which of the following statements is false regarding the root of the permanent maxillary lateral incisor?
   a. Has single root
   b. Root is about one and a half times the length of the crown
   c. Root length is greater in proportion to the crown length when compared to central incisor
   d. Apical third of root usually shows no curvature
10. Cross-section of the maxillary permanent lateral incisor root at cervix is:
    a. Triangular
    b. Oval
    c. Circular
    d. Diamond shaped

**Answers**

1. c    2. b    3. a    4. a    5. d    6. a    7. c    8. a
9. d    10. b

# The Permanent Mandibular Incisors

## INTRODUCTION

There are four mandibular incisors—two central and two lateral. Mandibular incisors are the first permanent teeth to erupt. They have smaller mesiodistal dimensions than all other teeth. Among mandibular incisors, the lateral is larger than the central. It can be remembered that in the maxillary arch, the central incisor is larger than the lateral incisor. The crowns of these teeth exhibit lingual inclination over the root base which can be appreciated from proximal aspects. These are the teeth that show very few developmental grooves and lines.

## PERMANENT MANDIBULAR CENTRAL INCISOR

- Mandibular central incisors are the smallest teeth in the permanent dentition.
- They are also among the first permanent teeth to erupt into the oral cavity along with the first molars around 6–7 years of age.
- The mandibular central incisors have their mesial surfaces in contact with each other just like their maxillary counterparts.

## DETAILED DESCRIPTION OF MANDIBULAR CENTRAL INCISOR FROM ALL ASPECTS (FIGURES 10.1 TO 10.3)

The chronology and measurement of the mandibular central incisor is given in **Table 10.1**.

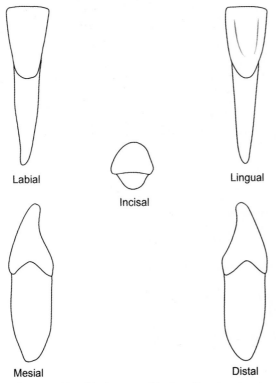

**Fig. 10.1:** Mandibular central incisor (line drawings).

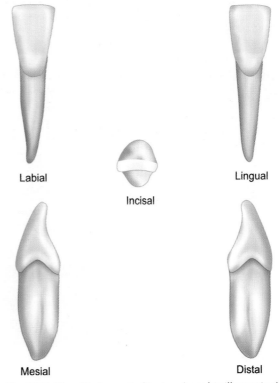

**Fig. 10.2:** Mandibular central incisor (graphic illustration).

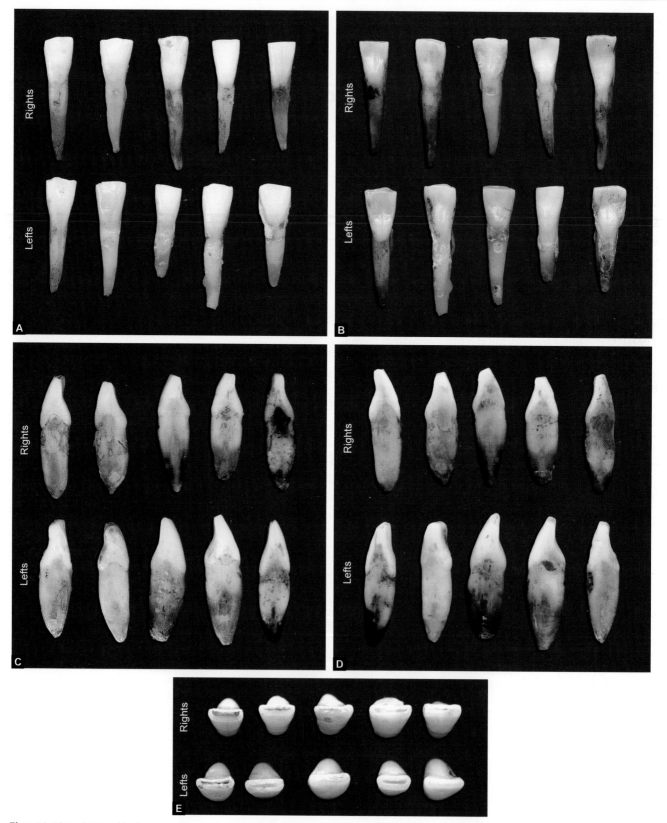

**Figs. 10.3A to E:** Mandibular central incisor—typical specimen from all aspects: (A) Labial aspect; (B) Lingual aspect; (C) Mesial aspect; (D) Distal aspect; (E) Incisal aspect.

**Table 10.1:** Mandibular central incisor—chronology and dimensions.

| Chronology | |
|---|---|
| First evidence of calcification | 3–4 months |
| Enamel completed | 4–5 years |
| Eruption | 6–7 years |
| Roots completed | 9 years |
| **Measurements** *Dimensions suggested for carving technique (in mm)* | |
| Cervicoincisal length of crown | 9.5 |
| Length of root | 12.5 |
| Mesiodistal diameter of crown | 5.0 |
| Mesiodistal diameter of crown at cervix | 3.5 |
| Labiolingual diameter of crown | 6.0 |
| Labiolingual diameter of crown at cervix | 5.3 |
| Curvature of cervical line—mesial | 3.0 |
| Curvature of cervical line—distal | 2.0 |

## CROWN

### Labial Aspect (Fig. 10.4)

*Geometric shape:* Trapezoid.

### Crown Outlines

- *Mesial and distal outlines* taper evenly from mesioincisal and distoincisal angles to the narrow cervix.
- Heights of contour of mesial and distal outlines are at incisal third. This places *both the contact areas at the same level.*
- *Incisal outline,* formed by the incisal ridge is straight and at right angles to the long axis of the crown. A newly erupted tooth shows *mamelons* on the incisal ridge **(Fig. 10.5)**.

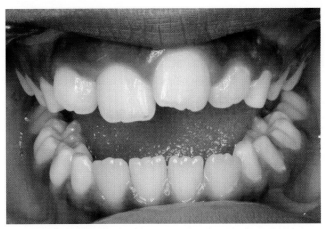

**Fig. 10.5:** Mamelons on erupting mandibular incisors.

- The *cervical line* on labial aspect is convex pointing apically.

### Labial Surface within the Outlines

- Labial surface is narrow and *bilaterally symmetrical.*
- The surface is smooth, convex in the cervical third and flattened in the incisal third.
- Both mesioincisal and distoincisal angles are sharp and at right angles.
- Both mesial and distal contact areas are at the same level—at the incisal third of crown near the mesial and distal incisal angles.

### Lingual Aspect (Fig. 10.6)

*Geometric shape:* Trapezoidal.

### Crown Outlines

Crown outlines are similar to that of the labial aspect.

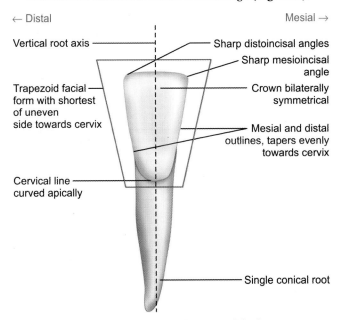

← Distal                                     Mesial →

- Vertical root axis
- Sharp distoincisal angles
- Sharp mesioincisal angle
- Trapezoid facial form with shortest of uneven side towards cervix
- Crown bilaterally symmetrical
- Mesial and distal outlines, tapers evenly towards cervix
- Cervical line curved apically
- Single conical root

**Fig. 10.4:** Mandibular central incisor—labial aspect.

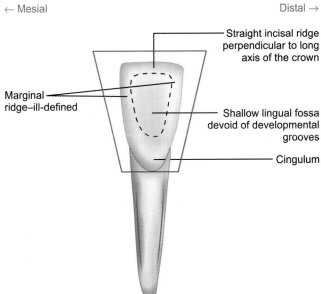

← Mesial                                     Distal →

- Straight incisal ridge perpendicular to long axis of the crown
- Marginal ridge–ill-defined
- Shallow lingual fossa devoid of developmental grooves
- Cingulum

**Fig. 10.6:** Mandibular central incisor—lingual aspect.

### Lingual Surface within the Outlines

- The lingual surface is narrower than the labial surface because of lingual convergence of the crown.
- The surface is smooth, flat in the incisal third and convex in the cervical portion near cingulum. The marginal ridges are ill defined.
- The lingual fossa between marginal ridges and cingulum is a smooth shallow concavity devoid of developmental grooves.

### Mesial Aspect (Fig. 10.7)

*Geometric shape:* Triangular

### Crown Outlines

- *Labial outline* is straight except at the cervical third, where it is convex. Height of contour of labial outline is at the cervical third
- *Lingual outline* is concavoconvex. Its height of contour is at cervical third on the cingulum
- *Incisal outline* is a small arc formed by the rounded incisal ridge. In a tooth with occlusal wear, there is a flat *incisal edge* sloping labially. Incisal surface of mandibular incisors have a labial slope and occlude with lingually sloping incisal edges of the maxillary incisors during mastication **(Fig. 10.8)**
- Cervical line on the mesial aspect shows a marked curvature towards incisal ridge.

### Mesial Surface within the Outlines

- The mesial surface is convex in the incisal third and becomes flat toward the middle third
- The tooth may exhibit a concavity in the cervical third above the cervical line
- The crown appears to be inclined lingually. The incisal ridge is placed lingual to a vertical line drawn through the center of the tooth

- The lingual inclination of crown is a feature of mandibular teeth to facilitate normal overjet.
- The *mesial contact area* is at incisal third of the crown.

### Distal Aspect (Fig. 10.9)

Distal aspect is similar to mesial aspect except that the extent of curvature of cervical line on distal aspect is 1 mm less than on the mesial.

### Incisal Aspect (Fig. 10.10)

*Geometric shape:* It is *oval* labiolingually.

### Relative Dimensions

- Labiolingual dimension is always greater than mesiodistal dimension.
- Bilateral symmetry of this tooth is easily appreciated from this aspect. Mesial half of the crown is equal to distal half.

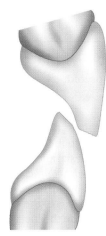

**Fig. 10.8:** Incisal edge—slopes lingually on maxillary incisors and slopes labially on mandibular incisors.

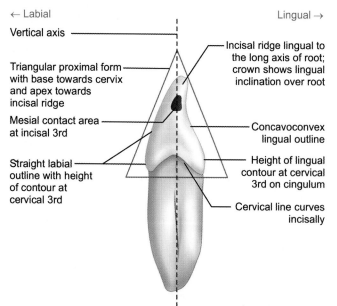

← Labial    Lingual →

Vertical axis

Triangular proximal form with base towards cervix and apex towards incisal ridge

Mesial contact area at incisal 3rd

Straight labial outline with height of contour at cervical 3rd

Incisal ridge lingual to the long axis of root; crown shows lingual inclination over root

Concavoconvex lingual outline

Height of lingual contour at cervical 3rd on cingulum

Cervical line curves incisally

**Fig. 10.7:** Mandibular central incisor—mesial aspect.

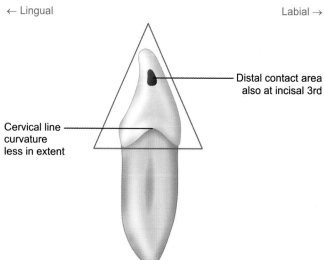

← Lingual    Labial →

Distal contact area also at incisal 3rd

Cervical line curvature less in extent

**Fig. 10.9:** Mandibular central incisor—distal aspect.

← Mesial          Distal →

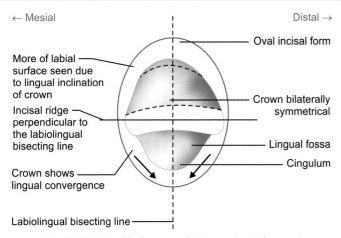

**Fig. 10.10:** Mandibular central incisor—incisal aspect.

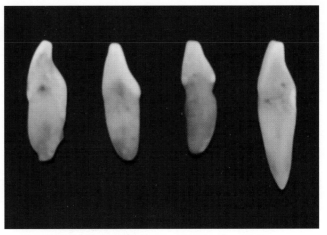

**Fig. 10.11:** Mandibular central incisor—variations.

- From this aspect, more of labial surface is seen than of the lingual surface because of lingual inclination of the crown. Labial surface is wider than lingual surface.

*Identification Features*

- When viewed incisally, the *incisal ridge is at right angles to the line bisecting the crown labiolingually.*
- This characteristic feature of central incisor helps in differentiating it from similarly looking mandibular lateral incisor. The incisal ridge of the mandibular lateral incisor is at an angle with the labiolingual bisecting line, and curves distally.

## ROOT

*Number:* Single root

*Size:* Maxillary permanent canine has the longest root of all teeth and its labiolingual thickness is greater than that of incisors.

*Form:*
- The root is conical in shape, narrower mesiodistally and wider labiolingually.
- Outlines of root are straight from cervix up to middle third. From this level the root tapers apically
- It is convex mesiodistally and flattened labiolingually
- Developmental grooves are seen on both mesial and distal surfaces of root and the groove is deeper on the distal surface

*Curvature:*
- Apical third of root usually is straight
- Sometimes, the root exhibits distal curvature.

*Apex:* Pointed apex

*Cross-section:* The cross-section of the root at cervix is oval.

## VARIATIONS (FIG. 10.11)

- Small tooth

- Short root
- Bifurcation of root.

## DEVELOPMENTAL ANOMALIES

- Talon's cusp
- Fusion between mandibular, central and lateral incisors.
 **Flowcharts 10.1 and 10.2** give a brief summary of mandibular central incisor anatomy. **Box 10.1** gives the tooth's identification features.

## PERMANENT MANDIBULAR LATERAL INCISORS

- Mandibular lateral incisor is very similar to the mandibular central in form as the two teeth function as a team
- It is slightly larger than the mandibular central incisor (unlike the case of maxillary incisors where the lateral is smaller than the central incisor)
- The crown of this tooth is slightly twisted on its root base to conform to the convexity of the mandibular arch.

---

**Box 10.1: Mandibular central incisor—identification features.**

- *Identification features of mandibular central incisor*
  - Smallest tooth in permanent dentition
  - The crown and root narrow mesiodistally and wider labiolingually
  - The crown is bilaterally symmetrical
  - Mesial and distal incisal angles are sharp
  - Mesial and distal contact areas are at same level near mesial and distal incisal angles
  - Viewed incisally, the incisal ridge is perpendicular to the line bisecting the crown labiolingually
- *Side identification*
  - Difficult to differentiate left and right mandibular central incisors since the tooth is bilaterally symmetrical
  - Developmental depression on root is deeper on distal surface
  - The root may show a distal curvature at the apex

**Flowchart 10.1:** Mandibular central incisor—major anatomic landmarks.

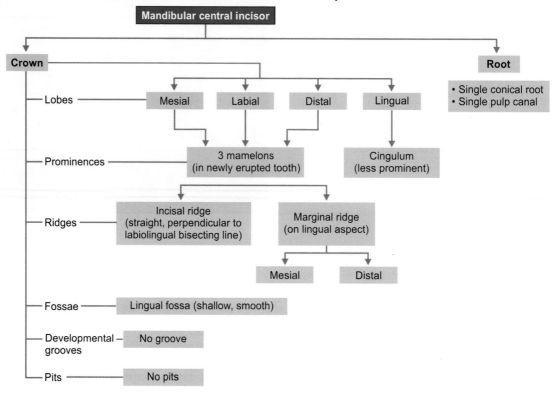

**Flowchart 10.2:** Mandibular central incisor (summary).

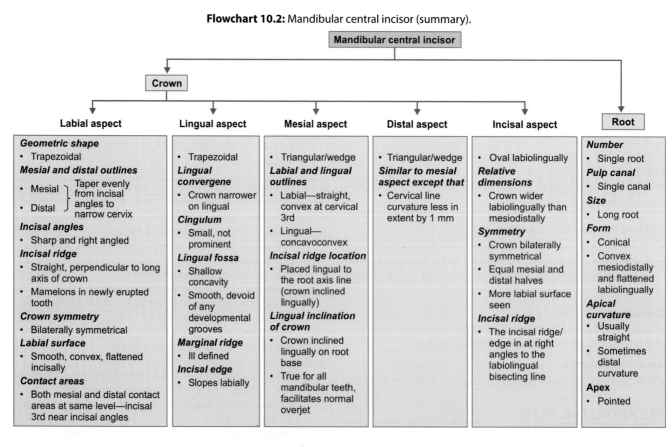

## DETAILED DESCRIPTION OF MANDIBULAR LATERAL INCISOR FROM ALL ASPECTS (FIGURES 10.12 TO 10.14)

The chronology and measurement of the mandibular lateral incisor is given in **Table 10.2**.

## CROWN

### Labial Aspect (Fig. 10.15)

*Geometric shape:* The crown is trapezoidal from labial aspect.

### Crown Outlines

- *Mesial outline* is almost straight, in line with mesial outline of the root. The maximum convexity of the mesial outline (mesial contact area) is at incisal third of crown
- *Distal outline* is straight near cervix and becomes slightly convex as it reaches the distoincisal angle. Its height of maximum convexity is also within incisal third
- *Incisal outline* formed by the incisal ridge is straight but has a tendency to slope cervically in adistal direction
- A newly erupted tooth may show mamelons **(Fig. 10.5)**. The *cervical line* is curved apically.

### Labial Surface within the Outlines

- The crown is not bilaterally symmetrical. Distal half of the crown is slightly larger
- The mesiodistal width of crown is approximately 1 mm more than that of mandibular central incisor

**Table 10.2:** Mandibular lateral incisor.

| Chronology | |
|---|---|
| First evidence of calcification | 3–4 months |
| Enamel completed | 4–5 years |
| Eruption | 7–8 years |
| Roots completed | 10 years |
| **Measurements** *Dimensions suggested for carving technique (in mm)* | |
| Cervicoincisal length of crown | 9.5 |
| Length of the root | 14.0 |
| Mesiodistal diameter of crown | 5.5 |
| Mesiodistal diameter of crown at cervix | 4.0 |
| Labiolingual diameter of crown | 6.5 |
| Labiolingual diameter of crown at cervix | 5.8 |
| Curvature of cervical line—mesial | 3.0 |
| Curvature of cervical line—distal | 2.0 |

- Mesioincisal angle forms at right angle, but the distoincisal angle is more rounded
- Labial surface is smooth, convex cervically and flattened incisally.

### Lingual Aspect (Fig. 10.16)

*Geometric shape:* Trapezoid

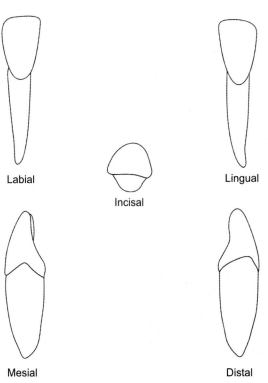

**Fig. 10.12:** Mandibular lateral incisor (line drawings)

Labial · Incisal · Lingual · Mesial · Distal

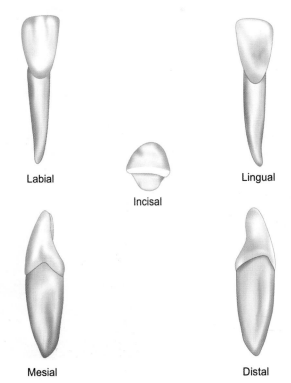

**Fig. 10.13:** Mandibular lateral incisor (graphic illustration).

Labial · Incisal · Lingual · Mesial · Distal

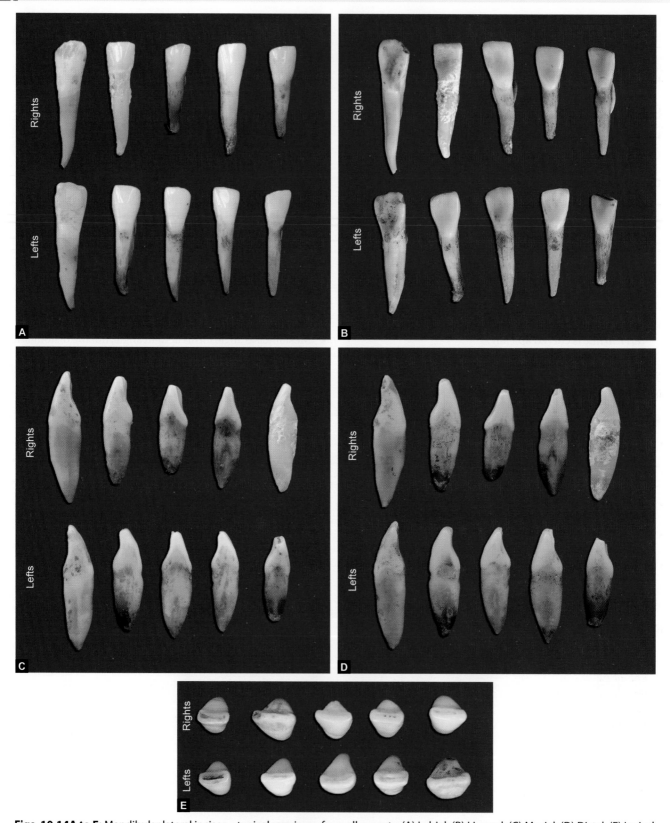

**Figs. 10.14A to E:** Mandibular lateral incisor—typical specimen from all aspects: (A) Labial; (B) Lingual; (C) Mesial; (D) Distal; (E) Incisal.

← Distal      Midline      Mesial →

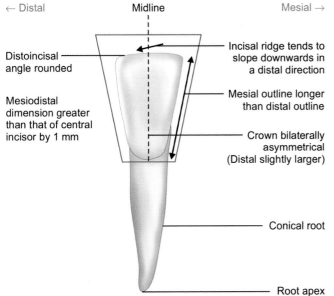

Distoincisal angle rounded

Mesiodistal dimension greater than that of central incisor by 1 mm

Incisal ridge tends to slope downwards in a distal direction

Mesial outline longer than distal outline

Crown bilaterally asymmetrical (Distal slightly larger)

Conical root

Root apex

**Fig. 10.15:** Mandibular lateral incisor—labial aspect.

← Mesial      Distal →

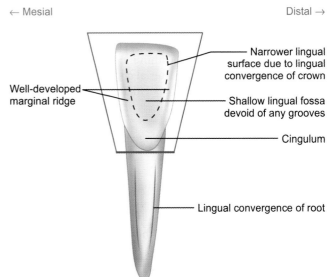

Narrower lingual surface due to lingual convergence of crown

Well-developed marginal ridge

Shallow lingual fossa devoid of any grooves

Cingulum

Lingual convergence of root

**Fig. 10.16:** Mandibular lateral incisor—lingual aspect.

## Crown Outlines

Outlines on lingual aspect are similar to that of labial aspect.

## Lingual Surface within the Outlines

- Lingual surface is similar to that of mandibular central incisor but is wider mesiodistally
- The crown tapers lingually making the lingual surface narrower than the labial surface
- The lingual surface is smooth, devoid of developmental grooves, and is convex near cingulum
- Lingual fossa is shallow and marginal ridges are relatively well-formed
- Sometimes the tooth may show deep cervicoincisal groove especially in Mongoloid race group.

## Mesial Aspect (Fig. 10.17)

***Geometric shape:*** Triangular

## Crown Outlines

- *Labial outline* is convex near cervical line and is straight from its height of contour up to incisal ridge. Height of labial contour is at cervical third.
- *Lingual outline* is straight in the incisal third, slightly concave in middle third and is convex at cervical third.
- Height of contour on lingual outline is also at cervical third on the cingulum.
- *Incisal outline* is formed by incisal ridge which is lingual to the root axis line. In a worn tooth, an incisal edge with a labial slope is seen.

← Labial      Lingual →

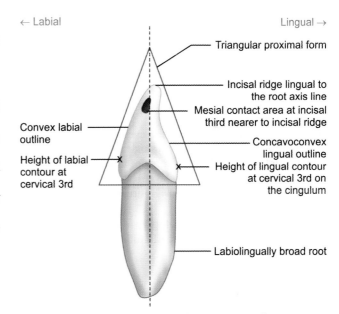

Triangular proximal form

Incisal ridge lingual to the root axis line

Mesial contact area at incisal third nearer to incisal ridge

Convex labial outline

Concavoconvex lingual outline

Height of labial contour at cervical 3rd

Height of lingual contour at cervical 3rd on the cingulum

Labiolingually broad root

**Fig. 10.17:** Mandibular lateral incisor—mesial aspect.

- The *cervical line* is convex pointing incisally.

## Mesial Surface within the Outlines

- Mandibular lateral incisor is broader buccolingually than the mandibular central incisor. It is convex and smooth.
- The crown shows lingual inclination it's the root base.
- The mesial surface is longer than the distal surface.
- *Mesial contact area* is at incisal third of the crown.

## Distal Aspect (Fig. 10.18)

Distal aspect is similar to mesial aspect except the following features:

- *Cervical* line on distal surface is less curved.
- *Distal contact area* is still within incisal third but is more cervically placed than the mesial contact area in order to reach the mesial contact area of mandibular canine.

## Incisal Aspect (Fig. 10.19)

***Geometric shape:*** It is *oval* labiolingually.

### Relative Dimension

Labiolingual dimension is greater than mesiodistal dimension.

### Symmetry

Unlike the mandibular centrals, the crown is not bilaterally symmetrical.

### Incisal Form

- The incisal aspect provides the identification feature of mandibular lateral incisor.
- The *incisal ridge is at an angle to the line bisecting the tooth labiolingually* rather than being perpendicular to it. This arrangement allows the incisal ridge to follow the curvature of mandibular arch.
- The crown of mandibular lateral incisor appears to be slightly twisted on its root base from this aspect.

## ROOT

- Mandibular lateral incisor has a single root which resembles the mandibular central incisor root in every aspect but is considerably longer.
- The root may sometimes show bifurcation onto buccal and lingual divisions.

  **Flowcharts 10.3 and 10.4** give a brief summary of mandibular central incisor. The identification features of the tooth are given in **Box 10.2**.

## VARIATIONS

- Two canals in a single root
- Bifurcation of root into labial and lingual divisions
- Long root
- Small size of tooth.

## DEVELOPMENTAL ANOMALIES

- Congenitally missing
- Fusion between mandibular central and lateral incisor.

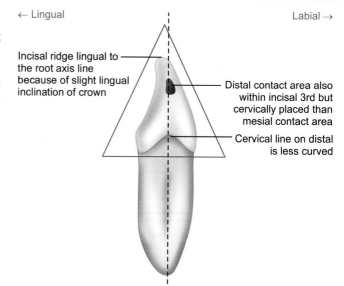

← Lingual　　　　　　　　　　　Labial →

Incisal ridge lingual to the root axis line because of slight lingual inclination of crown

Distal contact area also within incisal 3rd but cervically placed than mesial contact area

Cervical line on distal is less curved

**Fig. 10.18:** Mandibular lateral incisor—distal aspect.

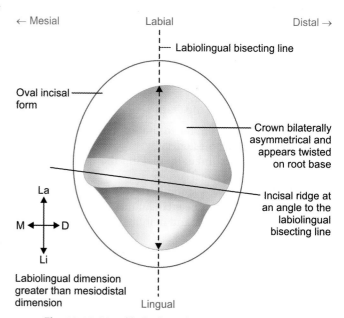

← Mesial　　　　　Labial　　　　　Distal →

Labiolingual bisecting line

Oval incisal form

Crown bilaterally asymmetrical and appears twisted on root base

Incisal ridge at an angle to the labiolingual bisecting line

La

M ←　→ D

Li

Labiolingual dimension greater than mesiodistal dimension

Lingual

**Fig. 10.19:** Mandibular lateral incisor—incisal aspect.

## Proximal Surface (Mesial and Distal Views)

No much difference between the two teeth.

## Incisal Aspect

*It is mainly from incisal view that the mandibular central and lateral incisors can be differentiated from one another.*

**Flowchart 10.3:** Mandibular lateral incisor—major anatomic landmarks.

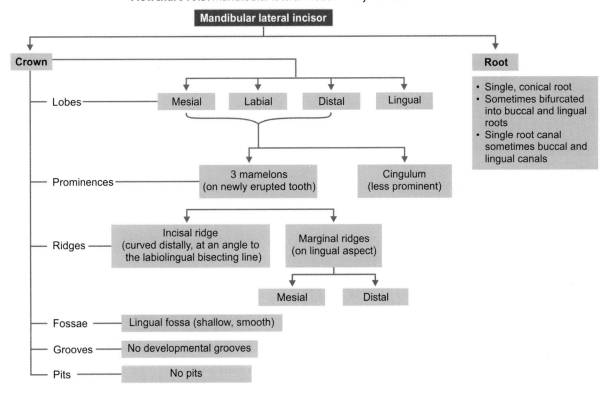

**Flowchart 10.4:** Mandibular lateral incisor (summary).

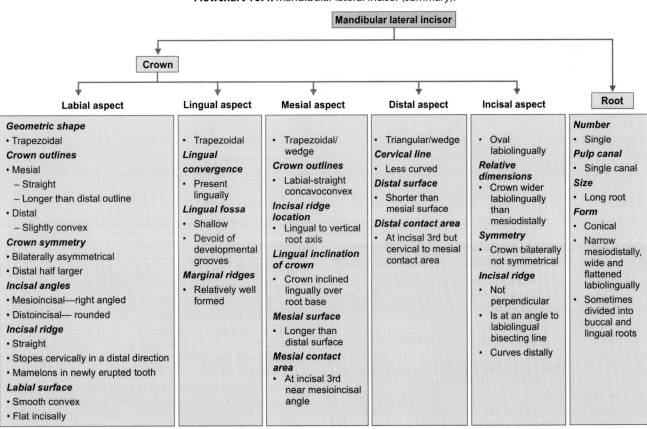

**Table 10.3:** Differences between mandibular permanent central and lateral incisors (type traits)*

| Characteristics | Mandibular permanent central incisor | Mandibular permanent lateral incisor |
|---|---|---|
| **Tooth nomenclature** | | |
| Universal system | Right 25; Left 24 | Right 26; Left 23 |
| **Zsigmondy/Palmer system** | | |
| FDI system | Right 41; Left 31 | Right 42; Left 32 |
| **Chronology** | | |
| Eruption | 6–7 years, first tooth to erupt along with 1st molar | 7–8 years |
| Root completion | 9 years | 10 years |
| Dimensions | Smallest tooth in permanent dentition | Slightly larger than the mandibular central incisor in all dimensions |
| **Crown** | | |
| *Labial aspect* | | |
| Crown width | Smallest tooth | Wider than the central incisor |
| Symmetry | Crown bilaterally symmetrical | Bilaterally asymmetrical |
| Mesial and distal outlines | Both mesial and distal outlines are straight | Straight mesial outline and slightly curved distal outline |
| *Incisal angles* | | |
| • Mesioincisal angle<br>• Distoincisal angle | Both incisal angles are sharp and right angled | • *Mesial:* Sharp and right angled<br>• *Distal:* Slightly rounded |
| Proximal contacts | Both contact areas are at same level, very near to incisal ridge in incisal third | Not exactly same level though still in incisal third. Contact areas are cervically located than those of central incisor |
| Incisal ridge | Straight | Slopes downwards distally |
| *Lingual aspect* | | |
| *No major differences seen except that the lateral incisor is wider* | | |
| Marginal ridge | Ill-defined | Well-defined |
| Incisal ridge/edge | Located lingual to the vertical root axis | Lingual to vertical root axis |
| Incisal ridge/edge | Is at right angles to the labiolingual bisecting line | Is at an angle to the labiolingual bisecting line. It is twisted distolingually on the root base to conform to the mandibular arch curvature |
| Cingulum | Cingulum is centered mesiodistally | Positioned distally (Cingulum is off center to distal) |
| **Root** | | |
| Number | Single | Single |
| Size | Shorter and smaller | Longer and larger |
| Developmental grooves | On both mesial and distal surfaces deeper on distal surface | On both mesial and distal surfaces |
| Pulp canals | Usually 1 canal | 1 canal |

*Mandibular central and lateral incisors appear very similar in form and could only be differentiated by examining them from incisal aspect.

---

**Box 10.2: Mandibular lateral incisor—identification features.**

- *Identification features of mandibular lateral incisor*
  - The mandibular lateral incisor is slightly larger than the mandibular central incisor
  - The crown is bilaterally asymmetrical
  - Mesioincisal angle is sharp, distoincisal angle is slightly rounded
  - Viewed incisally, the incisal ridge is placed at an angle to the line bisecting the tooth labiolingually
- *Side identification*
  - Mesioincisal angle is sharp
  - Distoincisal angle

## BIBLIOGRAPHY

1. Benjamin KA, Dowson J. Incidence of two canals in human mandibular incisor teeth. Oral Surg Oral Med Oral Pathol Oral Radiol Endod. 1974;38(1):122-6.
2. Brand RW, Isselhard DE. Anatomy of Orofacial Structures, 5th edition. St Louis: CV Mosby; 1994.
3. Kabak YS, Abbott PV. Endodontic treatment of mandibular incisors with two root canals: report of two cases. Aust Endod J. 2007;33:27-31.
4. Miyashita M, Kasahara E, Yasuda E, et al. Root canal system of the mandibular incisor. J Endod. 1997;23(8):479-84.
5. Rankine-Willson RW, Henry P. The bifurcated root canals in lower anterior teeth. J Am Dent Assoc. 1965;70:1162-5.

## MULTIPLE CHOICE QUESTIONS

1. The smallest tooth in permanent dentition is:
   a. Maxillary permanent lateral incisor
   b. Mandibular permanent lateral incisor
   c. Mandibular permanent central incisor
   d. Maxillary permanent central incisor

2. Which of the following statements is true:
   a. In maxillary arch, the central incisor is larger than the lateral
   b. In mandibular arch, also the central incisor is larger than the lateral
   c. In mandibular arch, the lateral incisor is larger than the central
   d. Both a and c

3. The crown of mandibular permanent central incisor is:
   a. Bilaterally asymmetrical from labial and lingual aspects
   b. Bilaterally symmetrical from labial, lingual and incisal aspects
   c. Bilaterally symmetrical from all aspects
   d. Bilaterally asymmetrical from all aspects

4. The geometrical shape of mandibular permanent central incisor from the labial aspect is:
   a. Triangular
   b. Hexagonal
   c. Octagonal
   d. Trapezoid

5. Mesioincisal angle of mandibular permanent central incisor is:
   a. Acute angled
   b. Obtuse angled
   c. Right angled
   d. None of the above

6. Distoincisal angle of mandibular permanent central incisor is:
   a. Acute angled
   b. Right angled
   c. Obtuse angled
   d. None of the above

7. In mandibular permanent central incisor, the mesial and distal contact area are:
   a. At the same level
   b. At different levels
   c. Absent one side
   d. Absent on both the sides

8. Mesial and distal contact area of mandibular permanent central incisor is located at:
   a. Middle third
   b. Cervical third
   c. Incisal third
   d. None of the above

9. The differences between mesial and distal surface of mandibular permanent central incisor is:
   a. Extent of curvature of cervical line on distal aspect is 1 mm less than on the mesial
   b. Extent of curvature of cervical line on mesial aspect is 1 mm less than on the distal
   c. Extent of curvature of cervical line on distal aspect is 4 mm more than on the mesial
   d. None of the above

10. In mandibular permanent central incisor, the labiolingual dimension is:
    a. Always smaller than mesiodistal dimension
    b. Always greater than mesiodistal dimension
    c. Both are exactly same
    d. None of the above

**Answers**

1. c    2. d    3. b    4. d    5. c    6. b    7. a    8. c
9. a    10. b

# The Permanent Canines

## INTRODUCTION

There are four permanent canines: two in each dental arch and only one member of its class in each quadrant. Permanent canines develop from four lobes, three labial and one lingual. The middle labial lobe in canine is highly developed incisally to form a strong, well-formed cusp.

The name "canine" is derived from Latin word for dog *canis,* as the corresponding teeth are very prominent members of the dentition of these animals. The canine teeth are prominent in other carnivores and also in primates (gorilla, chimpanzee, etc.). In human dentition, although canines have larger and stronger roots than other teeth, the crowns do not project much higher than the adjacent teeth. This permits wider range of side-to-side (lateral) jaw movements which is so characteristic of human dentition.

The maxillary permanent canines have other synonyms like:

- Cuspids
- Dog teeth
- Eye teeth
- Corner teeth
- Beauty teeth
- Corner stone of dental arches.

The four permanent canines are placed at the corners of the mouth; thus they sometimes are referred to as the *corner teeth* **(Fig. 11.1)**. Unlike incisors that have straight incisal ridges, the canine teeth have a well-formed pointed cusp developed from their middle labial lobe. Hence, they are also called as *cuspids.* Because of their shape and position in the arches maxillary and mandibular canines assist in guiding the teeth into intercuspal position by *canine guidance.*

The canines have longest and strongest roots of all teeth. The roots have excellent anchorage in the alveolar bone with an extra length and width. Alveolar bone over the roots of maxillary permanent canine, labially, is prominent and is called *canine eminence.* Maxillary and mandibular permanent canines help to establish normal facial expression at the corners of the mouth—with their position, form of canine

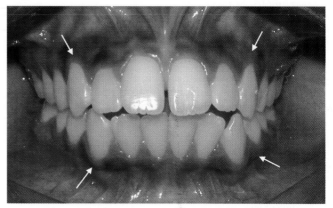

**Fig. 11.1:** Being at the corners of the mouth, the canines are sometimes referred to as the corner teeth.

eminence, and thus they are of high esthetic value. Facial profile changes when canines are lost due to some reason.

Extra anchorage of the long roots and self-cleansing convex surfaces of their crowns make the permanent canines highly stable teeth in the mouth. They are often the last ones to go. When one considers their longevity, crucial position in the arches, importance in establishment of occlusion and facial expression, the term *corner stone* of dental arches seems justified.

## FUNCTIONS

- The canines assist the permanent incisors and premolars in mastication.
- They are mainly used for tearing food.
- Help in seizing, slicing, and chewing food.
- In carnivores, the canines act as important tools during hunting and self-defense. They are used for prehension (seizing) of their prey.
- Canine teeth exhibit prominent sexual dimorphism, especially in lower animals (e.g. wild bear, etc.). The canine teeth are noticeably larger and longer in males than females in these animals.

## COMMON CHARACTERISTICS (CLASS TRAITS) OF PERMANENT CANINES

- The canines develop from four lobes: Three labial and one lingual.

- They are wider buccolingually than mesiodistally.
- Their middle labial lobe is highly developed into well-formed cusp.
- Their labial surfaces have a labial ridge extending from the cusp tip to the cervical line.
- Lingual aspect shows well-formed cingulum and a lingual fossa, which may be divided by a lingual ridge into two small fossae.
- Their distal cusp slope is longer than the mesial cusp slope.
- The canines typically have their contact areas at different levels cervico-occlusally. This is because the adjacent teeth of canines, with which they make contact, are of different classes, lateral incisor mesially and the first premolar distally.
- They have single root, longest and strongest of all teeth providing the best anchorage among anteriors.

## PERMANENT MAXILLARY CANINE

Maxillary permanent canine is the longest tooth of all and exhibits some of the characteristics of permanent maxillary incisors and some features of premolars. In many ways, it acts like a transition between anterior and posterior segments of the dental arch. In all mammals, the maxillary canine is the first tooth situated in the maxilla immediately behind the premaxillary suture. The chronology and measurement of the maxillary canine is given in **Table 11.1**.

### Detailed Description of Maxillary Canine from All Aspects (Figs. 11.2 to 11.4)

*Crown*

*Labial aspect* (**Fig. 11.5**):

*Geometric shape:* General shape of the crown from labial aspect is that of a *trapezoid or pentagonal* form.

**Table 11.1:** Maxillary canine—chronology and dimensions.

| Chronology | |
|---|---|
| First evidence of calcification | 4–5 months |
| Enamel completed | 6–7 years |
| Eruption | 11–12 years |
| Roots completed | 13–15 years |
| **Measurements** *Dimensions suggested for carving technique (in mm)* | |
| Cervicoincisal length of crown | 10.0 |
| Length of root | 17.0 |
| Mesiodistal diameter of crown | 7.5 |
| Mesiodistal diameter of crown at cervix | 5.5 |
| Labiolingual diameter of crown | 8.0 |
| Labiolingual diameter of crown at cervix | 7.0 |
| Curvature of cervical line—mesial | 2.5 |
| Curvature of cervical line—distal | 1.5 |

*Crown outlines:*
- *Mesial outline* is slightly convex. Maximum convexity of the mesial outline *(mesial contact area)* is at the junction of incisal and middle third of the crown.

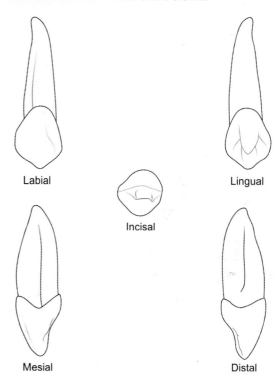

**Fig. 11.2:** Maxillary right canine—line drawings.

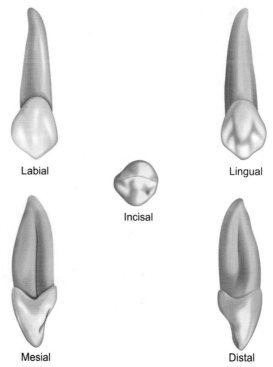

**Fig. 11.3:** Maxillary right canine—graphic illustration.

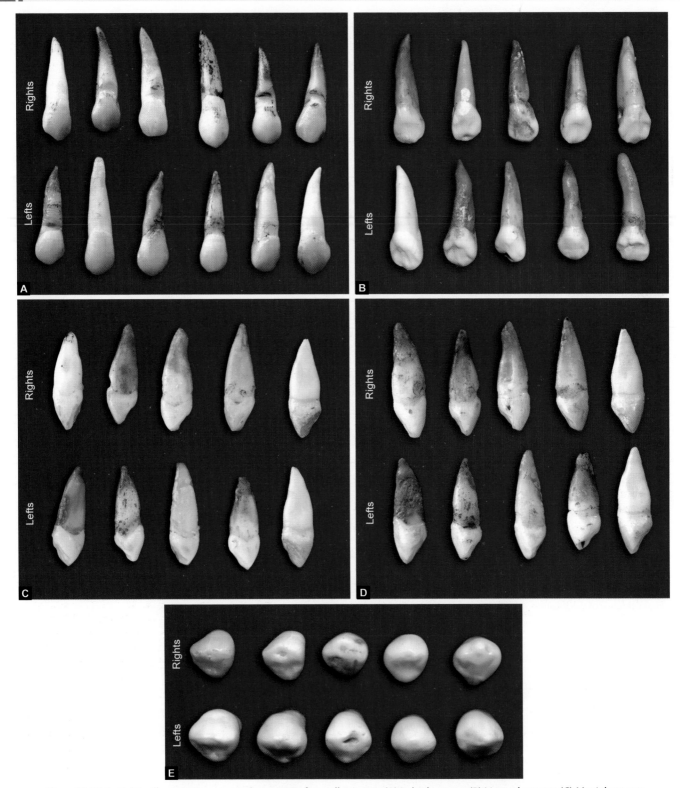

**Figs. 11.4A to E:** Maxillary canine—typical specimen from all aspects: (A) Labial aspect; (B) Lingual aspect; (C) Mesial aspect; (D) Distal aspect; (E) Incisal aspect.

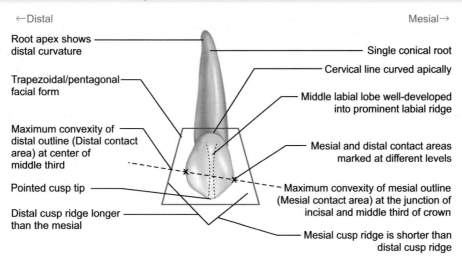

**Fig. 11.5:** Maxillary canine—labial aspect.

- *Distal outline* is more convex. Maximum convexity of the distal outline *(distal contact area)* is at the center of middle third of the crown.
- *Incisal outline* is formed by two slopes extending downwards from mesial and distal contact areas to meet the cusp tip at midline. These slopes are called as *mesial and distal cusp ridges.* The distal cusp ridge is longer and is slightly rounded, whereas the mesial cusp ridge is usually concave. The pointed cusp becomes flat over the time due to wearing away.
- The *cervical line* on the labial surface is smoothly convex pointing apically.

*Labial surface within the outlines:*
- From labial aspect the maxillary permanent canine resembles a premolar.
- The crown is narrower than the maxillary central incisor mesiodistally by 1 mm and much narrower at cervix.
- The middle labial lobe is well-developed than other lobes and forms a linear elevation extending from cervical line to the cusp tip. This feature is called as *labial ridge.*
- The mesial and distal contact areas are noticeably at different levels in maxillary canine and this can be easily appreciated from labial view.
- The labial surface is generally smooth and convex except for the shallow depressions on either side of the labial ridge.
- In a newly erupted tooth, two shallow developmental grooves separating the three labial lobes can be seen.

### Lingual aspect (Fig. 11.6):

*Geometric shape:* Trapezoidal or pentagonal

*Crown outlines:* These are similar to that of the labial aspect.

*Lingual surface within the outlines:*
- The lingual surface of maxillary permanent canine is narrower than the labial surface because of lingually converging proximal walls.

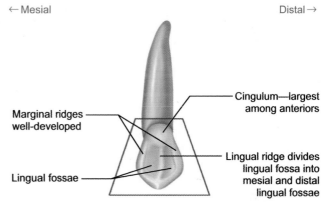

**Fig. 11.6:** Maxillary canine—lingual aspect.

- The cervical portion of lingual surface is occupied by a large, smooth, well-developed cingulum. The cingulum of maxillary canine is largest of all anteriors and sometimes it is pointed like a small cusp.
- The marginal ridges are strongly developed and along with cingulum they form the boundaries of lingual fossa.
- The lingual fossa is more concave and may be divided by a lingual ridge into two small concavities called mesial and distal lingual fossae.
- The lingual fossa is usually devoid of any developmental grooves.

### Mesial aspect (Fig. 11.7):

*Geometric shape:* The maxillary permanent canines appear *triangular or wedge-shaped* from proximal view like incisors but with more labiolingual bulk.

*Crown outlines:*
- The *labial outline* of maxillary permanent canine is more convex than that of maxillary permanent central incisor due to the presence of prominent labial ridge from cervical

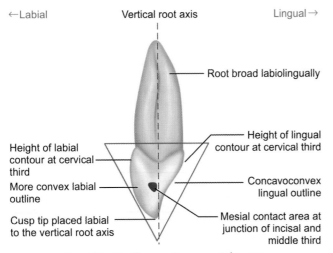

**Fig. 11.7:** Maxillary canine—mesial aspect.

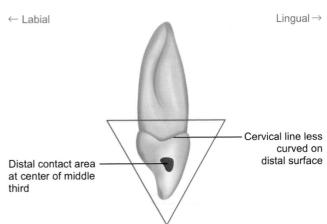

**Fig. 11.8:** Maxillary canine—distal aspect.

line to cusp tip. *Height of labial contour* is within cervical third but is placed more incisally than that of the maxillary permanent central incisor.

- The *lingual outline* is "S" shaped, follows the convexity of cingulum at the cervical third, concavity of lingual fossa in the center, and becomes convex again toward the incisal third. It is more convex in the cervical portion because of large cingulum. *Height of contour lingually* is at the cervical third, located on cingulum, and is incisally placed than that of the maxillary central incisor.
- *Incisal outline* forms a small arc representing the cusp tip. Pointed cusp tip may become flat due to occlusal wear.
- *Cervical line* on the mesial aspect is convex pointing toward the cusp tip.

*Mesial surface within the outlines:*

- Maxillary permanent canine has the greatest labiolingual width amongst anteriors. Thus, the tooth appears more bulkier from proximal aspects.
- The mesial surface is generally convex except for a small concavity in the cervical portion above the contact area.
- Unlike the incisal ridge of maxillary incisors, the cusp tip of maxillary canine is not centered over the root. It is placed labial to the vertical root axis.
- *Mesial contact area:* The mesial contact area is at the junction of incisal and middle third of the crown cervicoincisally, and is at the center labiolingually.

**Distal aspect (Fig. 11.8):** The distal aspect of maxillary permanent canine is similar to the mesial aspect except for the following features:

- The cervical line is less curved on the distal surface.
- The distal marginal ridge is strongly developed than the mesial.
- The distal surface shows more concavity apical to the distal contact area.
- The *distal contact area* is at the center of middle third of the crown.

**Incisal aspect (Fig. 11.9):**

*Geometric shape:* Diamond-shaped

From incisal aspect, the following features are noted:

- *Relative dimensions:* The labiolingual dimension of the crown of maxillary permanent canine is greater than the mesiodistal dimension.
- *Symmetry:* The crown is *asymmetrical* with distal half of the crown larger than the mesial half.
- *Position of cusp tip:* The cusp tip is located labial to the center of the crown labiolingually, and mesial to the center mesiodistally.
- *Labial ridge:* It appears prominent from incisal view, which is more convex at cervical third and gets flattened toward incisal third.
- *Cingulum:* It forms a shorter convex arc at the cervical portion of lingual surface.

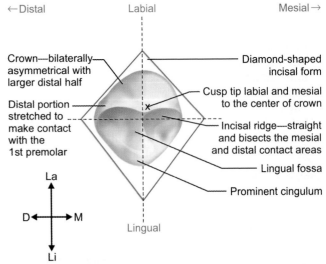

**Fig. 11.9:** Maxillary canine—incisal aspect.

- The lingual fossa, the lingual ridge, and the marginal ridges bordering the lingual fossa can be seen.
- *The distal portion* of the crown appears to be stretched to make contact with the first premolar.
- *The cusp ridges* form a straight line mesiodistally which bisects the contact areas.

### Root

Morphology of the root can be described under the following headings:

| | |
|---|---|
| *Number:* | Single root |
| *Size:* | Maxillary permanent canine has the longest root of all teeth and its labiolingual thickness is greater than that of incisors |
| *Form:* | • The root is conical in shape, narrower mesiodistally, and wider labiolingually |
| | • Similar to the crown, the root also exhibits lingual convergence |
| | • The labial and lingual surfaces are smoothly convex |
| | • The mesial and distal surfaces are flattened and exhibit *developmental depressions* for major part of the root |
| | • Developmental depression on the distal surface is deeper. These developmental depressions help to reinforce anchorage in alveolar bone |
| *Curvature:* | Apical third of the root usually shows distal curvature |
| *Apex:* | Apex of the root is relatively blunt |
| *Cross-section:* | The cross-section of the root at cervix is oval |

### Variations (Fig. 11.10)

Variations of maxillary permanent canine are listed below:
- Very long crown or long root
- Short crown or root.

### Developmental Anomalies

- Ectopic eruption
- Transposition **(Fig. 11.11)**.

### Clinical Considerations

- Maxillary canines are the most commonly impacted teeth after the third molars **(Fig. 11.12A)**.
- In the maxillary arch, the permanent canines erupt after the eruption of one or both the premolars. Hence, if space is not maintained until their eruption the maxillary permanent canines often erupt labially out of the arch causing malocclusion **(Fig. 11.12B)**.
- Maxillary permanent canines provide good support when utilized as abutments in prosthetic replacement of missing teeth.
- Deep concavity on the maxilla, posterior to the canine eminence, is called canine fossa. During surgical procedures, the maxillary sinus is often entered by an incision through canine fossa as the wall of the sinus is thin there.
- Canine guidance is important in establishment of occlusion.
- Maxillary permanent canine to mandibular canine relationship is observed for classifying malocclusions especially when the first molars are missing.
- Intercanine distance is often used as a gender trait in dental anthropology.

A brief summary of maxillary canine is given in **Flowcharts 11.1 and 11.2**.

**Box 11.1** shows the identification features of maxillary canine.

### PERMANENT MANDIBULAR CANINE

The mandibular canine closely resembles the maxillary canine. In comparison to its maxillary counterpart, the

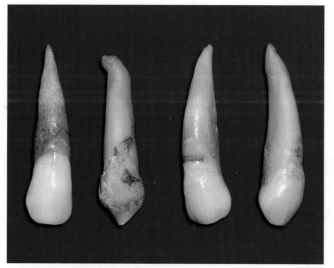

**Fig. 11.10:** Maxillary canine—variations.

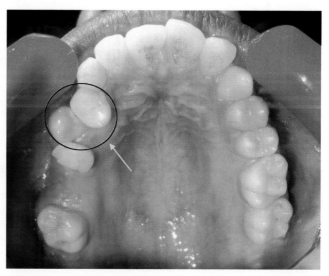

**Fig. 11.11:** Transposition of maxillary canine and first premolar.

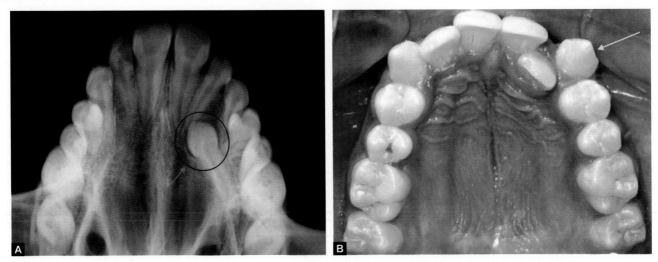

**Figs. 11.12A and B:** (A) Occlusal radiograph showing impacted maxillary canine; (B) Labially erupted upper canines causing malocclusion.

**Flowchart 11.1:** Maxillary canine—major anatomic landmarks.

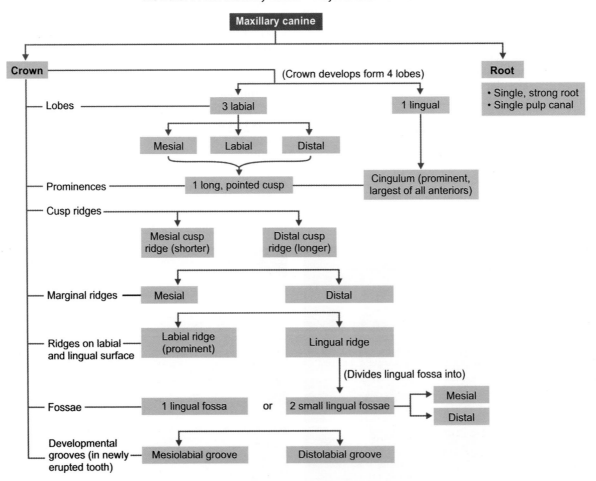

Flowchart 11.2: Maxillary canine—summary.

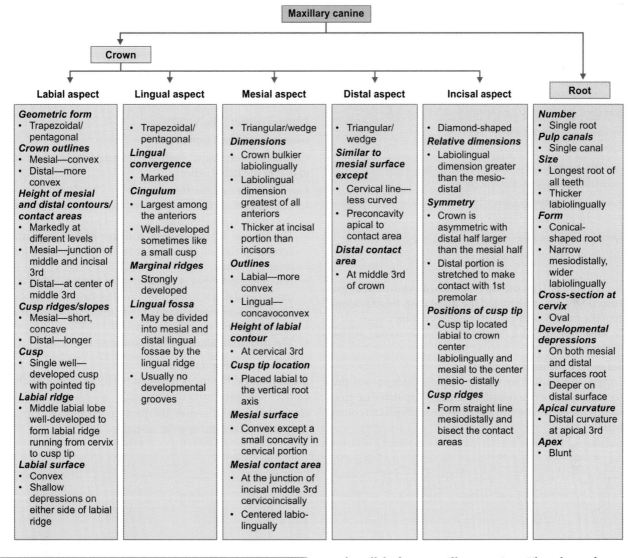

mandibular canine has a long narrow crown, shorter root, poorly developed cingulum, and less prominent cusp. The mandibular canine erupts prior to mandibular premolars

and well before maxillary canine. The chronology and measurement of the mandibular canine is given in **Table 11.2**.

## Detailed Description of Mandibular Canine from All Aspects (Figs. 11.13 to 11.15)

### Crown

*Labial aspect* (**Fig. 11.16**)*:*

*Geometric shape:* Trapezoidal or pentagonal

*Crown outlines:* The labial aspect reveals the major differences between the maxillary and mandibular canines.

- The *mesial outline* is almost straight, in line with the mesial outline of the root and it joins the mesial cusp. The maximum convexity of the mesial outline *(The mesial contact area)* is near the mesioincisal angle.
- *Distal outline* is less convex than that of maxillary canine. The *distal contact area* is more incisally located than that of maxillary canine.

**Table 11.2:** Mandibular canine—chronology and measurements.

| Chronology | |
|---|---|
| First evidence of calcification | 4–5 months |
| Enamel completed | 6–7 years |
| Eruption | 9–10 years |
| Roots completed | 12–14 years |
| **Measurements** *Dimensions suggested for carving technique (in mm)* | |
| Cervicoincisal length of crown | 11.0 |
| Length of root | 16.0 |
| Mesiodistal diameter of crown | 7.0 |
| Mesiodistal diameter of crown at cervix | 5.5 |
| Labiolingual diameter of crown | 7.5 |
| Labiolingual diameter of crown at cervix | 7.0 |
| Curvature of cervical line—mesial | 2.5 |
| Curvature of cervical line—distal | 1.0 |

- *Incisal outline:* The cusp tip is in line with vertical root axis. Cusp ridges are straight and the distal cusp ridge is longer than the mesial as in case of maxillary canine.
- *Cervical outline:* The cervical line on the labial surface curves apically.

*Labial surface within the outlines:*
- Crown of mandibular canine appears longer, not only because of its extra length of 1 mm, but also due to its narrow mesiodistal width and more incisally placed contact areas.

- Mesioincisal and distoincisal angles are well defined.
- The labial ridge running from cervix to the cusp tip is less prominent than that of the maxillary canine.
- The crown appears to be tilted distally on the root base because of its straight mesial outline and curved distal outline.
- When cusp tip is worn off, the tooth appears like a lateral incisor from labial aspect.

### Lingual aspect (Fig. 11.17)

*Geometric shape:* Trapezoidal

*Crown outlines:* Crown outlines of lingual surface are similar to that of the labial aspect.

*Lingual surface within the outlines:*
- The lingual surface is narrower than the labial surface as the crown tapers lingually.
- The lingual surface is less concave and more flattened similar to that of mandibular lateral incisor. The lingual fossa is shallow.
- When lingual ridge is present, there are two small fossae, mesial and distal lingual fossae. The lingual ridge is also less well developed than that of the maxillary canine.
- The cingulum is poorly developed.
- The marginal ridges are less prominent.

### Mesial aspect (Fig. 11.18):

Some major differences between maxillary and mandibular canines are noted from this aspect.

*Geometric shape:* The mesial aspect has a *triangular* form with its base at cervix and apex at cusp tip.

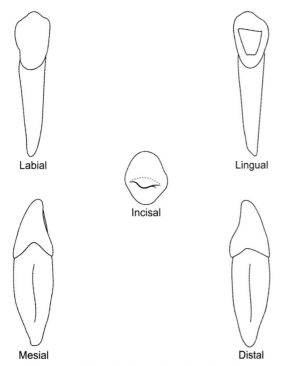

**Fig. 11.13:** Mandibular canine—line drawings.

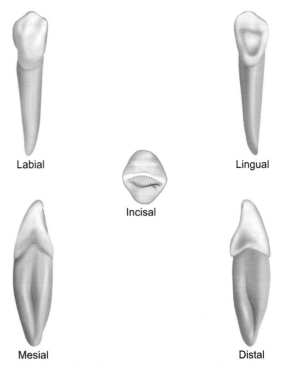

**Fig. 11.14:** Mandibular canine—graphic illustration.

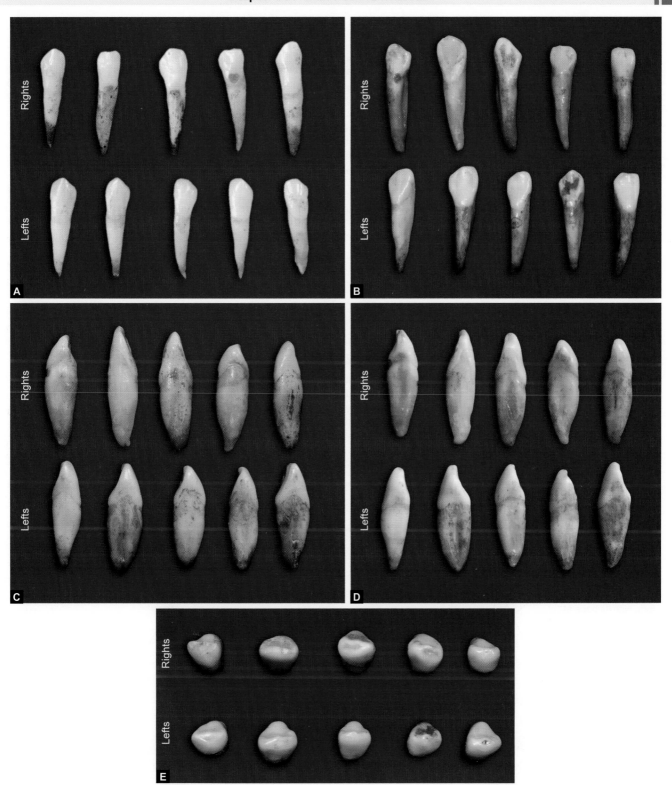

**Figs. 11.15A to E:** Mandibular canine—typical tooth specimen from all aspects: (A) Labial aspect; (B) Lingual aspect; (C) Mesial aspect; (D) Distal aspect; (E) Incisal aspect.

←Distal                                                Mesial→

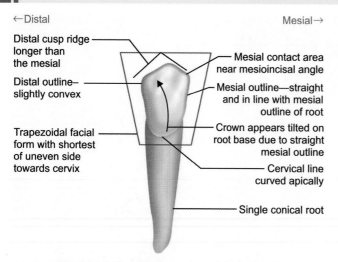

**Fig. 11.16:** Mandibular canine—labial aspect.

←Mesial                                                Distal→

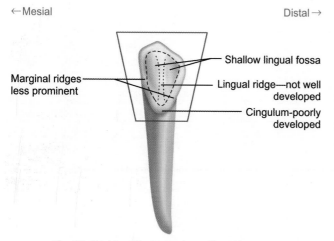

**Fig. 11.17:** Mandibular canine—lingual aspect.

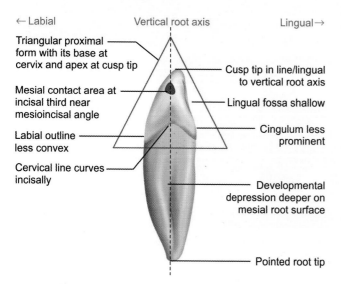

**Fig. 11.18:** Mandibular canine—mesial aspect.

*Crown outlines:*
- *Labial outline:* It is less convex especially near the cervical line.
- *Lingual outline:* It follows a less convex cingulum and less concave lingual fossa.
- *Incisal outline:* Cusp tip is thin, pointed and cusp ridge is thin labiolingually.
- *Cervical outline:* The cervical line shows more curvature incisally than that of the maxillary canine.

*Mesial surface within the outlines:*
- The cusp tip is in the center or lingual to the vertical root axis. It can be remembered that cusp tip of maxillary canine is labial to the vertical root axis.
- The lower teeth show a lingual inclination over the root base. This conforms to the general rule that the upper teeth overlap the lower teeth in occlusion.
- *Mesial contact area* is at incisal third near the mesioincisal angle.

***Distal aspect*** (Fig. 11.19)***:***
- It is similar to mesial aspect of mandibular canine except that the cervical line is less curved on distal surface.
- *Distal contact area* is at the junction of incisal and middle thirds.

***Incisal aspect*** (Fig. 11.20)***:***

*Geometric shape:* Oval

Incisal aspect is similar to that of maxillary canine except the following features:
- Mesial outline is less curved.
- Cingulum is smaller.
- Cusp tip and cusp ridges are lingually inclined. Whereas cusp ridges of maxillary canine extend straight to bisect the mesial and distal contact areas.

***Root***

Mandibular canine root differs from the root of maxillary canine in following ways:

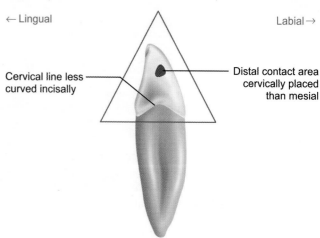

**Fig. 11.19:** Mandibular canine—distal aspect.

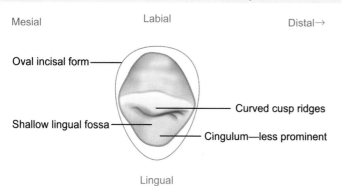

Mesial     Labial     Distal→

Oval incisal form

Shallow lingual fossa

Curved cusp ridges

Cingulum—less prominent

Lingual

**Fig. 11.20:** Mandibular canine—incisal aspect.

| | |
|---|---|
| *Number:* | Usually single, but bifurcated root is a common variation than the maxillary canine root |
| *Size:* | It is shorter by 1–2 mm |
| *Form:* | The root is thinner mesiodistally and its lingual surface is more narrower than that of maxillary canine. The developmental depression is more deeper on mesial surface of the root |
| *Apex:* | Mandibular canine has a more pointed root tip |
| *Curvature:* | The root is usually straight and sometimes shows mesial curvature at its apical third |

The differences between maxillary and mandibular canines (arch traits) are given in **Table 11.3**.

## Variations (Figs. 11.21A to C)

- Bifurcation of the root
- Long root
- Short root.

## Clinical Considerations

- The mandibular canine along with the maxillary canine establishes *canine guidance*.

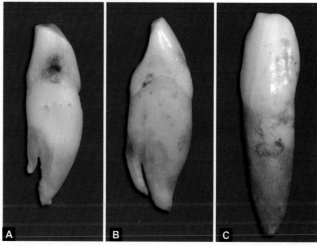

**Figs. 11.21A to C:** Mandibular canine with bifurcated root.

**Table 11.3:** Differences between maxillary and mandibular permanent canines.

| Characteristics | Maxillary permanent canine | Mandibular permanent canine |
|---|---|---|
| **Tooth nomenclature** | | |
| Universal system | Right 6; Left 11 | Right 27; Left 22 |
| **Zsigmondy/Palmer system** | Right 3⌋; Left ⌊3 | Right 3⌋; Left ⌊3 |
| FDI system | Right 13; Left 23 | Right 43; Left 33 |
| **Chronology** | | |
| Eruption | • 11–12 years<br>• Usually erupt after one or both the maxillary premolars | • 9–10 years<br>• Erupts before mandibular premolars and well before maxillary canine |
| Root completion | 13–15 years | 12–14 years |
| **General features:** | | |
| Lobes | Develops from 4 lobes middle labial lobe is very well developed into labial ridge | From 4 lobes<br>Middle labial lobe is not so well developed |
| General size | • Longest tooth of all<br>• Bulkier crown<br>• Longest root of all | • Second longest tooth<br>• Crown longer by 1 mm and slender<br>• Root shorter by 1 mm |
| **Crown** | | |
| *Labial aspect:* | | |
| Crown form | Pentagonal, resembles a premolar | Trapezoid, resembles lateral incisor |
| Mesiodistal width | Crown is broader and shorter | Crown is longer and narrower mesiodistally |
| Labial surface | The labial surface is more convex | Labial surface is convex |
| The cusp | • The cusp is sharp and very well developed.<br>• Incisal portion of cusp and cusp ridges occupy one-third of crown length | • The cusp is not so well developed<br>• Incisal portion occupies one-fifth of crown length |

*Contd...*

*Contd...*

| Characteristics | Maxillary permanent canine | Mandibular permanent canine |
|---|---|---|
| Cusp ridges | Mesial cusp ridge is usually concave, distal longer | Cusp ridges are straight, distal longer |
| Labial ridge | Labial ridge is very prominent | Labial ridge is less prominent |
| Crown tilt | Crown is upright on root base | From this aspect crown appears to be tilted distally on root base—since mesial crown outline is straight following mesial outline of root |
| Contact areas | Are markedly at dissimilar levels. <br> *Mesial*—at the junction of incisal and middle third <br> *Distal*—at center of middle third | Are within incisal third <br> Mesial—near mesioincisal angle <br> Distal—at the junction of incisal and middle third |
| *Lingual aspect*: | | |
| Lingual surface | Lingual surface is more irregular | Smooth and is similar to that of mandibular lateral incisors |
| Cingulum | The cingulum is large, very well developed; sometimes may even be pointed like a small cusp | The cingulum is smooth and poorly developed |
| Marginal ridges | Marginal ridges are strongly developed | Marginal ridges are thin and less distinct |
| Lingual fossa | Lingual fossa is more concave | Lingual fossa is shallow and smooth |
| Lingual ridge | Lingual ridge is more prominent | Lingual fossa is less prominent |
| *Proximal aspects*: | | |
| Crown bulk | Crown is more bulky labiolingually | Crown appears less bulkier |
| Lingual inclination of crown | Crown upright on root base | Crown lingually tilted on its root base |
| Position of cusp tip | Cusp tip is labial to the vertical root axis | Cusp tip is placed lingual to the vertical root axis |
| Incisal edge | Incisal edge is lingually sloping | Incisal edge is labially sloping |
| *Incisal aspect*: | | |
| Incisal form | Diamond-shaped | Oval |
| Dimension | Labiolingual dimension is greater among all the anteriors | Crown is less bulkier labiolingually |
| Crown symmetry | Crown appears asymmetrical with the mesial half of the crown bigger than the distal half | Crown is symmetrical |
| Cusp tip | Cusp tip is labial to the center of crown labiolingually and mesial to the center mesiodistally | Cusp tip is in the center or lingually placed |
| Cusp ridges | • Cusp ridges with contact area extensions form a straight line mesiodistally <br> • Large cingulum forms a more pronounced convexity of lingual surface <br> • Labial ridge prominently seen on labial surface <br> • Lingual ridge is more prominent | • Cusp ridges (especially distal) are inclined lingually <br> • Less convex lingual surface <br> • Labial ridge is less prominent <br> • Lingual ridge is less prominent |
| **Root** | | |
| Number | Single conical root and is never bifurcated | Usually single root may be bifurcated into buccal and lingual |
| Size | • Longest root with extra anchorage <br> • Lingual surface is narrower than labial | • Root is 1–2 mm shorter <br> • Lingual surface is much more narrower about ½ of the width of labial surface |
| Apex curvature | • Apex is blunt <br> • Apical third of the root shows distal curvature | • Apex is slightly sharp <br> • Root is usually straight, sometimes has mesial curvature |
| Developmental grooves | Developmental groove on distal surface of root is more deeper | Developmental groove on mesial surface is more pronounced |
| Pulp canals | Single canal | Single canal, 2 canals if bifurcated |

(FDI: Federation Dentaire Internationale)

- The relationship of maxillary canine to mandibular canine is an important consideration while classifying malocclusions. Frequent bifurcation of roots should be considered during root canal therapy.

**Flowcharts 11.3 and 11.4** give brief summary of mandibular canine morphology.

**Box 11.2** lists the tooth's identification features.

---

**Box 11.2: Mandibular canine—identification features.**

- *Identification features of mandibular canine*:
  - The mandibular permanent canine has a long and narrow crown with a sharp cusp
  - The labial ridge and cingulum are less prominent
  - The distal cusp slope is longer than the mesial
  - The crown appears to be tilted distally on the root base
  - The root is long and narrow
  - When viewed proximally, the cusp tip is lingual to the root axis line
- *Side identification*:
  - The distal cusp slope is longer
  - Developmental depression on the mesial surface of the root is deeper
  - When viewed labially, the mesial outline is straight and distal outline is rounded

---

**Flowchart 11.3:** Mandibular canine—major anatomic landmarks.

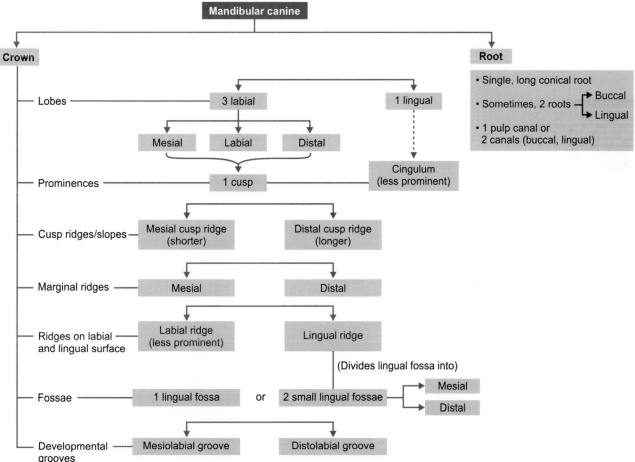

**Flowchart 11.4:** Mandibular canine—summary.

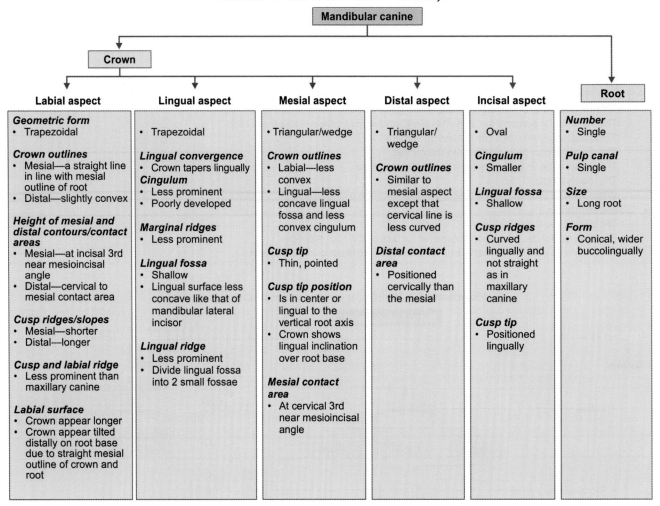

## BIBLIOGRAPHY

1. Babacan H, Kiliç B, Biçakçi A. Maxillary canine-1st premolar transposition in the permanent dentition. Angle Orthod. 2008;78(5):954-60.
2. Bedoya MM, Park JH. A review of the diagnosis and management of impacted maxillary canines. J Am Dent Assoc. 2009;140(12):1485-93.
3. Bishara SE. Impacted maxillary canines: A review. Am J Orthod Dentofac Orthoped. 1992;101(2):159-71.
4. Peck L, Peck S, Attia Y. Maxillary canine-1st premolar transposition, associated dental anomalies and genetic basis. Angle Orthod. 1993;63(2):99-109.
5. Segura JJ, Hattab F, Ríos V. Maxillary canine transpositions in two brothers and one sister: associated dental anomalies and genetic basis. ASDC J Dent Child. 2002;69(1): 54-8, 12.

## MULTIPLE CHOICE QUESTIONS

1. Synonyms of maxillary permanent canine are followings, except:
   a. Beauty tooth
   b. Corner stone of dental arch
   c. Cuspids
   d. Canivos teeth
2. The maxillary permanent canines are named because they:
   a. Closely resemble the tearing teeth of carnivores, especially those of dogs
   b. Are corner stones of arches
   c. Are four in number
   d. Are having longest roots
3. The maxillary permanent canine develops from:
   a. 2 lobes
   b. 3 lobes

c. 4 lobes

d. 5 lobes

4. Which of the following statements is false?

   a. The maxillary permanent canine has longest and strongest roots of all teeth

   b. The maxillary permanent canines are six in number

   c. The maxillary permanent canines are also called as cuspids

   d. Roots of maxillary permanent canines have excellent anchorage in the alveolar bone with an extra length and wider labiolingual width

5. The term canine eminence refers to:

   a. Alveolar bone over the roots of maxillary permanent canines, labially, is prominent and/or is prominent labial alveolar bone over the roots of maxillary permanent canines

   b. Prominent lingual alveolar bone over the roots of maxillary permanent canines

   c. Least prominent labial alveolar ridge/bone over the roots of maxillary permanent canines

   d. Least prominent labial alveolar ridge/bone over the roots of maxillary permanent canines

6. Following are the functions of maxillary permanent canines, except:

   a. They assist permanent incisors and premolars in mastication

   b. They are mainly used for tearing food

   c. They help in seizing, slicing, and chewing food

   d. They are esthetically not important

7. The characteristics of maxillary permanent canines are:

   a. Maxillary permanent canines exhibit some of the characteristics of maxillary permanent incisors

   b. Maxillary permanent canines exhibit some of the characteristics of permanent premolars

   c. Maxillary permanent canines exhibit longest root of all

   d. All of the above

8. The shape of the crown of maxillary permanent canine from the labial aspect is:

   a. Trapezoidal

   b. Pentagonal

   c. Hexagonal

   d. Both A and B

9. The mesial outline of the crown of maxillary permanent canine from the labial aspect is:

   a. Convex arc from cervix to the area where it joins the mesial cusp slope

   b. Concave arc from cervix to the area where it joins the mesial cusp slope

   c. Straight from cervix to the area where it joins the mesial cusp slope

   d. None of the above

10. The minimum convexity of the mesial outline of maxillary permanent canine from the labial aspect lies at:

    a. The junction of cervical and middle third of the crown

    b. The junction of incisal and middle third of the crown

    c. At the cervical third

    d. Near the gingival margin.

**Answers**

1. d     2. a     3. c     4. b     5. a     6. d     7. d     8. d

9. a     10. c

# 12

# The Permanent Maxillary Premolars

**Did you know?**

- Typical dental formula of primitive mammals had 4 premolars. Over the evolution, it reduced to 3 in primates and 2 premolars in humans with absence of *p1* and *p2*.
- **Carnassial teeth** in carnivores are blade-like upper last premolar and lower first molar evolved for slicing flesh like scissors.

## INTRODUCTION

There are eight premolars; four in each dental arch and two in each quadrant. The premolars are named so since they are located anterior to the molars in the permanent dentition **(Fig. 12.1)**. *There are no premolars in deciduous dentition and they succeed deciduous molars.* Premolars along with the molars occupy posterior segments of dental arches and are collectively referred to as "posterior teeth".

Premolars are often also called as "bicuspids" suggestive of having two cusps. However, the mandibular first premolar has only one functional cusp and the mandibular second premolar frequently has three cusps. Moreover, the premolar

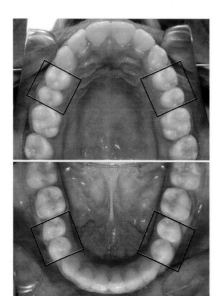

**Fig. 12.1:** "Premolars" are situated anterior to the molars. They together with the molars form the posteriors of the dental arch.

teeth in carnivorous animals exhibit varied occlusal anatomy, thus precluding the usage of "bicuspid" term. Hence the term premolar is generally preferred in both dental and comparative anatomy.

They have single root except the maxillary first premolar which has two roots—buccal and lingual.

## FUNCTIONS

- First premolars with their sharp cusps assist canines in tearing food.
- They grind food along with molars.
- Provide support to cheek near corners of mouth.
- They reinforce esthetics during smiling.

## COMMON CHARACTERISTICS (CLASS TRAITS) OF PREMOLARS

- The premolars develop from four lobes with an exception of the mandibular second premolar which develops from five lobes.
- They generally have two cusps, one buccal and one lingual except for mandibular second premolars which often carry three cusps.
- All premolars have single root except maxillary first premolars which are frequently bifurcated.
- Their buccolingual dimension is greater than the mesiodistal dimension.
- The contact areas are broader than that of the anterior and are placed nearly at the same level. Contact areas are buccal to center of the crowns buccolingually.
- Crests of buccal and lingual contours are more occlusal than seen on anterior teeth.
- Marginal ridges are at a higher level (occlusally placed) mesially than distally. Exception is in case of mandibular first premolar where the distal marginal ridge is more occlusally placed than mesial marginal ridge.

## MAXILLARY FIRST PREMOLAR

The maxillary first premolar has two cusps—buccal and lingual and frequently has two roots. Sometimes it can have a single root with two pulp canals. The buccal cusp is longer than the lingual cusp by 1 mm. The tooth resembles maxillary permanent canine from buccal aspect, but with a shorter crown and root. The crown is angular with prominent buccal line angles.

The maxillary first premolar develops from four lobes—three buccal lobes forming the buccal cusp and a single lingual lobe forming the lingual cusp. The chronology and measurements of the maxillary first premolar is given in **Table 12.1**.

## DETAILED DESCRIPTION OF MAXILLARY FIRST PREMOLAR FROM ALL ASPECTS (FIGS. 12.2 TO 12.4)

### Crown

### Buccal Aspect (Fig. 12.5A)

*Geometric shape:* Trapezoidal

*Crown outlines:*

*Mesial outline:*
- The mesial outline is slightly concave near cervical line and becomes convex as it joins the mesial cusp slope.
- Height of contour of mesial outline *(mesial contact area)* is occlusal to the center of crown cervico-occlusally.

*Distal outline:*
- Distal outline is straight and meets the distal cusp slope.
- Its height of contour *(distal contact area)* is broader and slightly occlusally placed than the mesial contact area.

*Occlusal outline:*
- Occlusal outline is formed by the cusp tip and cusp slopes of the buccal cusp.

**Table 12.1:** Maxillary first premolar—chronology and dimensions.

| Chronology | |
|---|---|
| First evidence of calcification | Years |
| Enamel completed | 5–6 years |
| Eruption | 10–11 years |
| Roots completed | 12–13 years |
| **Measurements** *Dimensions suggested for carving technique (in mm)* | |
| Cervico-occlusal length of crown | 8.5 |
| Length of root | 14.0 |
| Mesiodistal diameter of crown | 7.0 |
| Mesiodistal diameter of crown at cervix | 5.0 |
| Buccolingual diameter of crown | 9.0 |
| Buccolingual diameter of crown at cervix | 8.0 |
| Curvature of cervical line—mesial | 1.0 |

- Mesial cusp slope is straight or sometimes concave whereas distal cusp slope is more rounded.

*Cervical outline:* Cervical line slightly curves toward the root apex.

*Buccal surface within the outlines:*
- Tooth appears similar to maxillary canine from buccal aspect but the crown is shorter and narrower than that of maxillary canine **(Fig. 12.5B)**.

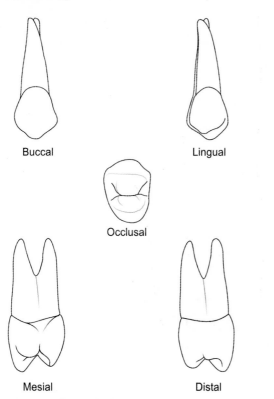

**Fig. 12.2:** Maxillary right first premolar—line drawings.

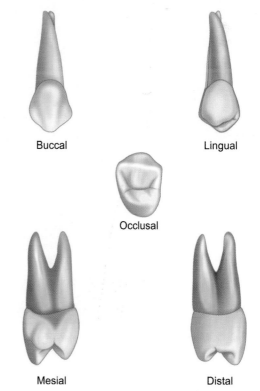

**Fig. 12.3:** Maxillary right first premolar—graphic illustrations.

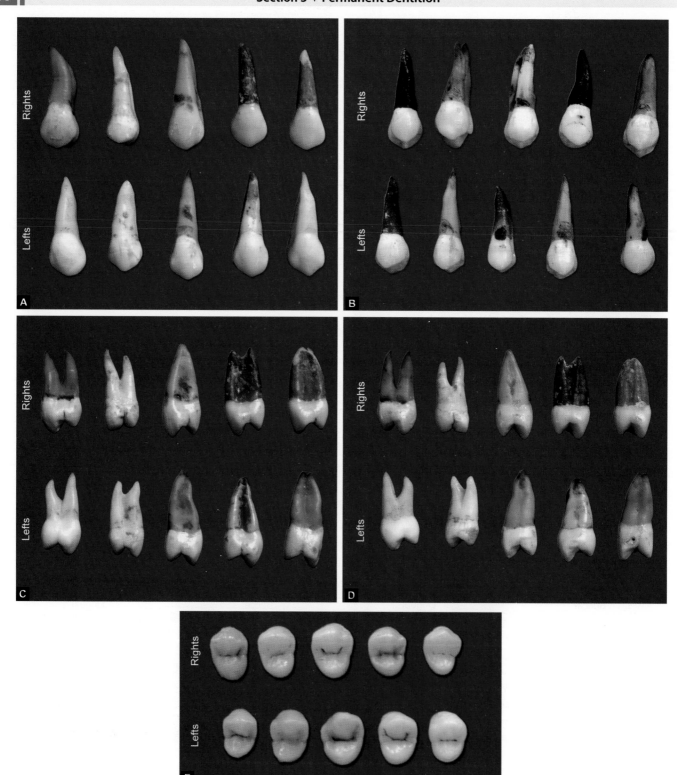

**Figs. 12.4A to E:** Maxillary first premolar—typical tooth specimen from all aspects: (A) Buccal aspect; (B) Lingual aspect; (C) Mesial aspect; (D) Distal aspect; (E) Occlusal aspect.

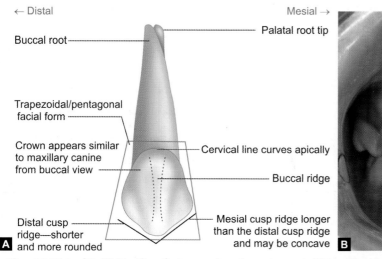

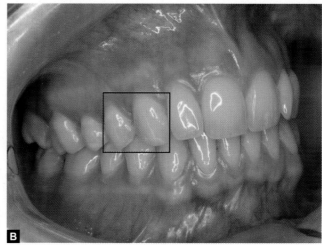

**Figs. 12.5A and B:** (A) Maxillary first premolar—buccal aspect; (B) Maxillary first premolar appears similar to the maxillary canine but with shorter and narrower crown.

- The middle buccal lobe is strongly developed than the other lobes and forms a continuous ridge from cusp tip to cervix called "buccal ridge".
- Mesial slope is longer than the distal slope (it can be remembered that distal cusp slope is generally longer in other teeth).
- The buccal surface is convex except the developmental depressions on either side of buccal ridge demarcating the three lobes.

## Palatal Aspect (Fig. 12.6)

**Geometric shape:** Trapezoidal

**Crown outlines:**

*Mesial outline*  
*Distal outline* } are similar to buccal aspect  
*Cervical outline*  
*Occlusal outline:*
- Lingual cusp is pointed with its cusp slopes meeting at right angles.
- Buccal cusp tip with its cusp slopes are seen because of a shorter lingual cusp.

**Lingual surface within the outlines:**
- Lingual surface is narrower than buccal surface as the proximal walls converge toward smaller lingual cusp.
- Lingual surface is smooth and more convex.
- Sometimes there can be lingual ridge.
- The lingual line angles are not as prominent as buccal line angles.

## Mesial Aspect (Fig. 12.7)

**Geometric shape:** The proximal aspects of all maxillary posteriors have a *trapezoid* outline with the longest of uneven sides toward cervical portion and shortest of uneven sides toward occlusal portion.

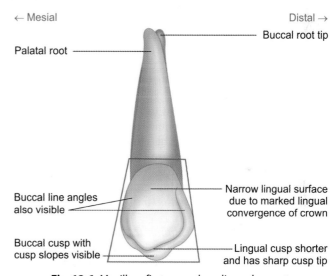

**Fig. 12.6:** Maxillary first premolar—lingual aspect.

**Crown outlines:**

*Buccal outline:*
- Buccal outline is convex near cervix and become straight as it reaches the buccal cusp tip.
- Height of buccal contour is at cervical third.

*Lingual outline:*
- Lingual outline is a convex arc from cervical line to the tip of lingual cusp.
- Its height of contour is at the center of middle third.

*Occlusal outline:*
- Occlusal outline is formed by mesial marginal ridge which is slightly concave.
- The triangular ridges of buccal and lingual cusp are also seen converging cervically toward the center of occlusal surface.

*Cervical outline:*
- The cervical line is slightly curved occlusally.

← Buccal                                                                                   Lingual →

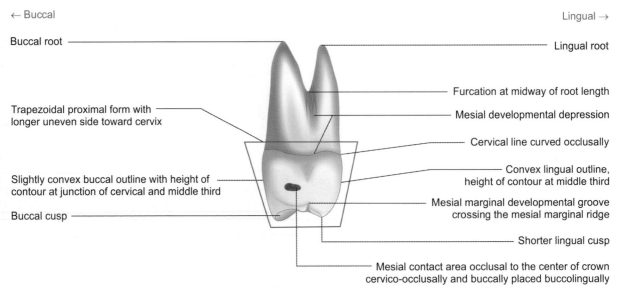

Buccal root ——————————————————————————————— Lingual root

————————— Furcation at midway of root length

Trapezoidal proximal form with ——————— Mesial developmental depression
longer uneven side toward cervix

————————— Cervical line curved occlusally

Slightly convex buccal outline with height of ———————— Convex lingual outline,
contour at junction of cervical and middle third    height of contour at middle third

Buccal cusp ————————————— Mesial marginal developmental groove
                                              crossing the mesial marginal ridge

————————— Shorter lingual cusp

Mesial contact area occlusal to the center of crown
cervico-occlusally and buccally placed buccolingually

**Fig. 12.7:** Maxillary first premolar—mesial aspect.

***Mesial surface within the outlines:***

- Mesial surface shows both the cusps and the cusp tips are well within the confines of the root trunk.
- The lingual cusp is shorter than the buccal cusp by 1 mm or more.
- A marked concavity located in the center of the mesial surface, cervical to the contact area is called as *mesial developmental depression.* This concavity extends apically crossing the cervical line and joins the developmental depression between the two roots.
- There is a deep developmental groove crossing the mesial marginal ridge called *mesial marginal developmental groove.*
- *Mesial marginal developmental groove and mesial developmental depression* are the identifying features of maxillary first premolar, and help to differentiate the tooth from maxillary second premolar.
- The *mesial contact area* is occlusal to the center of crown cervico-occlusally and more buccally placed buccolingually.

## Distal Aspect (Fig. 12.8)

***Geometric shape:*** Trapezoidal

***Crown outlines:***

Mesial outline ⎫
Distal outline ⎬ are similar to mesial aspect
Occlusal outline ⎭

*Cervical outline:* The cervical line on the lingual surface is straight rather than curving occlusally.

***Distal surface within the outlines:***

- The distal surface is generally convex.
- The distal marginal ridge is smooth; devoid of any grooves.
- *Distal contact area* is at the same level as mesial contact area but is more broader and more buccally placed buccolingually.

← Lingual                                          Buccal →

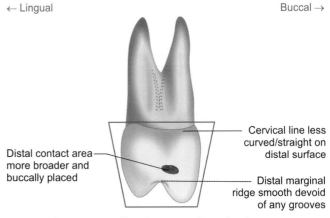

Cervical line less
curved/straight on
distal surface

Distal contact area
more broader and
buccally placed

Distal marginal
ridge smooth devoid
of any grooves

**Fig. 12.8:** Maxillary first premolar—distal aspect.

## Occlusal Aspect (Figs. 12.9A and B)

***Geometric shape:*** Occlusal aspect of this tooth has a *hexagonal shape with unequal sides.*

The six sides in clockwise direction are:

1. Mesiobuccal
2. Mesial
3. Mesiolingual
4. Distolingual
5. Distal
6. Distobuccal.

***Relative dimensions:*** From occlusal aspect, it is easily noted that the buccolingual dimension is greater than mesiodistal dimension. The crown is wider buccally than lingually.

*Position of cusp tips and contact area extensions:*

- The *buccal cusp* is placed slightly distal to the midline.
- The *lingual cusp* tip is located mesial to the midline.

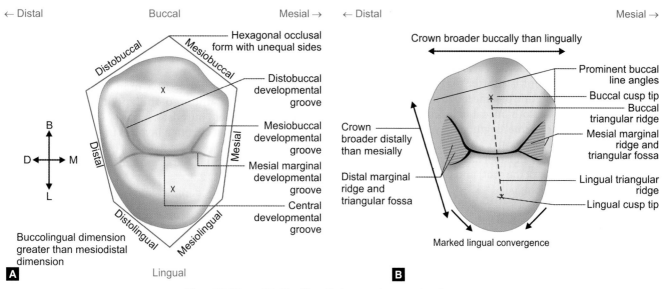

**Figs. 12.9A and B:** Maxillary first premolar—occlusal aspect.

*Boundaries of occlusal surface:*

*The occlusal surface is bounded by:*
- Mesial and distal cusp ridges of buccal and lingual cusps
- Mesial and distal marginal ridges

*Mesial and distal marginal ridges converge toward lingual cusp.*

*Occlusal surface within boundaries:*
- Cusps and cusp ridges
- Grooves and pits
- Marginal ridges and fossae.

*Cusps and cusp ridges:*

*Buccal cusp:*
- Among the two cusps, the buccal cusp is longer and well-formed.
- *Mesiobuccal and distobuccal cusp ridges* are well defined and make a relatively straight line.
- *Buccal triangular ridge* is well defined extending from buccal cusp tip lingually up to the central developmental groove in the center of the occlusal surface.
- Buccal cusp has inclined planes on either side of the triangular ridge sloping toward the central groove.

*Lingual cusp:*
- It is smaller and shorter than the buccal cusp.
- *Mesiolingual and distolingual cusp ridges* are more curved and form a semicircular outline merging with the marginal ridges
- A less prominent *lingual triangular ridge* extends from lingual cusp tip to the central groove.
- There are inclined planes on either side of triangular ridge.

*Grooves and pits:*

*Grooves:* There are four major grooves:
1. Central groove
2. Mesiobuccal groove

3. Distobuccal groove
4. Mesial marginal developmental groove.

- The *central developmental groove* running in a mesiodistal direction divides the occlusal surface evenly. This groove is at the bottom of central sulcus.
- Two small grooves join the central groove near mesial and distal marginal ridge buccally. These are called *mesiobuccal* and *distobuccal developmental grooves.*
- The *mesial marginal developmental groove* extends from the central groove mesially and crosses the mesial marginal ridge to reach the mesial surface. This is the important identifying feature of maxillary first premolar.

*Pits:* There are two pits—
1. *Mesial pit* is formed by convergence of:
   - Central developmental groove
   - Mesiobuccal developmental groove
   - Mesial marginal developmental groove.
2. *Distal pit* is formed by convergence of:
   - Central developmental groove
   - Distobuccal developmental groove.

*Marginal ridges and fossae:*

*Marginal ridges:* There are two marginal ridges:
1. *Mesial marginal ridge*: It is notched by mesial marginal developmental groove.
2. *Distal marginal ridge*: It is smooth.

*Fossae:* There are two triangular fossae:
1. *Mesial triangular fossa* is a small triangular depression with mesial marginal ridge forming the base and mesial pit forming the apex of the triangle. Mesial marginal groove runs across mesial triangular fossa.
2. *Distal triangular fossa* is a shallower triangular depression with distal marginal ridge forming the base and distal pit forming the apex of the triangle.

## Root

Morphology of the root can be described under the following headings:

*Number:* Two roots—buccal and lingual

*Size:* The root is shorter than that of maxillary canine and of same length as maxillary molar roots. Both buccal and lingual roots are of nearly same length.

*Form:* *Two root form:*
- Bifurcated root has a root trunk (undivided part of the root) and two branches: Buccal and lingual
- The root is narrow and convex mesiodistally, broader and flattened buccolingually
- The root is bifurcated for half its length and its bifurcation point is more nearer to cervical line on mesial aspect
- Developmental depression and groove is prominent on the mesial surface of the root
- Two pulp canals with two apical foramen

*Single root form:*
- The single root often shows deep developmental grooves and has two pulp canals

*Curvature:* Apical end of the root usually shows distal curvature

*Apex:* Buccal root apex is sharp and distal root has a blunt apex

### Variations (Fig. 12.10A)

- Single root (commonly seen)
- Short root
- Long root.

### Developmental Anomalies (Fig. 12.10B)

Dens evaginatus or Leong's premolar.

### Clinical Considerations

Maxillary and mandibular first premolars are the most common teeth to undergo therapeutic extraction for orthodontic treatment purposes.

Transposition of teeth often involves maxillary canine and maxillary premolar.

Anatomy of maxillary first premolar is summarized in **Flowcharts 12.1 and 12.2**.

**Box 12.1** shows the identification features of the tooth.

## MAXILLARY SECOND PREMOLAR

The maxillary second premolar closely resembles maxillary first premolar and assists the latter in function. When compared to maxillary first premolars, it is less angular, exhibits a more rounded appearance, and has two cusps of nearly same size **(Fig. 12.11)**.

The maxillary second premolar is more variable in its size and has a single root. However, average dimensions of both the premolars are same **(Table 12.2)**.

## DETAILED DESCRIPTION OF MAXILLARY SECOND PREMOLAR FROM ALL ASPECTS (FIGS. 12.12 TO 12.14)

### Crown

*Buccal Aspect (Fig. 12.15)*

***Geometric shape:*** Trapezoid with narrow cervix.

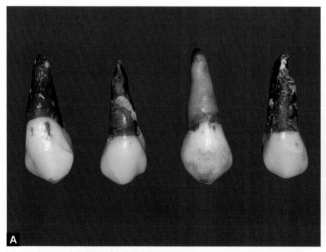
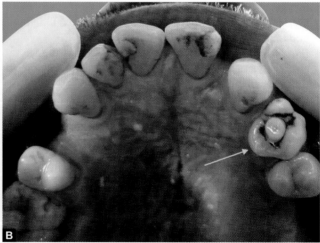

**Figs. 12.10A and B:** (A) Maxillary first premolar—variations; (B) Dens evaginatus or Leong's premolar.

**Flowchart 12.1:** Maxillary first premolar—major anatomic landmarks.

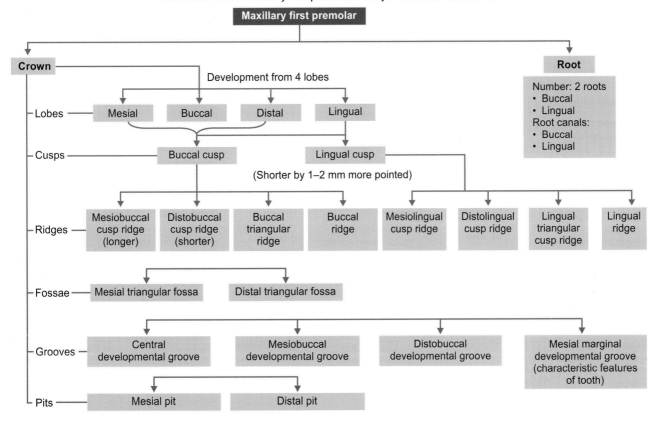

- *Identification features of maxillary first premolar*:
  - Tooth has two cusps, lingual cusp is shorter
  - It frequently has two roots and sometimes single root with deep developmental grooves
  - Mesial developmental depression on mesial surface of crown which may extend onto root surface
  - Mesial marginal developmental groove is the distinguishing feature of maxillary second premolar
- *Side identification*:
  - Presence of mesial marginal developmental groove on the mesial side
  - Deep developmental depression on mesial surface of the root

**Table 12.2:** Maxillary second premolar—chronology and measurements.

| Chronology | |
|---|---|
| First evidence of calcification | 2–2¼ years |
| Enamel completed | 6–7 years |
| Eruption | 10–12 years |
| Roots completed | 12–14 years |
| **Measurements** *Dimensions suggested for carving technique (in mm)* | |
| Cervico-occlusal length of crown | 8.5 |
| Length of root | 14.0 |
| Mesiodistal diameter of crown | 7.0 |
| Mesiodistal diameter of crown at cervix | 5.0 |
| Buccolingual diameter of crown | 9.0 |
| Buccolingual diameter of crown at cervix | 8.0 |
| Curvature of cervical line—mesial | 1.0 |
| Curvature of cervical line—distal | 0.0 |

**Crown outlines:**

*Mesial outline:* It is slightly convex from cervix to the point where it joins the mesial slope of the buccal cusp.

*Distal outline:* It is more convex than the mesial outline.

*Cervical outline:* Cervical line curves in an apical direction.

**Flowchart 12.2:** Maxillary first premolar—summary.

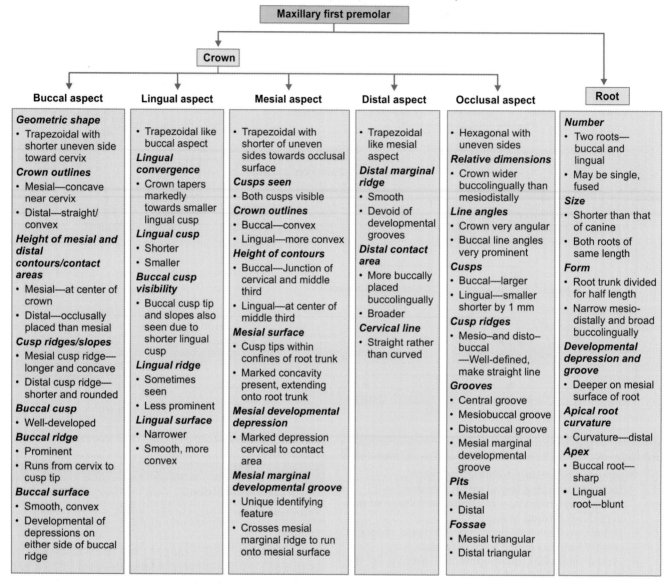

| Buccal aspect | Lingual aspect | Mesial aspect | Distal aspect | Occlusal aspect | Root |
|---|---|---|---|---|---|
| **Geometric shape**<br>• Trapezoidal with shorter uneven side toward cervix<br>**Crown outlines**<br>• Mesial—concave near cervix<br>• Distal—straight/convex<br>**Height of mesial and distal contours/contact areas**<br>• Mesial—at center of crown<br>• Distal—occlusally placed than mesial<br>**Cusp ridges/slopes**<br>• Mesial cusp ridge—longer and concave<br>• Distal cusp ridge—shorter and rounded<br>**Buccal cusp**<br>• Well-developed<br>**Buccal ridge**<br>• Prominent<br>• Runs from cervix to cusp tip<br>**Buccal surface**<br>• Smooth, convex<br>• Developmental of depressions on either side of buccal ridge | • Trapezoidal like buccal aspect<br>**Lingual convergence**<br>• Crown tapers markedly towards smaller lingual cusp<br>**Lingual cusp**<br>• Shorter<br>• Smaller<br>**Buccal cusp visibility**<br>• Buccal cusp tip and slopes also seen due to shorter lingual cusp<br>**Lingual ridge**<br>• Sometimes seen<br>• Less prominent<br>**Lingual surface**<br>• Narrower<br>• Smooth, more convex | • Trapezoidal with shorter of uneven sides towards occlusal surface<br>**Cusps seen**<br>• Both cusps visible<br>**Crown outlines**<br>• Buccal—convex<br>• Lingual—more convex<br>**Height of contours**<br>• Buccal—Junction of cervical and middle third<br>• Lingual—at center of middle third<br>**Mesial surface**<br>• Cusp tips within confines of root trunk<br>• Marked concavity present, extending onto root trunk<br>**Mesial developmental depression**<br>• Marked depression cervical to contact area<br>**Mesial marginal developmental groove**<br>• Unique identifying feature<br>• Crosses mesial marginal ridge to run onto mesial surface | • Trapezoidal like mesial aspect<br>**Distal marginal ridge**<br>• Smooth<br>• Devoid of developmental grooves<br>**Distal contact area**<br>• More buccally placed buccolingually<br>• Broader<br>**Cervical line**<br>• Straight rather than curved | • Hexagonal with uneven sides<br>**Relative dimensions**<br>• Crown wider buccolingually than mesiodistally<br>**Line angles**<br>• Crown very angular<br>• Buccal line angles very prominent<br>**Cusps**<br>• Buccal—larger<br>• Lingual—smaller shorter by 1 mm<br>**Cusp ridges**<br>• Mesio–and disto–buccal—Well-defined, make straight line<br>**Grooves**<br>• Central groove<br>• Mesiobuccal groove<br>• Distobuccal groove<br>• Mesial marginal developmental groove<br>**Pits**<br>• Mesial<br>• Distal<br>**Fossae**<br>• Mesial triangular<br>• Distal triangular | **Number**<br>• Two roots—buccal and lingual<br>• May be single, fused<br>**Size**<br>• Shorter than that of canine<br>• Both roots of same length<br>**Form**<br>• Root trunk divided for half length<br>• Narrow mesio-distally and broad buccolingually<br>**Developmental depression and groove**<br>• Deeper on mesial surface of root<br>**Apical root curvature**<br>• Curvature—distal<br>**Apex**<br>• Buccal root—sharp<br>• Lingual root—blunt |

*Occlusal outline:*
- The tip of the buccal cusp is less pointed than that of maxillary first premolar
- Distal slope of buccal cusp is longer than the mesial slope. This feature is similar in all the permanent canines and premolars. One exception is maxillary first premolar in which the mesial slope is longer than the distal slope.

***Buccal surface within the outlines:*** The tooth is thicker at cervical portion than the maxillary first premolar. Its buccal ridge is not as prominent as that of maxillary first premolar. The buccal surface is generally convex.

### Lingual Aspect (Fig. 12.16):

***Geometric shape:*** Trapezoidal like buccal aspect.

*Crown outlines:*

Mesial outline ⎫
Distal outline ⎬ are similar to buccal aspect
Cervical outline ⎭

*Occlusal outline:*
- Lingual cusp tip and its cusp slopes form the occlusal outline.
- As the lingual cusp is nearly as long as the buccal cusp, only a part of buccal profile may be seen.

***Lingual surface within the outlines:*** Lingual surface appears broader and longer than that of maxillary permanent first premolar.

### Mesial Aspect (Fig. 12.17):

***Geometric shape:*** Trapezoid with narrow occlusal table.

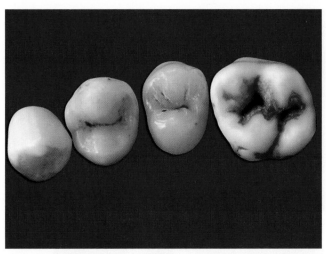

**Fig. 12.11:** Compared to maxillary first premolar, the maxillary second premolar is less angular with oval occlusal form, two cusps of equal size, and a single root.

*Crown outlines:* Buccal and lingual outlines are convex from cervix to the respective cusp tips.

*Occlusal outline:*
- The mesial marginal ridge is horizontal to the long axis of tooth.
- Buccal and lingual triangular ridges are seen inclining toward the center of occlusal surface.

*Cervical outline:* The cervical outline is slightly curved occlusally.

*Mesial surface within the outlines:*
- From mesial aspect, it is noted that both buccal and lingual cusps are of the same length. The distance between the cusp tips is wider than seen in maxillary first premolar.
- The mesial surface is smoothly convex and there is no developmental groove crossing the mesial marginal ridge.
- *Mesial contact area* is broader than that of the maxillary first premolar though located at the same level.

## Distal Aspect (Fig. 12.18)

Distal aspect of maxillary second premolar is similar to mesial aspect except that the cervical line is rather straight than curved.

## Occlusal Aspect (Fig. 12.19)

*Geometric shape:*
- The crown appears oval rather than hexagonal from occlusal aspect.
- The crown is less angular and more rounded with less prominent buccal line angles.

*Cusps and ridges:*
- Lingual cusp is as large as buccal cusp and their tips are less pointed than that of maxillary first premolar cusps.
- Mesial and distal cusp ridges of both the cusps are less well defined.
- The crown tapers lingually to a lesser extent than the maxillary first premolar, since both buccal and lingual cusps are of similar size.

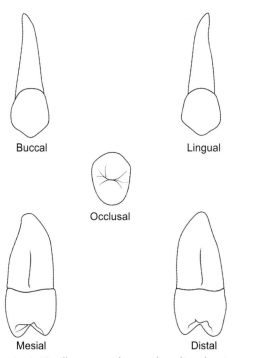

**Fig. 12.12:** Maxillary second premolar—line drawings.

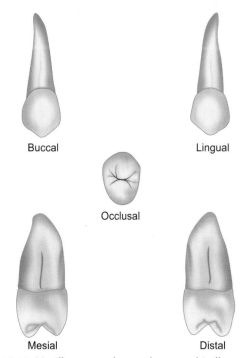

**Fig. 12.13:** Maxillary second premolar—graphic illustrations.

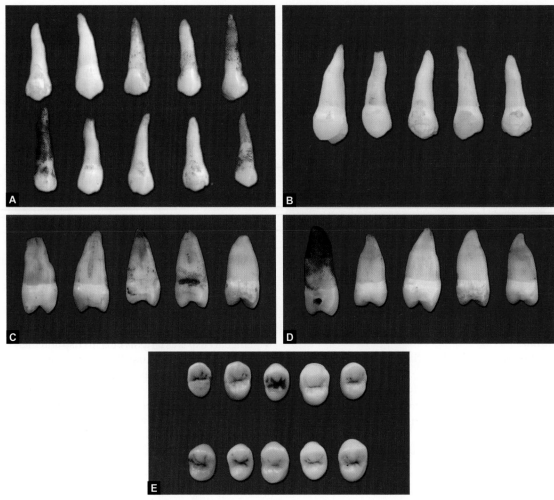

**Figs. 12.14A to E:** Maxillary second premolar—typical tooth specimen from all aspects: (A) Buccal aspect; (B) Lingual aspect; (C) Mesial aspect; (D) Distal aspect; and (E) Occlusal aspect.

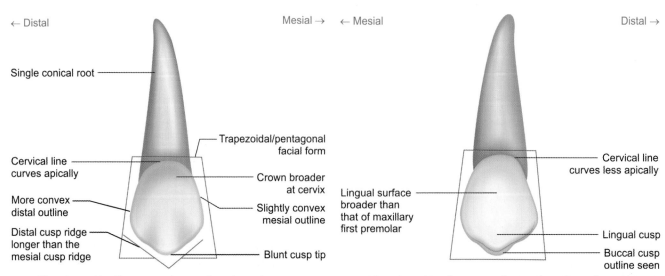

← Distal      Mesial →      ← Mesial      Distal →

Single conical root

Cervical line curves apically

More convex distal outline

Distal cusp ridge longer than the mesial cusp ridge

Trapezoidal/pentagonal facial form

Crown broader at cervix

Slightly convex mesial outline

Blunt cusp tip

**Fig. 12.15:** Maxillary second premolar—buccal aspect.

Lingual surface broader than that of maxillary first premolar

Cervical line curves less apically

Lingual cusp

Buccal cusp outline seen

**Fig. 12.16:** Maxillary second premolar—lingual aspect.

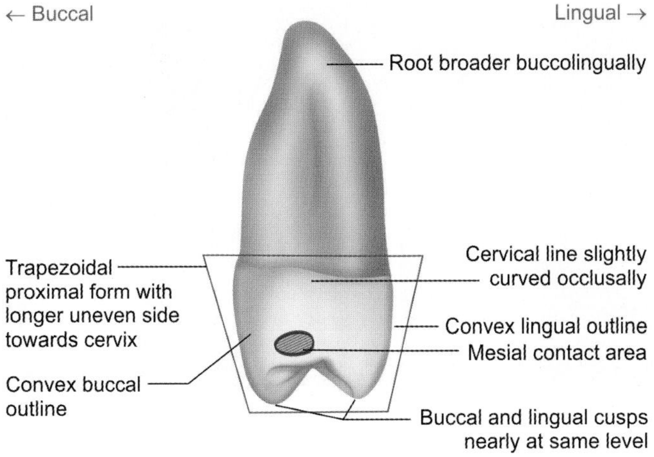
← Buccal
Lingual →
Root broader buccolingually
Trapezoidal proximal form with longer uneven side towards cervix
Cervical line slightly curved occlusally
Convex lingual outline
Mesial contact area
Convex buccal outline
Buccal and lingual cusps nearly at same level

**Fig. 12.17:** Maxillary second premolar—mesial aspect.

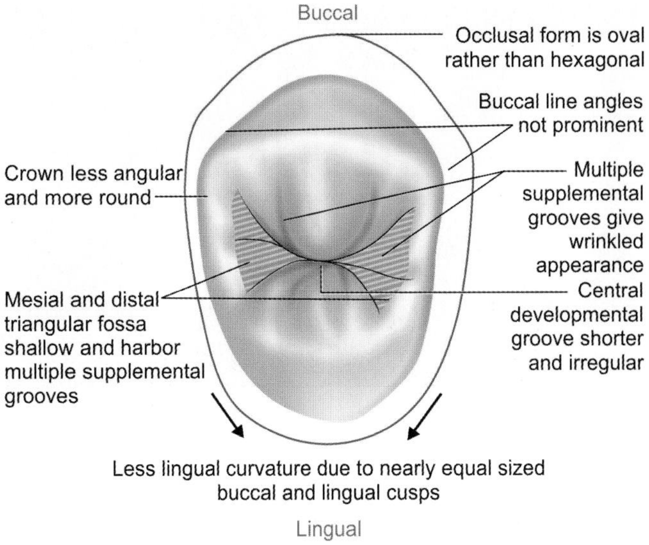
Buccal
Occlusal form is oval rather than hexagonal
Buccal line angles not prominent
Crown less angular and more round
Multiple supplemental grooves give wrinkled appearance
Mesial and distal triangular fossa shallow and harbor multiple supplemental grooves
Central developmental groove shorter and irregular
Less lingual curvature due to nearly equal sized buccal and lingual cusps
Lingual

**Fig. 12.19:** Maxillary second premolar—occlusal aspect.

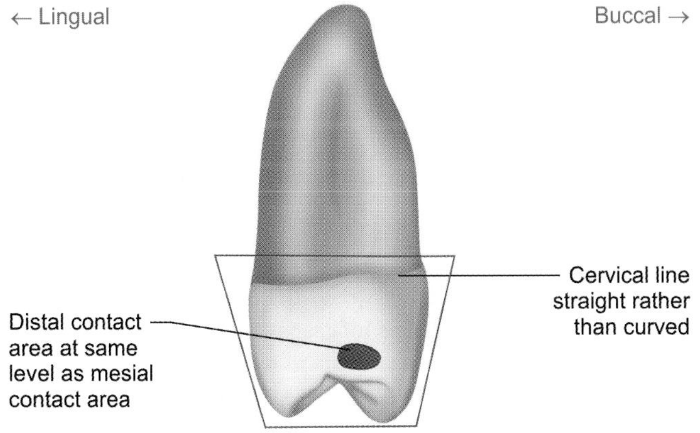
← Lingual
Buccal →
Cervical line straight rather than curved
Distal contact area at same level as mesial contact area

**Fig. 12.18:** Maxillary second premolar—distal aspect.

***Grooves and pits:***

*Grooves:*

- The *central developmental groove* is shorter and irregular.
- *Multiple supplementary grooves* radiate from the central developmental groove giving a *wrinkled appearance* to the occlusal surface.

*Pits:* The *mesial and distal pits* are placed less apart as the central developmental groove is shorter.

***Marginal ridges and fossae:***

- Both mesial and distal marginal ridges are strong and well developed.
- Mesial and distal triangular fossae are shallow and harbor supplemental grooves.

## Root

Morphology of the root can be described under the following headings:

| | |
|---|---|
| *Number* | Single root with a single pulp canal. |
| *Size* | The root is of the same length or a little longer than maxillary first premolar root. |
| *Form* | • The root is narrow mesiodistally and broader buccolingually<br>• It tapers evenly from cervix to the apex when viewed from buccal and lingual aspects.<br>• When viewed from proximal aspects, the apical half of the root appears to taper buccally |
| *Developmental depressions* | • Developmental depression is deeper on distal surface of the root<br>• Whereas in maxillary first premolar the developmental depression is deeper on the mesial surface |
| *Curvature* | Apical third of the root may show a distal curvature |
| *Apex* | Relatively blunt. |

## Variations (Figs. 12.20A to C)

The tooth varies in its size; the crown of maxillary second premolar may be smaller or bigger than the maxillary first premolar. Root may be bifurcated at its apex having two canals and two apical foramina.

## Developmental Anomalies

- Parapremolars
- Dens evaginatus.

## Clinical Considerations

Maxillary and mandibular second premolars are sometimes therapeutically extracted during orthodontic treatment and malocclusions.

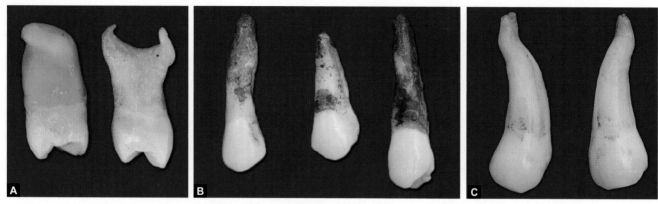

**Figs. 12.20A to C:** Maxillary second premolar—variations.

Anatomy of maxillary second premolar is summarized in **Flowcharts 12.3 and 12.4**.

**Box 12.2** shows identification features of the tooth.

The differences between maxillary first and second premolars (type traits) are given in **Table 12.3**.

**Flowchart 12.3:** Maxillary second premolar—major anatomic landmarks.

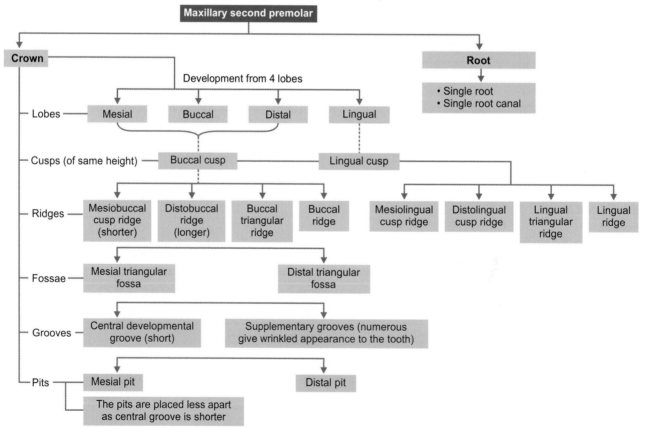

**Flowchart 12.4:** Maxillary second premolar—summary.

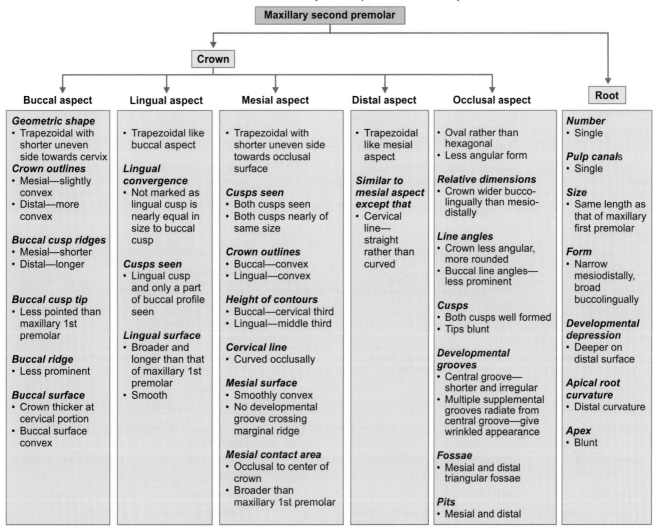

- *Identification features of maxillary second premolar*:
    - Both the cusps are of almost equal size
    - Tooth has a single root and single pulp canal
    - The crown is less angular and more rounded from occlusal view
    - There are no developmental grooves crossing the marginal ridges
    - Central developmental groove is shorter and occlusal surface has a wrinkled appearance because of multiple supplementary grooves
- *Side identifications*:
    - Distal slope or cusp ridge of buccal cusp is longer than that of mesial
    - Root may show distal curvature at its apical third
    - Developmental depression deeper on distal surface of root

**Table 12.3:** Differences between maxillary first and second premolars (maxillary premolar type traits).

| Characteristics | Maxillary first permanent premolar | Maxillary second permanent premolar |
|---|---|---|
| ***Tooth nomenclature*** | | |
| Universal system | Right 5, Left 12 | Right 4; Left 13 |
| Zsigmondy/Palmer system | Right 4⌋; Left ⌊4 | Right 5⌋; Left ⌊5 |
| FDI system | Right 14; Left 24 | Right 15; Left 25 |
| ***Chronology*** | | |
| Eruption | 10–11 years | 10–12 years |
| Lobes | From 4 lobes | Also from 4 lobes |
| General tooth size and form | No much variation in tooth size. More angular and lingual cusp is shorter | Crown may be smaller or bigger than the first premolar. Root may be slightly longer. Crown is less angular. Both the cusps are of almost same size |
| ***Crown*** | | |
| *Buccal aspect:* | | |
| Crown width | Crown is narrow at cervix | Crown appears thicker at cervical portion |
| Crown height | Larger and longer | Smaller and shorter crown |
| Cusp tip | More pointed with sharp angle between cusp slopes (105°) | Less pointed, blunt. Cusp angle (125°) |
| Slopes or ridges of buccal cusp | Mesial slope is longer than the distal | Distal slope is longer |
| Buccal line angles | Crown is more angular. Buccal line angles are sharp | Crown is more rounded and less angular |
| Buccal surface | More convex | Less convex |
| *Lingual aspect:* | | |
| Lingual cusp | It is shorter and narrower than the buccal cusp | Lingual cusp is of the same length and width as buccal cusp |
| Crown length | The crown appears shorter from lingual aspect | Crown appears comparatively longer from lingual aspect |
| Lingual surface | Less convex | More convex |
| Lingual convergence | Marked lingual convergence present. Crown tapers more toward lingual aspect because of smaller lingual cusp | Crown does not tapers much lingually |
| *Proximal aspects:* | | |
| Cusps height | Lingual cusp is shorter by 1–2 mm | The two cusps are same height |
| Intercuspal width | Distances between buccal and lingual cusp tip is less | Distances between the two cusp tips is more |
| Cusp tips | More sharp | More blunt |
| *Height of contour:* | | |
| • Buccal | At cervical third | At cervical third |
| • Lingual | At middle third | At middle third |
| Developmental depression | Marked concavity present in the center of mesial surface called *"mesial developmental depression"*. This mesial concavity extends onto root trunk | No developmental depression, mesial surface is smoothly convex |
| Developmental grooves | *Mesial marginal developmental grooves* extending from central groove of occlusal surface crosses the mesial marginal ridge to reach the mesial surface of crown | No developmental groove crossing the mesial marginal ridge |

*Contd...*

*Contd...*

| Characteristics | Maxillary first permanent premolar | Maxillary second permanent premolar |
|---|---|---|
| Contact areas | Contact area is narrower on mesial surface rather than on the distal surface as the tooth contacts with maxillary canine mesially | Both the contact areas are broader. As it is in contact with posterior teeth on both sides |
| Cervical line | Less curved | Less curved |
| Distal contact area | Broader than mesial | Both contacts are broader |
| *Occlusal aspect:* | | |
| General shape | Hexagonal outline | Oval outline |
| Line angles | Crown is angular with well-defined buccal line angles | Crown appears more rounded with less pronounced buccal line angles |
| Occlusal table | The occlusal table is smaller buccolingually because of a lesser distance between the cusp tips | Wider occlusal table because a greater distance between the cusp tips |
| Location of cusp tips | Lingual cusp tip positioned off center to the mesial | Both cusp tips centered mesiodistally |
| Crown width (mesiodistal) | Crown is wider buccally than lingually because of a smaller lingual cusp | Crown is equally wide both buccally and lingually |
| Crown width buccolingual | Wider distally than mesially. Crown appears to curve mesially due to mesial marginal developmental groove | Equally wide, mesially and distally |
| Marginal ridges | Mesial marginal ridge is shorter | Both marginal ridges equal length |
| Central developmental groove | Longer | Shorter |
| Supplementary grooves | Very few supplementary grooves. Occlusal surface is more regular | Multiple supplementary grooves radiate from central distal groove giving the occlusal surface a *"wrinkled appearance"* |
| **Root** | | |
| Number | Two roots: Buccal and lingual. Sometimes single | One root |
| Size | Comparatively shorter. Both buccal and lingual roots are of same length | Root is often slightly longer than the maxillary first premolar |
| Root form | Long root trunk with bifurcation at middle third of the root. The two roots diverge from bifurcation point and later face each other at apical ends | Conical root tapers evenly from cervix to apex |
| Developmental grooves and depressions | More deeper on mesial surface | More deeper on distal side |
| Variations | Root form is variable. The root is frequently bifurcated but can be single or laminated (fused bifurcated roots) | Root formed is less variable |
| Root canals | Two canals | One canal |

(FDI: Federation Dentaire Internationale)

## BIBLIOGRAPHY

1. Kartal N, Ozçelik B, Cimilli H. Root canal morphology of maxillary premolars. J Endod. 1998;24(6):417-9.
2. Pécora JD, Saquy PC, Sousa Neto MD, et al. Root form and canal anatomy of maxillary 1st premolars. Braz Dent J. 1992;2(2):87-94.
3. Peck L, Peck S, Attia Y. Maxillary canine first premolar transposition, associated dental anomalies and genetic basis. Angle Orthod. 1993;63:99-109.

## MULTIPLE CHOICE QUESTIONS

1. Which of the following statements is false regarding the maxillary premolars?
   a. There are eight premolars, four in each arch and two in each quadrant
   b. There are no premolars in deciduous dentition and they succeed deciduous molars
   c. Premolars along with molars occupy posterior segment of dental arches and are collectively referred to as posterior teeth

d. Premolars are often also called as tricuspids

2. Which of the following premolars has only one functional cusp?
   a. Mandibular first premolar
   b. Mandibular second premolar
   c. Maxillary first premolar
   d. Maxillary secind premolar

3. Which of the following premolar can have three cusps?
   a. Mandibular first premolar
   b. Mandibular second premolar
   c. Maxillary first premolar
   d. Maxillary second premolar

4. Generally, premolars develop from four lobes, except:
   a. Mandibular first premolar
   b. Mandibular second premolar
   c. Maxillary first premolar
   d. Maxillary second premolar

5. Which of the following teeth shows wrinkled occlusal surface?
   a. Maxillary 2nd premolar
   b. Mandibular 2nd premolar
   c. Maxillary 1st premolar
   d. Mandibular 1st premolar

6. Which of the following premolars generally has two roots?
   a. Mandibular first premolar
   b. Mandibular second premolar
   c. Maxillary first premolar
   d. Maxillary second premolar

7. Which of the following premolars has a single root?
   a. Mandibular first premolar
   b. Mandibular second premolar
   c. Maxillary second premolar
   d. All of the above

8. The following are the functions of premolars, except:
   a. They grind the food along with molar
   b. They provide support to check near corner of mouth
   c. They reinforce esthetics during smiling
   d. None of the above

9. Which of the following statements is false regarding maxillary first premolar?
   a. The maxillary first premolar has two cusps and frequently has one root with one pulp canal
   b. The maxillary first premolar has two cusps and two roots; buccal and lingual
   c. Sometimes they can have a single root with two pulp chamber
   d. The crown is angular with prominent buccal line angle

10. In maxillary first premolar:
    a. The buccal cusp is longer than the lingual cusp by 1–2 mm
    b. The lingual cusp is longer than the buccal cusp
    c. Both the cusps are equal sized
    d. Either (a) or (b)

**Answers**

1. d    2. a    3. b    4. b    5. a    6. c    7. d    8. d
9. a    10. a

# The Permanent Mandibular Premolars

## INTRODUCTION

The mandibular premolars differ from each other in their development and form. Among mandibular premolars, the first premolar is always smaller, developing from four lobes; whereas the second premolar is larger, developing from five lobes **(Fig. 13.1)**. The crowns of both the teeth are inclined lingually on their root bases. They have single root.

## MANDIBULAR FIRST PREMOLAR

The mandibular first premolar develops from four lobes: Mesial, distal, buccal, and lingual; and has two cusps: buccal and lingual. The buccal cusp is well developed and is the only functional cusp occluding with the maxillary teeth. The lingual cusp is very small and nonfunctional. The chronology and measurements of the mandibular first premolar are given in **Table 13.1**.

The mandibular first premolar shows resemblance to both of its neighboring teeth; the mandibular canine and second premolar.

The features that resemble those of the mandibular canine are:
- Viewed buccally, the buccal cusp is long and sharp. It is the only functional cusp.
- From the proximal view, the buccolingual measurement is similar to that of the canine.
- The occlusal table slopes lingually because of very small lingual cusp.
- Viewed occlusally, the occlusal outline of the crown resembles the incisal outline form of the mandibular canine.

The characteristics that resemble those of the second mandibular premolar are:
- The tooth has two cusps like the second premolar.

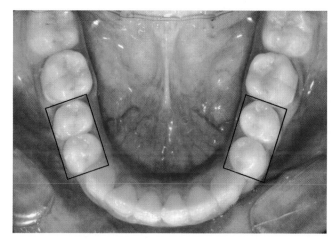

**Fig. 13.1:** Among mandibular premolars, first premolar is smaller than the second premolar.

**Table 13.1:** Mandibular first premolar—chronology and dimensions.

| Chronology | |
|---|---|
| First evidence of calcification | 1¾–2 years |
| Enamel completed | 5–6 years |
| Eruption | 10–12 years |
| Roots completed | 12–13 years |
| **Measurements** *Dimensions suggested for carving technique (in mm)* | |
| Cervico-occlusal length of crown | 8.5 |
| Length of root | 14.0 |
| Mesiodistal diameter of crown | 7.0 |
| Mesiodistal diameter of crown at cervix | 5.0 |
| Buccolingual diameter of crown | 7.5 |
| Buccolingual diameter of crown at cervix | 6.5 |
| Curvature of cervical line—mesial | 1.0 |
| Curvature of cervical line—distal | 0.0 |

- Viewed buccally, the crown and root form resemble that of the second premolar.
- Both the contact areas on mesial and distal surfaces are the same level. This feature is common to all posteriors.
- The curvature of cervical line mesially and distally is similar.

## DETAILED DESCRIPTION OF MANDIBULAR FIRST PREMOLAR FROM ALL ASPECTS (FIGS. 13.2 TO 13.4)

### Crown

#### Buccal Aspect (Fig. 13.5)

***Geometric shape:*** Crown is *trapezoidal* from buccal aspect and appears bilaterally symmetrical.

***Crown outlines:***

*Mesial outline:*
- Mesial outline is convex except near the cervical line where it is slightly concave.
- Height of contour (representing the *mesial contact area)* is just occlusal to the center of the crown cervico-occlusally.

*Distal outline:*
- It is concave near the cervix and becomes convex as it joins the occlusal outline.
- The *distal contact area* is broader and is at the same level as the mesial contact area.

*Occlusal outline:*
- The buccal cusp tip is sharp and the mesiobuccal and distobuccal cusp ridges are slightly concave on unworn premolar.
- Distal cusp ridge is longer than the mesial cusp ridge.

*Cervical outline:*
- The cervical line on buccal surface is curved apically.

***Buccal surface within the outlines:***
- The crown appears broader with a narrow cervix.
- The middle buccal lobe is well developed into a long buccal cusp and prominent buccal ridge.
- The buccal cusp tip is pointed and is placed slightly mesial to the center of the crown.
- The buccal surface is smooth and convex.

#### Lingual Aspect (Fig. 13.6)

***Geometric shape:*** *Trapezoidal* like that of buccal aspect.

***Crown outlines:***

*Mesial outline*
*Distal outline* } are similar to buccal aspect
*Cervical outline*

*Occlusal outline:*
- Occlusal boundary of lingual surface is formed by the cusp tip and cusp ridges of the lingual cusp.
- The occlusal outline is notched by a groove passing between mesial marginal ridge and mesiolingual cusp ridge.
- Because of a much shorter lingual cusp, buccal cusp tip and cusp ridges are visible from lingual aspect.

***Lingual surface within the outlines:***
- There is marked lingual convergence of the crown resulting in a much narrower lingual surface.
- Consequently, most of the mesial and distal surfaces can be seen from lingual aspect.

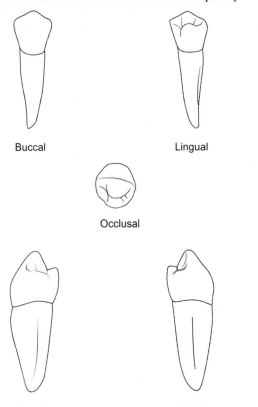

Buccal    Lingual

Occlusal

Mesial    Distal

**Fig. 13.2:** Mandibular first premolar—line drawings.

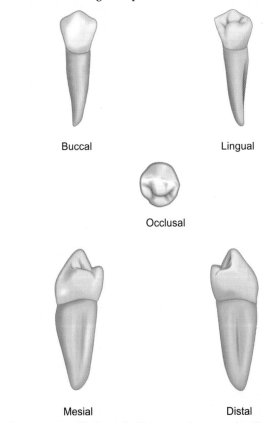

Buccal    Lingual

Occlusal

Mesial    Distal

**Fig. 13.3:** Mandibular right first premolar—graphic illustrations.

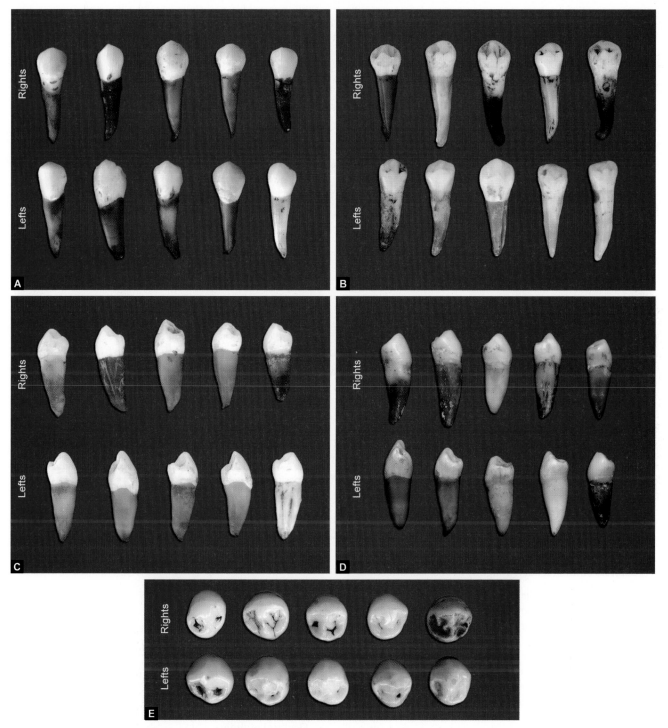

**Figs. 13.4A to E:** Mandibular first premolar—typical tooth specimen from all aspects: (A) Buccal aspect; (B) Lingual aspect; (C) Mesial aspect; (D) Distal aspect; (E) Occlusal aspect.

- Thus, most of the occlusal surface is visible because of shorter lingual cusp.
- The lingual cusp tip is pointed and is in line with the buccal triangular ridge which is clearly seen from this aspect.

- The characteristic feature of mandibular first premolar is the *mesiolingual developmental groove* extending from mesial developmental groove of occlusal surface onto the lingual surface mesially.

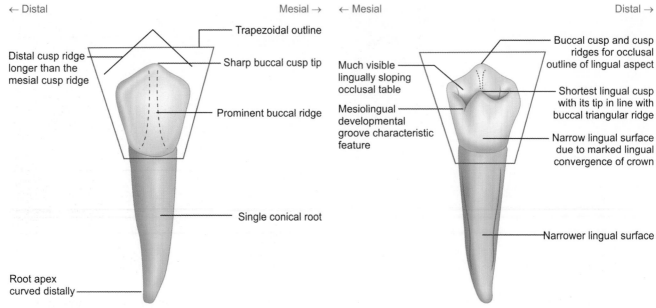

**Fig. 13.5:** Mandibular first premolar—buccal aspect.

**Fig. 13.6:** Mandibular first premolar—lingual aspect.

### Mesial Aspect (Fig. 13.7)

***Geometric shape:*** Crown appears *rhomboidal* which is true for proximal aspect of all mandibular posterior teeth.

***Crown outlines:***
- Buccal outline: It is markedly convex from cervix to buccal cusp tip. Height of buccal contour is at the cervical third of the crown.
- Lingual outline: It is convex stretching out of the confines of the root base and thus, creating an overhang above the root trunk lingually. Its height of contour is at the middle third of crown, near to lingual cusp tip.
- Occlusal outline: It is a concave arc sloping lingually.
- Cervical outline: It curves slightly in occlusal direction.

***Mesial surface within the outlines:***
- Mesial surface is smoothly convex except for the mesiolingual developmental groove and a concavity just above the cervical line. The buccal cusp tip is centered over the root base. In other words, it is in line with the vertical root axis.
- Lingual cusp tip is in line with lingual outline of root.
- The mesial marginal ridge slopes prominently in a lingual direction.
- Some part of occlusal surface with buccal and lingual triangular ridges can be seen from mesial aspect.
- *Mesial contact area*: It is occlusal to the center of crown, and is in line with the buccal cusp tip.

### Distal Aspect (Fig. 13.8)

***Geometric shape:*** Rhomboidal

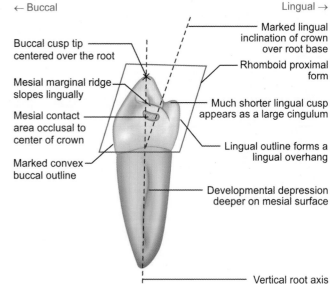

**Fig. 13.7:** Mandibular first premolar—mesial aspect.

***Crown outlines:***
- Buccal outline
- Lingual outline      } are similar to mesial aspect
- Occlusal outline
- Cervical outline: The cervical line on the distal surface is nearly a straight line.

***Distal surface within the outlines:***
- Distal marginal ridge is at a higher level than mesial marginal ridge from the cervix and is perpendicular to the long axis of tooth rather than sloping lingually.

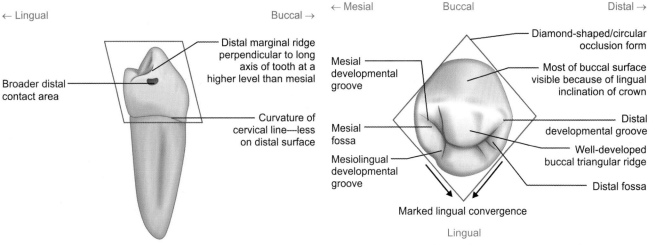

**Fig. 13.8:** Mandibular first premolar—distal aspect.

**Fig. 13.9:** Mandibular first premolar—occlusal aspect.

- The distal surface is smooth except for a small linear concavity just above the cervical line.
- The *distal contact area* is at the same level but broader than the mesial contact area.

### Occlusal Aspect (Fig. 13.9)

*Geometric shape:* Diamond-shaped or circular

*Relative dimensions:* Buccolingual dimension is only 0.5 mm greater than mesiodistal dimension, thus the crown appears circular rather than oval. Because of lingual inclination of the crown, most of the buccal surface and very little of lingual surface can be seen from occlusal aspect.

*Cusp and cusp ridges:*
- Buccal cusp is large making the major bulk of the crown and the lingual cusp is much smaller. The crown converges sharply toward lingual surface.
- Mesiobuccal and distobuccal cusp ridges are stronger than the mesiolingual and distolingual cusp ridges.
- Buccal triangular ridge is well developed whereas the lingual triangular ridge is less defined.
- There are inclined planes on either side of triangular ridges.

*Fossae:*
- Mandibular first premolar has two fossae: *(i) mesial (ii) distal fossa.*
- The fossae near marginal ridges are irregular rather than triangular and thus named as *mesial* and *distal fossae.*

*Grooves and pits:*
*Grooves:* There are three types—
1. Mesial developmental groove: It is located in the mesial fossa; is short and extends buccolingually.

2. Distal developmental groove: It is in the distal fossa and is longer.
3. Mesiolingual developmental groove: It is continuous from mesial groove and it extends between mesial marginal ridge and mesiolingual cusp ridge onto the lingual surface mesially. This groove is the *characteristic feature of mandibular first premolar.*

*Pit:* The distal fossa may have a pit in its center.

*Marginal ridges:*
- *Mesial marginal ridge* is shorter and is constricted because of mesiolingual developmental groove. It slopes sharply lingually in a cervical direction.
- *Distal marginal ridge* is confluent with the distolingual cusp ridge.

### Root

Morphology of the root can be described under the following headings:

| | |
|---|---|
| *Number:* | Single root |
| *Size:* | Slightly shorter than the mandibular second premolar root and 3–4 mm shorter than that of mandibular canine |
| *Form:* | • Conical in shape, tapering evenly from cervix to apex |
| | • The root is wider buccolingually than mesiodistally |
| | • Buccal and lingual surfaces are convex and proximal surfaces are flat |
| | • The root tapers acutely toward lingual surface |
| | • Lingual convergence of the root is exaggerated |

| *Developmental groove and depression* | • A deep developmental groove is often present on the mesial surface of root running longitudinally<br>• Developmental depression on the mesial surface of the root is deeper than on the distal surface |
|---|---|
| *Curvature* | Apical third of the root is often curved distally |
| *Apex* | Pointed |

### Variations (Fig. 13.10)

- Bifurcation of the root into buccal and lingual divisions is a fairly common variation.
- Long root.

### Developmental Anomalies

- Supernumerary tooth in the premolar region **(Fig. 13.11)**
- Dens evaginatus or Leong's premolar.

### Clinical Considerations

- A possibility of bifurcated roots must be considered during root canal therapy.
- Lingual inclination of the crown should be kept in mind during crown preparation and access cavity opening.

Identification of mandibular first premolar is given in **Box 13.1**.

The tooth's morphology is summarized in **Flowcharts 13.1 and 13.2**.

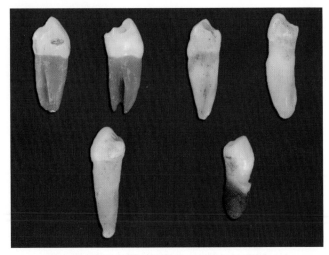

**Fig. 13.10:** Mandibular first premolar—variations.

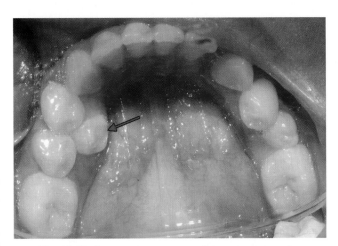

**Fig. 13.11:** Supernumerary premolars or parapremolar.

---

### MANDIBULAR SECOND PREMOLAR

The mandibular second premolar is larger than the mandibular first premolar and it resembles the latter only from buccal aspect. It has a broad occlusal table and assists mandibular molars in grinding the food. The crown shows wide variation in occlusal anatomy. It has a single root that resembles the root of mandibular first premolar in form although it is longer. Mandibular second premolar is the only premolar developing from five lobes: three buccal (mesial, buccal, distal lobes) and two lingual lobes (mesiolingual and distolingual lobes). **Table 13.2** shows the chronology and measurements of mandibular second premolar.

There are two common forms of mandibular second premolar **(Figs. 13.12A to C)**.
1. Three cusp form ("Y" groove pattern)—frequently seen
2. Two cusp form ("U" and "H" groove pattern).

### DETAILED DESCRIPTION OF MANDIBULAR SECOND PREMOLAR FROM ALL ASPECTS (FIGS. 13.13 TO 13.15)

### Crown

*Buccal Aspect (Fig. 13.16)*

**Geometric shape:** Trapezoidal

> **Box 13.1: Mandibular first premolar—identification features.**
>
> - *Identification features of mandibular first premolar:*
>   - Large pointed buccal cusp and a very small lingual cusp
>   - Marked lingual inclination of crown on its root base as observed from proximal view
>   - The buccal cusp tip is centered over the root trunk as seen from proximal view
>   - *Mesiolingual developmental groove* between mesial marginal ridge and mesiolingual cusp ridge, crossing onto the mesial portion of lingual surface is the characteristic feature of the tooth
>   - It has a single root
> - *Side identification:*
>   - Mesiolingual developmental groove is located on the lingual surface toward mesial portion of the crown
>   - Developmental groove is deeper on the mesial surface of the root

**Flowchart 13.1:** Mandibular first premolar—major anatomic landmarks.

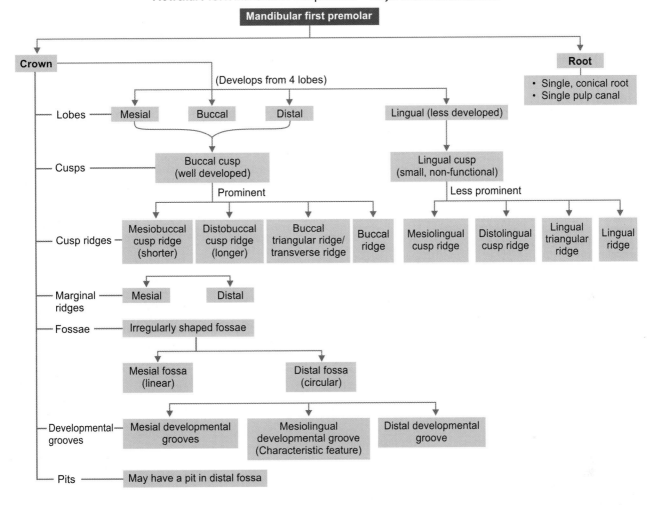

**Table 13.2:** Mandibular second premolars—chronology and measurements.

| Chronology | |
|---|---|
| First evidence of calcification | 2¼–2½ years |
| Enamel completed | 6–7 years |
| Eruption | 11–12 years |
| Roots completed | 13–14 years |
| **Measurements** *Dimensions suggested for carving technique (in mm)* | |
| Cervico-occlusal length of crown | 8.0 |
| Length of root | 14.5 |
| Mesiodistal diameter of crown | 7.0 |
| Mesiodistal diameter of crown at cervix | 5.0 |
| Buccolingual diameter of crown | 8.0 |
| Buccolingual diameter of crown at cervix | 7.0 |
| Curvature of cervical line—mesial | 1.0 |
| Curvature of cervical line—distal | 0.0 |

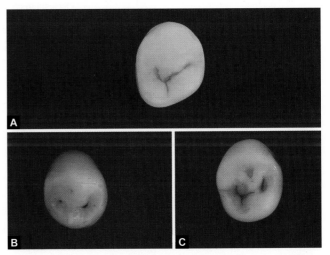

**Figs. 13.12A to C:** Mandibular second premolars have diverse occlusal anatomy: (A) With three cusps ("Y" groove pattern); (B) With two cusps ("U" groove pattern); (C) With two cusps ("H" groove pattern).

**Flowchart 13.2:** Mandibular first premolar—summary.

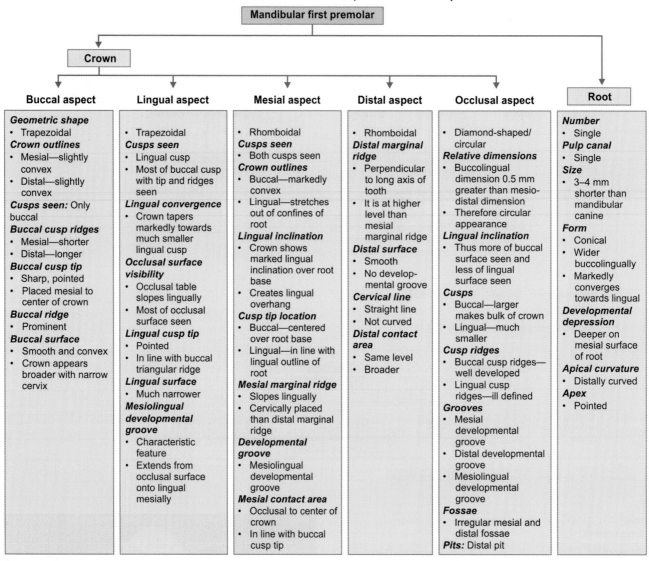

| Buccal aspect | Lingual aspect | Mesial aspect | Distal aspect | Occlusal aspect | Root |
|---|---|---|---|---|---|
| **Geometric shape**<br>• Trapezoidal<br>**Crown outlines**<br>• Mesial—slightly convex<br>• Distal—slightly convex<br>**Cusps seen:** Only buccal<br>**Buccal cusp ridges**<br>• Mesial—shorter<br>• Distal—longer<br>**Buccal cusp tip**<br>• Sharp, pointed<br>• Placed mesial to center of crown<br>**Buccal ridge**<br>• Prominent<br>**Buccal surface**<br>• Smooth and convex<br>• Crown appears broader with narrow cervix | • Trapezoidal<br>**Cusps seen**<br>• Lingual cusp<br>• Most of buccal cusp with tip and ridges seen<br>**Lingual convergence**<br>• Crown tapers markedly towards much smaller lingual cusp<br>**Occlusal surface visibility**<br>• Occlusal table slopes lingually<br>• Most of occlusal surface seen<br>**Lingual cusp tip**<br>• Pointed<br>• In line with buccal triangular ridge<br>**Lingual surface**<br>• Much narrower<br>**Mesiolingual developmental groove**<br>• Characteristic feature<br>• Extends from occlusal surface onto lingual mesially | • Rhomboidal<br>**Cusps seen**<br>• Both cusps seen<br>**Crown outlines**<br>• Buccal—markedly convex<br>• Lingual—stretches out of confines of root<br>**Lingual inclination**<br>• Crown shows marked lingual inclination over root base<br>• Creates lingual overhang<br>**Cusp tip location**<br>• Buccal—centered over root base<br>• Lingual—in line with lingual outline of root<br>**Mesial marginal ridge**<br>• Slopes lingually<br>• Cervically placed than distal marginal ridge<br>**Developmental groove**<br>• Mesiolingual developmental groove<br>**Mesial contact area**<br>• Occlusal to center of crown<br>• In line with buccal cusp tip | • Rhomboidal<br>**Distal marginal ridge**<br>• Perpendicular to long axis of tooth<br>• It is at higher level than mesial marginal ridge<br>**Distal surface**<br>• Smooth<br>• No developmental groove<br>**Cervical line**<br>• Straight line<br>• Not curved<br>**Distal contact area**<br>• Same level<br>• Broader | • Diamond-shaped/circular<br>**Relative dimensions**<br>• Buccolingual dimension 0.5 mm greater than mesio-distal dimension<br>• Therefore circular appearance<br>**Lingual inclination**<br>• Thus more of buccal surface seen and less of lingual surface seen<br>**Cusps**<br>• Buccal—larger makes bulk of crown<br>• Lingual—much smaller<br>**Cusp ridges**<br>• Buccal cusp ridges—well developed<br>• Lingual cusp ridges—ill defined<br>**Grooves**<br>• Mesial developmental groove<br>• Distal developmental groove<br>• Mesiolingual developmental groove<br>**Fossae**<br>• Irregular mesial and distal fossae<br>**Pits:** Distal pit | **Number**<br>• Single<br>**Pulp canal**<br>• Single<br>**Size**<br>• 3–4 mm shorter than mandibular canine<br>**Form**<br>• Conical<br>• Wider buccolingually<br>• Markedly converges towards lingual<br>**Developmental depression**<br>• Deeper on mesial surface of root<br>**Apical curvature**<br>• Distally curved<br>**Apex**<br>• Pointed |

***Crown outlines:***

*Mesial outline:*
- It is convex for a short distance near the cervical line.
- Its height of contour *(mesial contact area)* is at the middle third of the crown.

*Distal outline:*
- It is more convex.
- Its height of contour *(distal contact area)* is also at the middle third.

*Occlusal outline:* Buccal cusp tip is blunt with the mesial and distal buccal cusp ridges meeting at a more obtuse angle.

*Cervical outline:* It is slightly curved apically.

***Buccal surface within the outlines:***
- The crown appears short and bulky from buccal aspect. The buccal surface is smooth and convex.

- The buccal ridge extending from cervical line to the buccal cusp tip is very prominent.

### Lingual Aspect (Fig. 13.17)

***Geometric shape:*** Trapezoidal like the buccal aspect.

***Crown outlines:***

*Mesial outline*
*Distal outline* } are similar to buccal aspect
*Cervical outline*

*Occlusal outline:*
- Occlusal outline is formed by the lingual cusp tip and cusp ridges of lingual cusp or cusps (depending on cusp type).
- A part of buccal cusp is seen since the lingual cusp is not as long as the buccal cusp.

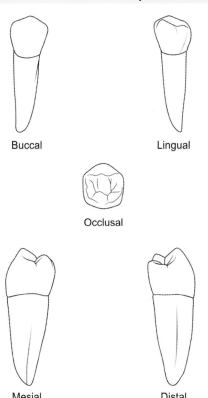

Buccal    Lingual

Occlusal

Mesial    Distal

**Fig. 13.13:** Mandibular right second premolar—line drawings.

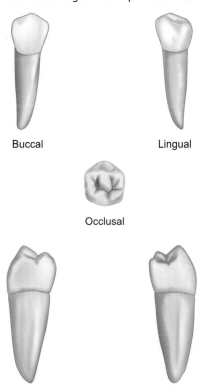

Buccal    Lingual

Occlusal

Mesial    Distal

**Fig. 13.14:** Mandibular right second premolar—graphic illustrations.

*Lingual surface within the outlines:*
- The crown appears bulky from lingual aspect too.
- The crown does not taper much lingually and thus, very little of proximal surfaces can be seen. In the three cusps type, there are two lingual cusps: *mesiolingual* and *distolingual.*
- The lingual cusp or cusps are well developed and are of nearly the same length as that of buccal cusp. A part of occlusal surface may be seen from lingual aspect.
- The lingual surface is smooth and spheroidal.

## Mesial Aspect (Fig. 13.18)

***Geometric shape:*** It is *rhomboidal* similar to proximal aspect of all mandibular posteriors.

***Crown outlines:***

*Buccal outline:* It is convex and the height of contour is at the middle third of crown.

*Lingual outline:*
- It is less convex and its height of contour is at the occlusal third of the crown.
- The lingual outline is out of confines of the root base.

*Occlusal outline:*
- It is concave.
- The mesial marginal ridge is at right angle to the long axis of the tooth.

*Cervical outline:* This outline curves occlusally.

***Mesial surface within the outlines:***
- The crown is lingually inclined on its root base but not to the extent of mandibular first premolar.
- The buccal cusp tip is blunt and is buccal to the vertical root axis.
- The lingual cusp tip is in line with lingual outline of the root.
- The mesial surface is smoothly convex and devoid of any developmental groove.
- *Mesial contact area*: It is at the middle third of the crown and centered buccolingually.

## Distal Aspect (Fig. 13.19)

***Geometric shape:*** Rhomboidal

***Crown outlines:***
- Buccal outline
- Lingual outline    } are similar to mesial aspect
- Cervical outline
- Occlusal outline: The distal marginal ridge is also at right angle to the long axis but is at a lower level than the mesial marginal ridge.

***Distal surface within the outlines:***
- Distal surface is also smoothly convex.
- More of occlusal surface can be seen than from mesial aspect, as distal marginal ridge is at a lower level. Distal contact area is at the same level as the mesial contact area, but is broader.

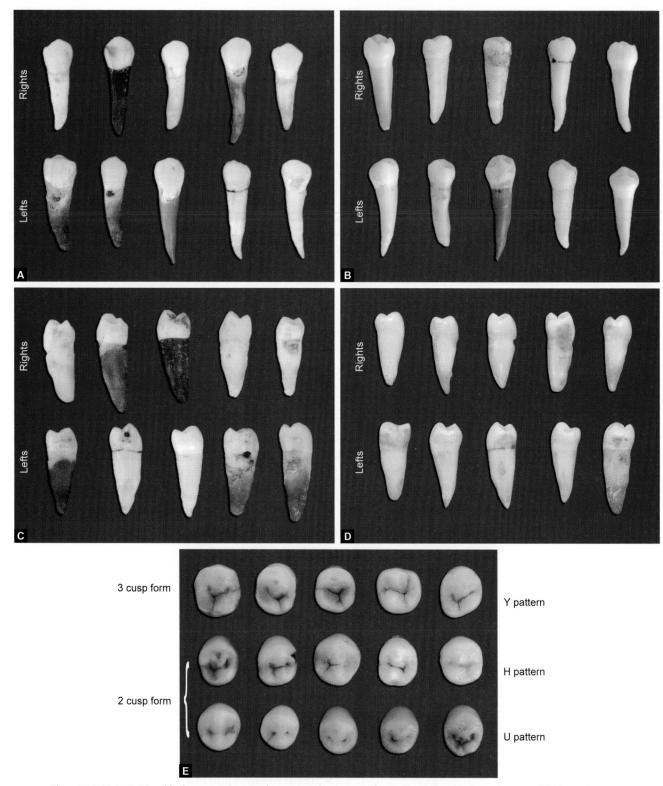

**Figs. 13.15A to E:** Mandibular second premolar—typical specimen from all aspects: (A) Buccal aspect; (B) Lingual aspect; (C) Mesial aspect; (D) Distal aspect; (E) Occlusal aspect.

← Distal                                        Mesial →

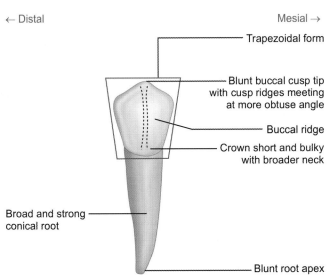

Trapezoidal form

Blunt buccal cusp tip
with cusp ridges meeting
at more obtuse angle

Buccal ridge

Crown short and bulky
with broader neck

Broad and strong
conical root

Blunt root apex

**Fig. 13.16:** Mandibular second premolar—buccal aspect.

← Buccal                                        Lingual →

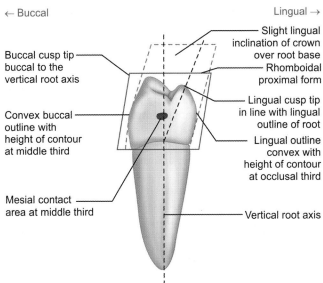

Buccal cusp tip
buccal to the
vertical root axis

Convex buccal
outline with
height of contour
at middle third

Mesial contact
area at middle third

Slight lingual
inclination of crown
over root base

Rhomboidal
proximal form

Lingual cusp tip
in line with lingual
outline of root

Lingual outline
convex with
height of contour
at occlusal third

Vertical root axis

**Fig. 13.18:** Mandibular second premolar—mesial aspect.

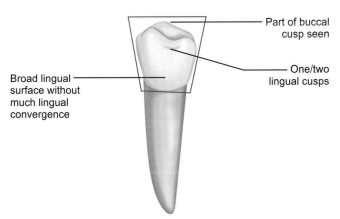

Part of buccal
cusp seen

One/two
lingual cusps

Broad lingual
surface without
much lingual
convergence

**Fig. 13.17:** Mandibular second premolar—lingual aspect.

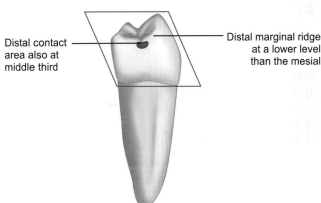

Distal contact
area also at
middle third

Distal marginal ridge
at a lower level
than the mesial

**Fig. 13.19:** Mandibular second premolar—distal aspect.

## Occlusal Aspect (Fig. 13.20)

Occlusal morphology varies in mandibular second premolar. There are two common forms:
1. Three cusps type with a "Y" groove pattern
2. Two cusps type with a "U" or "H" groove pattern.

### Three cusps type (more common):

*Geometric shape:* Square-shaped with nearly equal mesiodistal crown width buccally and lingually.

*Cusp and cusps ridges:* There are three cusps—
1. Buccal cusp is the largest one, followed by mesiolingual cusp and distolingual cusp in that order.
2. The lingual lobes are well developed.

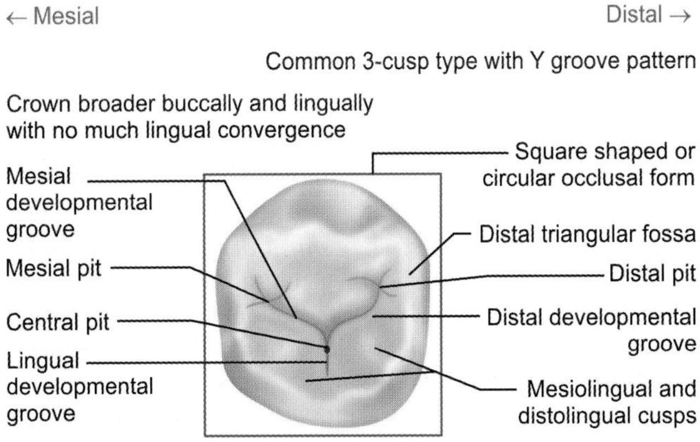

← Mesial                                        Distal →

Common 3-cusp type with Y groove pattern

Crown broader buccally and lingually
with no much lingual convergence

Mesial
developmental
groove

Mesial pit

Central pit

Lingual
developmental
groove

Square shaped or
circular occlusal form

Distal triangular fossa

Distal pit

Distal developmental
groove

Mesiolingual and
distolingual cusps

**Fig. 13.20:** Mandibular second premolar—occlusal aspect.

3. Each cusp has mesial and distal cusp ridges of its own, and a triangular ridge sloping from cusp tip toward the center of the occlusal surface.

### Grooves and pits:

*Grooves:* There are three developmental grooves converging at a central pit and thus, forming a *"Y"-shaped pattern.* Few supplementary grooves radiate from developmental grooves in the triangular fossa.

1. Mesial developmental groove: It is long and runs from the central pit mesiobuccally and ends in the mesial triangular fossa.
2. Distal developmental groove: It is a shorter groove running from the central pit to the distal triangular fossa.
3. Lingual developmental groove:
   – It runs in a lingual direction between two lingual cusps and ends on the lingual surface of the crown. It is usually centered over the root.
   – The mesiolingual cusp is wider than distolingual cusp; the lingual groove is placed slightly distal to the center of the crown.
   – In three cusp type, there is no central developmental groove.

*Pits:* There are three pits—
1. Central pit is located in the center of occlusal surface buccolingually and slightly distal to the center mesiodistally.
2. Mesial pit is in the mesial triangular fossa.
3. Distal pit is in the distal triangular fossa.

**Marginal ridges:** Both the marginal ridges are strongly developed. Sometimes supplementary grooves can cross them.

### Fossae:
- There are two small triangular fossae—mesial and distal.
- Triangular fossae harbor mesial or distal developmental grooves, mesial or distal pits, and some supplemental grooves.

### Two cusps type:

*Geometric shape:* Circular in outline.

*Cusps and ridges:*
- The two cusps are *buccal* and *lingual.*
- Buccal cusp is larger and lingual cusp is also well developed though it is slightly smaller.
- The crown tapers slightly toward lingual aspect.
- The cusps have mesial and distal cusp ridges and occlusally converging triangular ridges.

*Grooves and pits grooves:* The *central developmental groove* extends mesiodistally across the occlusal surface and ends in mesial and distal fossae. It may be straight or crescent shaped and separates the triangular ridges of buccal and lingual cusps. There are two groove patterns:
1. "U" pattern: Where central groove is crescent shaped.
2. "H" pattern: Where central groove is straight connecting mesial and distal fossa.

*Pits:*
- There may be mesial and distal pits located in the mesial and distal fossae.
- In two cusps type, there is no central pit.

*Marginal ridges and fossae:*
- Mesial and distal marginal ridges are strongly developed.
- The fossae near marginal ridges are irregular rather than triangular and are called as *mesial* and *distal occlusal fossae.*

## Root

Morphology of the root can be described under the following headings:

| | |
|---|---|
| *Number:* | Single root almost never bifurcated |
| *Size:* | The root is broader, stronger, and longer than that of the mandibular first premolar |
| *Form* | • The root is conical tapering from cervix to apex |
| | • It is wider mesiodistally and does not taper much toward lingual aspect |
| | • Buccal surfaces are convex and proximal surfaces are flat |
| *Curvature:* | The root may be straight or its apical end may have a distal curvature |
| *Apex:* | Blunt |

### Variations (Fig. 13.21)
- Very long or very short root.
- A developmental groove may be seen on buccal surface of the root.

### Developmental Anomalies
- Dens evaginatus (Leong's premolar) **(Fig. 13.22)**
- Supernumerary premolars.

### Clinical Considerations

Whether it is of three cusp type or two cusp type has to be noted while restoring this tooth.

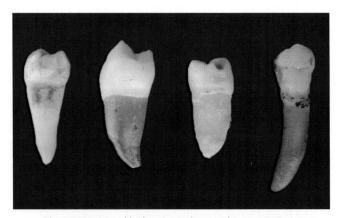

**Fig. 13.21:** Mandibular second premolar—variations.

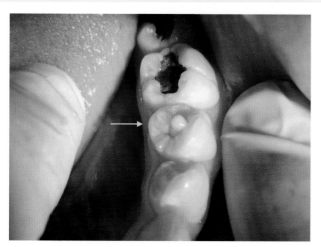

**Fig. 13.22:** Dens evaginatus (Leong's premolar).

The mandibular second premolar anatomy is summarized in **Flowcharts 13.3 and 13.4**. **Box 13.2** shows the identification features of this tooth.

**Box 13.2: Mandibular permanent second premolar—identification features.**

- *Identification features of mandibular second premolar:*
  – Lingual lobes are well developed into one or two lingual cusps
  – It is the only premolar with three cusps
  – The lingual cusps are almost at the same height as that of buccal cusps
  – Lingual inclination of crown on root base
  – The three cusps type has "Y"-shaped groove pattern on occlusal surface
  – On two cusp type, "U"- or "H"-shaped groove pattern is seen
  – Crown and root have very slight lingual convergence
  – Mesiolingual developmental groove is not present
  – Single root with less tendency for bifurcation
- *Side identification:*
  – Apical third of the root may show a distal curvature
  – In three cusp type, mesiolingual cusp is larger than the distolingual cusp

**Flowchart 13.3:** Mandibular second premolar—major anatomic landmarks.

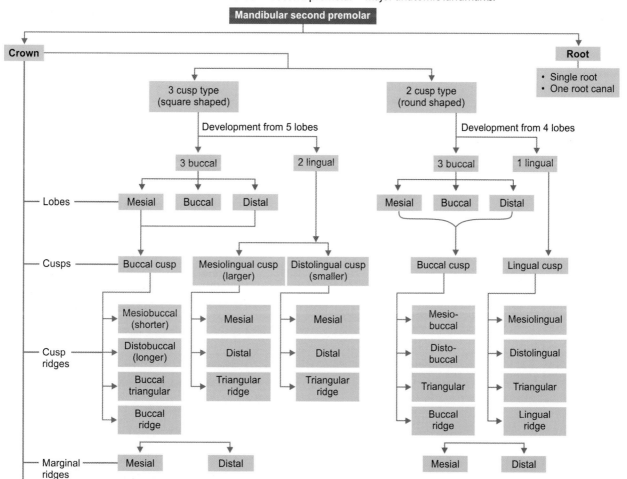

*Contd...*

*Contd...*

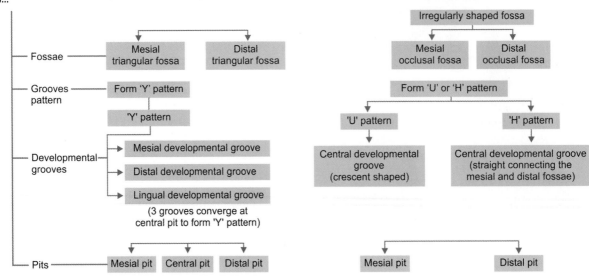

**Flowchart 13.4:** Mandibular second premolar—summary.

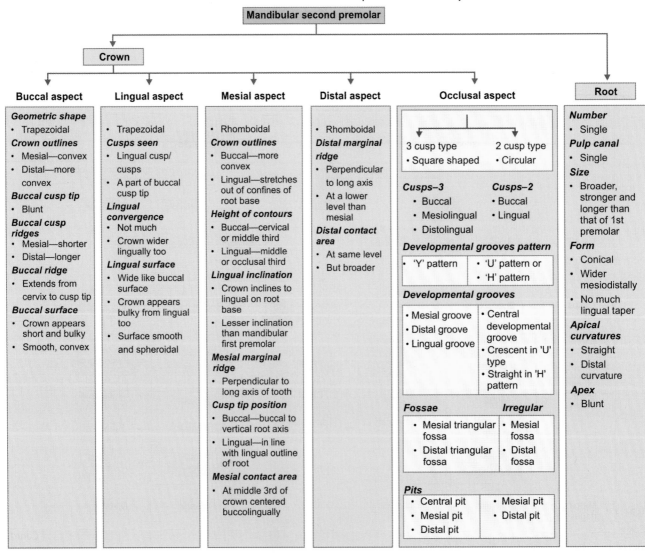

The Differences between maxillary and mandibular premolars (arch traits) are given in **Table 13.3** and Differences between mandibular first and second premolars (type traits) are given in **Table 13.4**.

**Table 13.3:** Differences between maxillary and mandibular premolars (arch traits).

| Characteristics | Maxillary permanent premolars | Mandibular permanent premolars |
|---|---|---|
| ***Tooth nomenclature*** | | |
| Universal system | Right 4, 5; left 12, 13 | Right 28, 29; left 20, 21 |
| Zsigmondy/Palmer system | Right 4⌋, 5⌋; Left ⌊4, ⌊5 | Right 4⌋, 5⌋; Left ⌊4, ⌊5 |
| FDI system | Right 14, 15; left 24, 25 | Right 44, 45; left 34, 35 |
| ***General features*** | | |
| Eruption sequence | Usually erupt before maxillary permanent canine | Erupt after mandibular permanent canine |
| Lobes | Develop from 4 lobes | 4 lobes—for first permanent premolar and 5 lobes—for second permanent premolars |
| Number of cusps | Two | Two—first premolar<br>3 common for second premolar, or two cusps |
| Number of roots | Two—first premolar<br>One—second premolar | Usually one |
| Sizes of cusps: | • Buccal and lingual cusps are almost equal in size and height<br>• Buccal and lingual cusps nearly equally well developed and of equal prominence | • Lingual cusps much shorter, especially in mandibular first premolar which is nonfunctional<br>• Buccal and lingual cusps of uneven development and prominence |
| Crown form | • First and second premolars are similar in form | • First and second premolars are widely different in form |
| ***Buccal aspect*** | | |
| Buccal cusp tip | Mesial and distal cusp ridges at the cusp tip meet at sharp angle | Cusp ridges meet at more obtuse angle |
| Buccal ridge | More prominent on maxillary premolars (especially on first premolar) | Less prominent on mandibular premolars |
| Buccal cusp slope or ridge | First premolar—mesial cusp slope is longer<br>Second premolar—distal cusp slope is longer | Distal cusp slope is longer in both premolars |
| ***Lingual aspect*** | | |
| Lingual convergence | Maxillary premolars show marked lingual convergence, especially the first premolars | Lingual convergence not present, especially in second premolar |
| ***Proximal aspects*** | | |
| Geometric form | Trapezoidal | Rhomboidal |
| Crown inclination | Crown nearly upright on root base | Crown shows marked lingual inclination on root base |
| Cusp height | Buccal and lingual cusps nearly of equal height | Lingual cusp much shorter and small in first premolar. It is nonfunctional cusp |
| Cusp tips spacing | Buccal and lingual cusp tips wide apart | Buccal and lingual cusps are more nearer |
| Buccal cusp tip location | Buccal cusp located buccal to the vertical root axis | Buccal cusp is centered over root base, because lingual tilt of crowns, the buccal cusp tip is in line with the vertical root axis |
| Lingual cusp tip | Located lingual to the root axis line | On or lingual to the lingual confines of root |
| Crown outlines | Buccal and lingual crown outlines well within confines of root base | Lingual crown outline out of confines of root base |
| ***Occlusal aspect*** | | |
| Crown dimension | Much wider buccolingually than mesiodistally | Buccolingual and mesiodistal dimensions nearly same |
| Geometric form | Ovoid or oblong | Round or squarish |
| Tapers to lingual | Marked in first premolars | Marked in first premolars |
| Cusps | Relatively wider buccolingually | Wider mesiodistally |

(FDI: Federation Dentaire Internationale)

**Table 13.4:** Differences between mandibular first and second premolars (mandibular premolar type traits).

| Characteristics | Mandibular first permanent premolar | Mandibular second permanent premolar |
|---|---|---|
| ***Tooth nomenclature*** | | |
| Universal system | Right 28, left 21 | Right 29; left 20 |
| Zsigmondy/Palmer system | Right 4⌋; Left ⌊4 | Right 5⌋; Left ⌊5 |
| FDI system | Right 44; left 34 | Right 45; left 35 |
| ***Chronology*** | | |
| Developmental lobes | 4 lobes, 3 labial, and 1 lingual lobe<br>Lingual lobe is not well developed | 5 lobes—frequently (3 labial and 2 lingual lobes) or 4 lobes<br>Lingual lobe is well developed |
| Eruption | 10–12 years | 11–12 years |
| Root completion | 12–13 years | 13–14 years |
| Variation in form | No much variation in form | Three cusp type or two cusp type |
| ***Crown*** | | |
| *Buccal aspect:* | | |
| Crown height | Longer crown | Shorter crown |
| Crown width | Narrow | Wider and bulky crown |
| Neck of the tooth | Narrow at cervix | Crown wider at cervix |
| Buccal ridge | More prominent | Less prominent |
| Contact area | Mesial contact area cervically located than distal | Distal contact area cervically located than the mesial |
| *Lingual aspect:* | | |
| Number of lingual cusps | 1 lingual cusp | 1 or 2 lingual cusps (mesiolingual cusp is wider than distolingual cusp) |
| Lingual cusp(s) | Very small, nonfunctional lingual cusp | Functional lingual cusp or cusps |
| Lingual cusp height | Very short | Nearly of same height as buccal cusp |
| Lingual convergence | Marked lingual convergence of crown due to small lingual cusp | Crown on lingual is as wide as buccal (very little lingual convergence) |
| Visibility of buccal profile and proximal surfaces | All of buccal profile<br>Proximal walls of crown are visible from lingual view | Only buccal cusp tip and part of proximal walls seen |
| Occlusal surface visibility | Most of occlusal surface visible along with buccal triangular ridge and marginal ridges | No much occlusal surface visible |
| Developmental grooves | *Mesiolingual developmental groove* extends from occlusal surface onto lingual surface mesially | No mesiolingual grove<br>A short lingual developmental groove separating two lingual cusps may be seen (In three cusp type) |
| Lingual surface | Narrow, notched by mesiolingual groove mesially | Broad and smooth spheroidal |
| *Proximal aspects:* | | |
| Similarity to canine | Appears similar to canine from proximal view | No similarity to canine |
| Lingual inclination of crown | Crown more lingually inclined on root base | Lingual tilt not so pronounced |
| Lingual cusp | Much shorter than buccal cusp | Lingual cusps are slightly shorter than buccal cusp |
| Occlusal plane | Tilted lingually due to very small lingual cusp | Horizontal, no lingual tilt |
| Lingual overhang on root | Lingual outline stretches out of confines of root. Creates overhang over root trunk | Lingual overhang of crown not so pronounced |
| *Marginal ridges:* | | |
| Length | Mesial marginal ridge is shorter than distal | Both marginal ridges of same size |
| Tilt | Marginal ridges lingually tilted | Marginal ridges are horizontal |

*Contd...*

*Contd...*

| Characteristics | Mandibular first permanent premolar | Mandibular second permanent premolar |
|---|---|---|
| Location | Mesial marginal ridge more cervically placed than distal (in general, distal marginal ridge is more cervically located in all teeth, mandibular first premolar is an exception) | Distal marginal ridge is more cervically placed than the mesial |
| Visibility of occlusal surface | More of occlusal surface is visible from mesial aspect | More of occlusal surface visible from distal aspect |
| *Cusp tip:* | | |
| Buccal cusp tip | In line with vertical root axis (centered over root base) | Buccal to the vertical root axis |
| Lingual cusp tip | In line with lingual outline of root | In line with or lingual to the lingual outline of root |
| Proximal surfaces | Mesial surface has mesiolingual groove | Smooth |
| Distal marginal ridge | At higher level than mesial ridge | At lower level than mesial ridge |
| Cervical line | Less curved | Less curved |
| *Occlusal aspect:* | | |
| Geometric form | Diamond-shaped | Square-shaped (three cusp type); circular (two cusp type) |
| Occlusal table | Small, nonfunctional occlusal surface | Large functional occlusal surface |
| Mesiodistal crown dimension | Greater buccally than lingually | Nearly equal buccally and lingually<br>Can be wider on lingually than buccally (three cusp type) |
| Visibility of buccal and lingual surfaces | Because of lingual crown tilt, most of buccal surface and very little lingual surface visible from occlusal view | Less of buccal and lingual surfaces are visible |
| Occlusal anatomy | Do not vary much | Varies according to 3 cusp type or 2 cusp type |
| Cusps | Large buccal and small nonfunctional lingual cusp | Buccal and 1 lingual or 2 lingual cusps (mesiolingual and distolingual) |
| Transverse ridge | Present | Not present |
| Occlusal groove pattern | No variability | Varies "Y" pattern—three cusp type "U" or "H" pattern—two cusp type |
| Developmental grooves | • Mesial developmental groove<br>• Distal developmental groove<br>• Mesiolingual developmental groove | In three cusp type:<br>1. Mesial developmental groove<br>2. Distal developmental groove<br>3. Lingual developmental groove<br>In two cusp type:<br>• Mesial developmental groove<br>• Distal developmental groove<br>• Central developmental groove |
| Fossae | Circular fossae near marginal ridges called mesial and distal fossae | In three cusp type: Mesial and distal triangular fossae<br>In 2 cusp type: Mesial and distal irregular fossae |
| Marginal ridges | Mesial marginal ridge is shorter and constricted because of mesiolingual developmental groove | Both mesial and distal marginal ridge equally well developed |
| **Root** | | |
| Number | Single (sometimes bifurcated) | Single |
| Size | Narrow and relatively wider buccolingually than mesiodistally | Broader, stronger, and longer than that of mandibular first premolars (wider buccolingually than mesiodistally) |
| Lingual taper | Root shows marked lingual taper | No much lingual tapering |
| Apex curvature | Pointed often distal curvature | Straight or distal curvature |
| Pulp canals | 1 canal | 1 canal |

(FDI: Federation Dentaire Internationale)

## BIBLIOGRAPHY

1. Ash MM, Nelson SJ. Wheeler's Dental Anatomy, Physiology and Occlusion, 8th edition. Saunders: St Louis; 2003.
2. Awawdeh LA, Al-Qudah AA. Root form and canal morphology of mandibular premolars in a Jordanian population. Int Endod J. 2008;41(3):240-8.
3. Cleghorn BM, Christie WH, Dong CC. The root and root canal morphology of the human mandibular 2nd premolar: a literature review. J Endod. 2007;33(9):1031-7.

## MULTIPLE CHOICE QUESTIONS

1. Mandibular permanent premolars differ from each other in their:
   a. Development
   b. Form
   c. Both A and B
   d. Neither A nor B
2. Mandibular permanent first premolar develops from:
   a. 4 lobes
   b. 5 lobes
   c. 3 lobes
   d. 2 lobes
3. Mandibular permanent second premolar develops from:
   a. 4 lobes
   b. 5 lobes
   c. 3 lobes
   d. 2 lobes
4. Compared to mandibular second premolar the mandibular first premolar is:
   a. Smaller
   b. Larger
   c. Same size
   d. None
5. Grooves seen in the mandibular permanent first premolar are _____

a. Mesial developmental groove
b. Distal developmental groove
c. Mesiolingual developmental groove
d. All of the above

6. Mandibular permanent first premolar has:
   a. Two cusps
   b. Three cusps
   c. Four cusps
   d. One cusp
7. Functional cusp of mandibular permanent first premolar is:
   a. Buccal cusp
   b. Lingual cusps
   c. Both A and B
   d. Neither A nor B
8. Nonfunctional cusp of mandibular first premolar is:
   a. Buccal cusp
   b. Lingual cusp
   c. Both A and B
   d. Neither A nor B
9. The largest cusp of mandibular permanent first premolar is:
   a. Lingual cusp
   b. Buccal cusp
   c. Accessory cusp
   d. None
10. Which of the following is true about mandibular first premolar?
    a. Mesial and distal contact areas at same level
    b. Buccolingual measurement is similar to that of mandibular canine
    c. Occlusal surface slopes drastically lingually in a cervical direction
    d. All of the above

**Answers**

1. c    2. a    3. b    4. a    5. d    6. a    7. a    8. b
9. b    10. d

# The Permanent Maxillary Molars

## INTRODUCTION

There are six molars in each arch and three in each quadrant. They occupy the most posterior segment of the dental arch **(Fig. 14.1)**. The molars are the largest and the strongest teeth owing to their greater crown bulk and excellent anchorage of their multiple roots. The maxillary molars generally have three roots; two buccal and one palatal, whereas the mandibular molars have two roots; mesial and distal. The third molars and some second molars may have fused roots.

The molar teeth do not succeed any deciduous teeth but erupt distal to the deciduous second molars. Thus, the permanent molars are not succedaneous teeth as they do not have any predecessors. The permanent first molars erupt at about 6 years of age, thus are sometimes called as *six year*

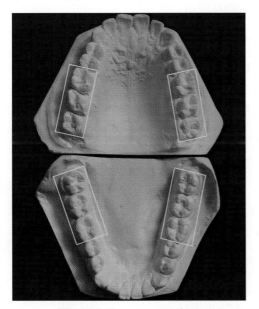

**Fig. 14.1:** Permanent molars.

*molars.* The third molars are present only in the permanent dentition and are commonly referred to as *wisdom teeth.* Third molars are the last teeth to erupt into oral cavity at around 18–21 years of age.

## COMMON CHARACTERISTICS (CLASS TRAITS) OF MOLARS

- The molars develop from four to five lobes: One lobe for each cusp. They are generally the largest teeth in both the arches.
- Their crowns are shorter cervico-occlusally although they are wider in all other aspects. Usually the distal halves of the crowns are shorter.
- The molars have four or five cusps and two or three roots.
- The bifurcated or trifurcated roots are strong, well formed, and are usually well spaced to have the best anchorage.
- The crowns usually taper from mesial to distal aspect so that the buccolingual width of the mesial half is greater than that of the distal half.
- The mesial and distal contact areas are broader and are at the same level.
- Usually, their distal marginal ridge is at a lower level than the mesial marginal ridge.
- The cervical line on proximal and other surfaces is rather straight without much curvature.
- The crest of curvature of the crowns on buccal surface is at the cervical third, whereas that of the lingual curvature in the middle third of the crown.
- The lingual cusps (especially, the mesiolingual cusp) are longer than the buccal cusps. Their occlusal tables are wide and best suited for comminution of food.

## FUNCTIONS OF MOLARS

Molars have widest occlusal tables and are the main teeth used for trituration and comminution of food. They give support to the cheeks.

## PERMANENT MAXILLARY FIRST MOLAR

Permanent maxillary first molar is the largest tooth in the maxillary arch. It develops from five lobes, has a large

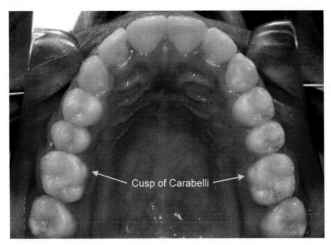

**Fig. 14.2:** Cusp of Carabelli of permanent maxillary first molar.

**Table 14.1:** Maxillary first molar—chronology and measurements.

| Chronology | |
|---|---|
| First evidence of calcification | At birth |
| Enamel completed | 2½–3 years |
| Eruption | 6–7 years |
| Roots completed | 9–10 years |
| **Measurements** *Dimensions suggested for carving technique (in mm)* | |
| Cervico-occlusal length of crown | 7.5 |
| Length of root | Buccal–12.0, lingual–13.0 |
| Mesiodistal diameter of crown | 10.0 |
| Mesiodistal diameter of crown at cervix | 8.0 |
| Buccolingual diameter of crown | 11.0 |
| Buccolingual diameter of crown at cervix | 10.0 |
| Curvature of cervical line—mesial | 1.0 |
| Curvature of cervical line—distal | 0.0 |

crown and three well-formed roots. The tooth has four well-developed cusps and a small supplemental cusp. The four cusps are mesiobuccal, distobuccal, mesiolingual, and the distolingual. The small, nonfunctional cusp found lingual to the mesiolingual cusp, is called the "*cusp/ tubercle of Carabelli*" or simply as the *fifth cusp* (**Fig. 14.2**). The presence of a well-developed fifth cusp or any trace of its development *(Carabelli's trait)* is the characteristic feature of maxillary first molars. The Carabelli's trait has varied expression; it can be in the form of a well-developed fifth cusp or in the form of a groove, depression or pit on the mesial portion of the lingual surface (**Figs. 14.3A and B**).

The trifurcated root provides an excellent anchorage in the alveolar bone and its tripod design is best suited to resist the oblique occlusal forces. The three roots are mesiobuccal, distobuccal, and lingual. The lingual root is the longest among the three roots.

The maxillary first molars begin to calcify at birth and erupt around 6 years of age. The chronology and measurements are given in **Table 14.1**.

## DETAILED DESCRIPTION OF MAXILLARY FIRST MOLAR FROM ALL ASPECTS (FIGS. 14.4 TO 14.6)

### Crown

#### *Buccal aspect (Fig. 14.7)*

**Geometric shape:** Trapezoidal

#### *Crown outlines:*

*Mesial outline:* The mesial outline is straight for most its course and becomes slightly convex as it joins the occlusal outline. The maximum convexity of mesial outline (*mesial contact area*) is at the occlusal third of the crown.

*Distal outline:*
- The distal outline is a more convex arc from cervix up to the point where it joins the occlusal outline.
- Its maximum convexity (*distal contact area*) is at the middle third of the crown.

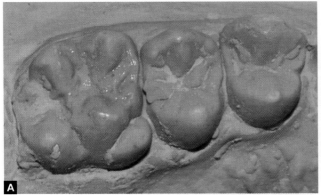
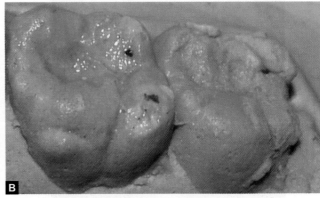

**Figs. 14.3A and B:** Varied expressions of Carabelli's trait.

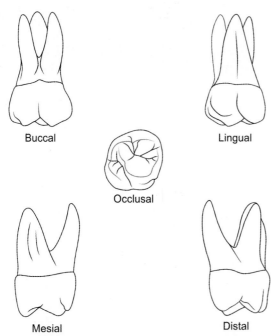

Fig. 14.4: Maxillary first molar—line drawings.

Buccal

Lingual

Occlusal

Mesial

Distal

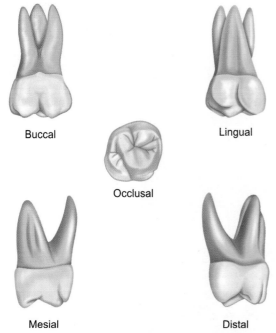

Buccal

Lingual

Occlusal

Mesial

Distal

Fig. 14.5: Maxillary first molar—graphic illustrations.

*Occlusal outline:*
- The occlusal outline is formed by the mesiobuccal and distobuccal cusp tips and their cusp slopes.
- The cusp slopes of mesiobuccal cusp make an obtuse angle, whereas the cusp slopes of distobuccal cusp meet at right angle.

- The occlusal outline is interrupted in midway by the buccal developmental groove.

*Cervical outline:* The cervical line on buccal surface of the crown is irregular and curves slightly in an apical direction.

***Buccal surface within the outlines:***
- All the cusps (most of buccal cusps and part of lingual cusps) are visible from buccal aspect.
- Some portion of distal surface can also be seen from this aspect as the crown tapers distally from mesial surface. Among the two buccal cusps, the mesiobuccal cusp is wider than the distobuccal cusp which is more pointed.
- Both the buccal cusps are nearly of same length though the mesiobuccal cusp may be longer.
- The *buccal developmental groove* separating the buccal cusp runs for half the length of buccal surface and ends in the buccal pit.
- The buccal surface is more convex in the cervical third, slightly concave or flattened in the middle third and is convex again in the occlusal third of the crown.

## Lingual Aspect (Fig. 14.8)

***Geometric shape:*** Trapezoidal like buccal aspect.

***Crown outlines:***
- Mesial outline: The mesial outline assumes a straight course dropping down from cervical area in a mesio-occlusal direction and joins the mesial slope of mesiolingual cusp at right angles.
- Distal outline: The distal outline forms a semicircular arc by merging smoothly with the distolingual cusp.
- Occlusal outline: The slopes of mesiolingual cusp are longer and meet at an obtuse angle. The *lingual developmental groove* interrupts the occlusal outline.

***Cervical outline:*** The cervical outline on lingual surface is nearly straight.

***Lingual surface within the outlines:***
- Only lingual cusps can be seen from the lingual aspect as the shorter buccal cusps are obscured. The mesiolingual cusp is much larger than the distolingual cusp which is smooth and spheroidal.
- The *lingual development groove* separating the two lingual cusps is confluent with the distolingual cusp, and extends mesiocervically to end at the center of lingual surface.
- The characteristic feature of lingual surface of maxillary 1st molar is the presence of some expression of *Carabelli's trait*. The fifth cusp may be well developed into a large cusp or may show traces of its development in the form of grooves, depressions or pits.
- When well developed, the fifth cusp ridge is cervically placed than the cusp ridge of mesiolingual cusp. It is usually separated by the mesiolingual cusp by a groove.
- A developmental depression begins at the center of lingual surface just cervical to the lingual developmental groove

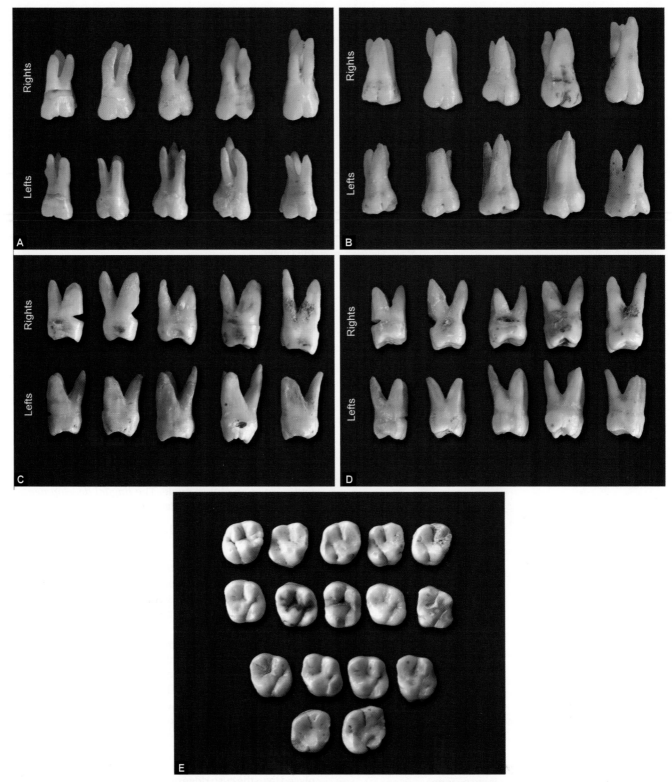

**Figs. 14.6A to E:** Maxillary first molar—typical specimen from all aspects: (A) Buccal aspect; (B) Lingual aspect; (C) Mesial aspect; (D) Distal aspect; (E) Occlusal aspect.

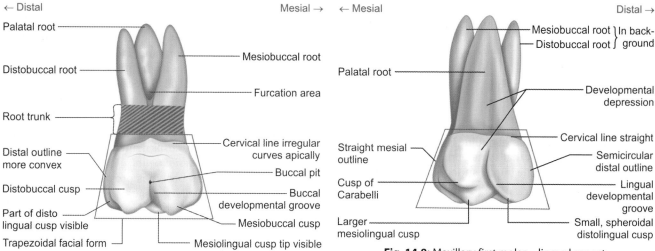

← Distal                                          Mesial →

Palatal root

Distobuccal root

Mesiobuccal root

Furcation area

Root trunk

Cervical line irregular curves apically

Distal outline more convex

Buccal pit

Distobuccal cusp

Buccal developmental groove

Part of disto lingual cusp visible

Mesiobuccal cusp

Trapezoidal facial form

Mesiolingual cusp tip visible

**Fig. 14.7:** Maxillary first molar—buccal aspect.

← Mesial                                          Distal →

Mesiobuccal root ⎫ In back-
Distobuccal root ⎬ ground

Palatal root

Developmental depression

Straight mesial outline

Cervical line straight

Semicircular distal outline

Cusp of Carabelli

Lingual developmental groove

Larger mesiolingual cusp

Small, spheroidal distolingual cusp

**Fig. 14.8:** Maxillary first molar—lingual aspect.

and extends beyond the cervical line onto the lingual surface of the lingual root to fade out at the middle third of the root.

### Mesial Aspect (Fig. 14.9)

***Geometric shape:*** It is *trapezoidal* like proximal aspect of all maxillary posteriors with shorter uneven side toward the occlusal portion.

#### Crown outlines:

*Buccal outline:* It is convex in cervical third and flattens out as it runs occlusally. Height of buccal contour is within the cervical third.

*Lingual outline:*
- It is a more convex arc from cervical line to the tip of mesiolingual cusp.
- Height of lingual contour is at the middle third of the crown.

- It curves inwards when a well-developed fifth cusp is present.

*Occlusal outline:* It is formed by the mesial marginal ridge along with the triangular ridges of mesiobuccal and mesiolingual cusps toward the center of the occlusal surface.

*Cervical outline:* Cervical outline on mesial surface curves occlusally up to 1 mm.

#### Mesial surface within the outlines:
- The mesiobuccal, mesiolingual, and fifth cusps are seen from mesial aspect.
- The cusp tips of mesiolingual and mesiobuccal cusp are within the confines of the root trunk.
- The mesiolingual cusp tip is on line with the long axis of the lingual root. The mesiobuccal cusp tip is on line with the buccal outline of the mesiobuccal root.
- There is a concavity cervical to the contact area which may extend onto the cervical portion of root trunk.

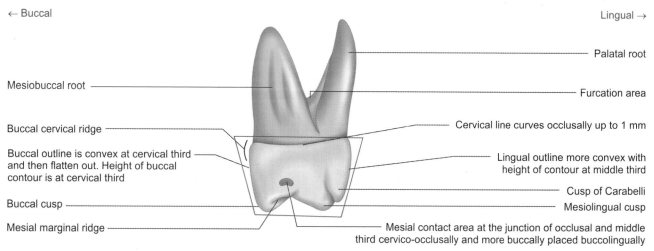

← Buccal                                                                                    Lingual →

Palatal root

Mesiobuccal root

Furcation area

Buccal cervical ridge

Cervical line curves occlusally up to 1 mm

Buccal outline is convex at cervical third and then flatten out. Height of buccal contour is at cervical third

Lingual outline more convex with height of contour at middle third

Cusp of Carabelli

Buccal cusp

Mesiolingual cusp

Mesial marginal ridge

Mesial contact area at the junction of occlusal and middle third cervico-occlusally and more buccally placed buccolingually

**Fig. 14.9:** Maxillary first molar—mesial aspect.

- The *mesial contact area* is at the junction of occlusal and middle third of the crown and is more buccally placed buccolingually.

### Distal Aspect (Fig. 14.10)

*Geometric shape:* Trapezoidal
The distal aspect has four outlines as mesial aspect.

***Crown outlines:***
- Buccal outline: The buccal outline is similar to that of the mesial aspect, except that some portion of buccal surface can also be seen as the buccal surface of the crown slants distally.
- Lingual outline: The lingual outline is smoothly convex from cervix to the distolingual cusp tip.
- Occlusal outline: The distal marginal ridge is shorter and at a lower level than the mesial marginal ridge. Thus, some part of occlusal surface with triangular ridges of distal cusps may be seen.
- Cervical outline: The cervical line on distal surface is nearly a straight line without much curvature.

***Distal surface within the outlines:***
- Only distobuccal and distolingual cusps are seen from distal aspect.
- The distal surface is narrower than the mesial surface as the crown tapers toward distal aspect.
- The distal surface is smoothly convex.
- The *distal contact area* is at the center of the crown both cervico-occlusally and buccolingually.

### Occlusal Aspect (Figs. 14.11A and B)

*Geometric shape:* The occlusal aspect of the maxillary first molar is *rhomboidal* with—
- Two acute angles—mesiobuccal and distolingual
- Two obtuse angles—distobuccal and mesiolingual.

***Relative dimensions:***
- The buccolingual dimension of the crown is greater than the mesiodistal dimension by about 1 mm.

- The crown tapers distally, thus it can be noted that the crown is wider mesially than distally.
- The crown does not show lingual convergence which is generally seen in most permanent teeth.
- In fact, mesiodistal dimension of the crown lingually is greater than its mesiodistal dimension buccally.

### Maxillary Molar Primary Cusp Triangle (Fig. 14.12)

- From the developmental point of view, the maxillary molars have only three primary cusps namely, the *mesiobuccal, the distobuccal, and the mesiolingual.*
- The distolingual cusp becomes progressively smaller on second and third maxillary molars.

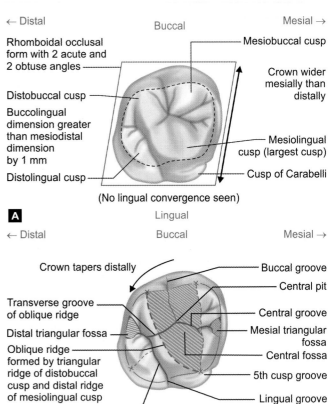

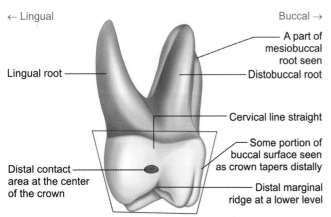

Fig. 14.10: Maxillary first molar—distal aspect.

Figs. 14.11A and B: Maxillary first molar—occlusal aspect.

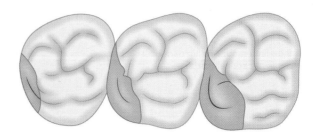

Fig. 14.12: Maxillary molar primary cusp triangle.

- The cusp of Carabelli present only in the first molar is considered as a secondary cusp.
- A triangular outline can be visualized by tracking the cusp ridges of three primary cusps, the mesial marginal ridge, and oblique ridge.
- These three primary cusps can be seated on the root trunk divided into three roots.
- This triangular arrangement of the three primary cusps is characteristic of all maxillary molars and is called as the *maxillary molar primary cusp triangle*. The design of the maxillary molar primary cusp triangle becomes progressively more evident from first molar to the third molar.

### Boundaries of the Occlusal Surface

The occlusal surface in the center of occlusal aspect is bounded by:
- Mesial and distal cusp ridges of four major cusps
- Mesial and distal marginal ridges.

### Occlusal Surface Within Boundaries

*The occlusal surface exhibits:* cusps and cusp ridges; grooves and pits; and fossae and marginal ridges.

**Cusps and cusp ridges:** The maxillary first molar has four major cusps and a supplemental fifth cusp (cusp of Carabelli), which may or may not be well developed.
- The cusps in the decreasing order of size are: mesiolingual (largest cusp) > mesiobuccal > distobuccal > distolingual > fifth cusp.
- Each cusp has mesial and distal cusp ridges and a triangular ridge of its own sloping toward the center of the occlusal surface.
- There are inclined planes on either side of each triangular ridge
- There is an additional ridge crossing the occlusal surface obliquely, called the *oblique ridge*
- *The oblique ridge is formed by the union of the triangular ridge of the distobuccal cusp and the distal ridge of the mesiolingual cusp. It is at the same level as the marginal ridges and is sometimes crossed by a developmental groove.*

### Grooves and pits:

#### Grooves
The maxillary first molar exhibits several developmental and supplemental grooves on its occlusal surface. The developmental grooves are situated at the bottom of deep long sulci traversing across the occlusal surface in different directions. The developmental grooves are:

*1. Buccal developmental groove:* It runs buccally from the central pit located in the central fossa and continues onto the buccal surface of the crown separating the two buccal cusps.

*2. Central developmental groove:* It runs in a mesial direction from central pit and ends at the apex of mesial triangular fossa where it is joined by supplemental grooves. This groove separates the triangular ridges of mesiobuccal and mesiolingual cusps.

*3. Transverse groove of oblique ridge:* It runs in a distolingual direction from the central pit and crosses the oblique ridge to reach the distal fossa.

*4. Distal oblique groove:* It is irregular and runs in an oblique direction; parallel to the oblique ridge. This groove separates the distolingual cusp from the rest of the occlusal surface which forms the primary triangle of maxillary molars.

*5. Lingual groove:* The distal oblique groove joins the lingual developmental groove which runs on the lingual surface separating the two lingual cusps.

*6. Fifth cusp groove:* It separates the fifth cusp from the mesiolingual cusp. When the fifth cusp is not well developed, there is some trace of fifth cusp development in the form of a developmental groove which is also called as fifth cusp groove.

*Multiple supplemental grooves:* There are several supplementary grooves especially at the apices of mesial and distal triangular fossae. Some of these supplemental grooves may cross the marginal ridges.

#### Pits
Three pits can be noted on the occlusal surface of maxillary first molar.
- *Central pit:* It is a pin point depression in the central fossa. Three major developmental grooves originate from the central pit and run in three different directions. The three grooves are at obtuse angles to each other. They are:
  1. The buccal developmental groove radiating in a buccal direction.
  2. The central developmental groove running mesially.
  3. Transverse groove of oblique ridge running distally.
- *Mesial pit:* It is at the apex of mesial triangular fossa and the central developmental groove terminates at this pit.
- *Distal pit:* It is at the apex of the distal triangular fossa and the distal oblique groove ends at this pit.

### Fossae and marginal ridges:
- There are two major and two minor fossae.
- The two major fossae are *central fossa* and the *distal fossa*.
- The two minor fossae are *mesial* and *distal triangular fossae*.

#### Major fossae:
- The *central fossa* is a large triangular depression in the center of the occlusal surface mesial to the oblique ridge.
- The central fossa is bounded by the distal slope of the mesiobuccal cusp, mesial slope of the distobuccal cusp, the crests of the oblique ridge and the crests of triangular ridge of mesiobuccal and mesiolingual cusps.

- It has the central pit at its center and three major developmental grooves run across it.
- The *distal fossa* is small linear developmental depression distal to the oblique ridge. It has distal oblique developmental groove at its deepest position.

*Minor fossae:*

- Mesial triangular fossa is a triangular depression having mesial marginal ridge at its base and mesial pit at its apex. Supplemental grooves radiate from the mesial pit forming the side of the triangle.
- The distal triangular fossa has the distal marginal ridge at its base and distal pit at its apex. Supplemental grooves radiate from the distal pit forming the sides of triangle.

*Marginal ridges:* The mesial and distal marginal ridges are well developed. The distal marginal ridge is shorter and is at a lower level than the mesial marginal ridge.

### Root

Morphology of the root can be described under the following headings:

| | |
|---|---|
| *Number:* | Three well-formed roots—mesiobuccal, distobuccal, and lingual or palatal |
| *Size:* | Roots are about twice the length of the crown. The palatal root is the longest and the largest and the two buccal roots are of nearly same length. The mesiobuccal root is larger than the distobuccal root |
| *Form:* | • The roots are strongly developed and designed to withstand the occlusal forces. The root trunk is about one-third the root length and is well within the confines of the crown |
| | • The root soon divides into three branches with the level of furcation nearest to the cervical line on the mesial surface |
| | • The palatal root is wider mesiodistally but narrower buccolingually. It extends lingually and stretches out of the confines of the crown before bending back in a buccal direction at its apical third |
| | • The mesiobuccal root is broader buccolingually than mesiodistally. The distobuccal root is the smallest root |
| | • The two buccal roots diverge from the root trunk for half their length and face each other again at their apical halves |
| | • The distobuccal root is more distally tilted whereas the mesiobuccal root has relatively straight long axis |
| *Developmental groove and depression:* | • There is a deep developmental groove beginning at the bifurcation of the buccal roots and runs toward the cervical line |
| | • There is a developmental depression at the bifurcation point of mesiobuccal and |

| | |
|---|---|
| | lingual root which extends lingually toward the cervical line |
| *Curvature:* | Buccal roots tend to tilt distally. The palatal root has a vertical axis and its apical third is curved buccally |
| *Apex:* | All three roots have bluntly rounded apices |

### Variations

Morphology of maxillary first molar does not vary much except for the widely varied expression of the Carabelli's trait.

### Developmental Anomalies (Figs. 14.13A and B)

- Supernumerary roots (tooth may have extra roots)
- Dilaceration of root (sharp bend in the root)
- Concrescence (fusion of two adjacent teeth by cementum).

### Clinical Considerations

- The anteroposterior position of maxillary and mandibular first molars is observed to establish Angle's key of occlusion. Angle's key of occlusion is used to classify malocclusion of teeth **(Figs. 14.14A to C)**.
- As the three roots provide excellent anchorage, left and right maxillary first molars are used for anchorage in orthodontic treatment **(Figs. 14.15A and B)**.
- The oblique ridge has to be restored during conservative and prosthetic procedures on the maxillary first molar.
- Carabelli's trait is used in anthropology for distinguishing the different population groups. Cusp of Carabelli is much more frequently seen in white population and less frequent in Mongoloid and Negroid race groups.
- The maxillary first molar anatomy is summarized in **Flowcharts 14.1 and 14.2**.

**Box 14.1** shows the identification features of this tooth.

---

### PERMANENT MAXILLARY SECOND MOLAR

The permanent maxillary second molar resembles the permanent maxillary first molar closely and supplements the latter in function. The crown of maxillary permanent second molar is slightly shorter than that of maxillary

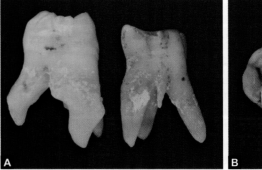
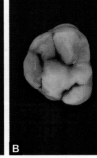

**Figs. 14.13A and B:** Maxillary first molar—developmental anomalies.

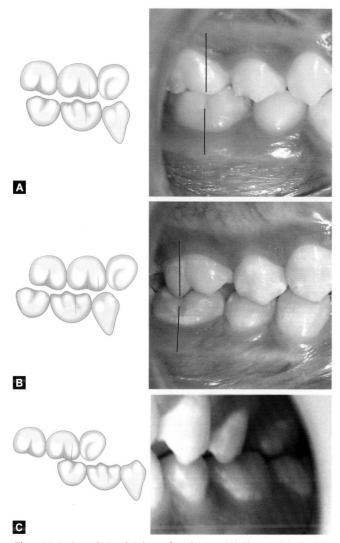

**Figs. 14.14A to C:** Angle's key of occlusion: (A) Class 1; (B) Class 2; (C) Class 3.

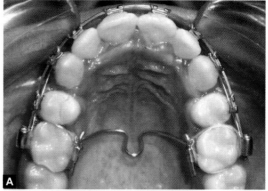

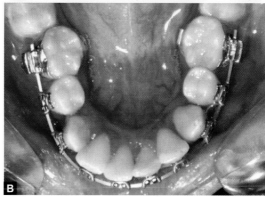

**Figs. 14.15A and B:** Permanent maxillary first molars are often used as intraoral anchorage units during orthodontic treatment. The irregular teeth are pulled back into normal alignment using the first molars as steady pillars of anchorage.

---

**Box 14.1: Maxillary first molar—identification features.**

- *Identification features of maxillary first molar:*
  - The tooth has a large crown and three roots
  - The crown is wider buccolingually than mesiodistally
  - Its occlusal aspect is rhomboidal
  - The cusp of Carabelli is a unique feature of maxillary molar, present lingual to the mesiolingual cusp
  - Another characteristic feature of maxillary molar is the oblique ridge running obliquely from the mesiolingual cusp to the distobuccal cusp
- *Side identification:*
  - When viewed occlusally, the crown is wider mesially than distally
  - By locating the cusp of Carabelli, which is present lingual to the mesiolingual cusp
  - The buccal roots tend to have a distal inclination

---

permanent first molar, although the roots are as long as the roots of maxillary permanent first molar. The roots are not as divergent as seen in maxillary permanent first molar. The distobuccal cusp is somewhat less developed than that in maxillary first molar. The distolingual cusp is smaller leaving the maxillary molar primary cusp triangle more prominent.

There are two forms of maxillary second molar depending on their occlusal anatomy (**Figs. 14.16A and B**):

1. *Four cusp type* with *rhomboidal occlusal design*: This type is more common and resembles maxillary first molar in occlusal form.
2. *Three cusp type* with *pear or heart-shaped occlusal aspect* resembling maxillary third molar.

The maxillary and mandibular second molars begin to calcify by 2½ years and erupt around 12 years of age. The maxillary and mandibular second molars are thus sometimes referred to as the *12-year molars*.

The chronology and measurements of maxillary second molar are given in **Table 14.2**.

**Flowchart 14.1:** Maxillary first molar—major anatomic landmarks.

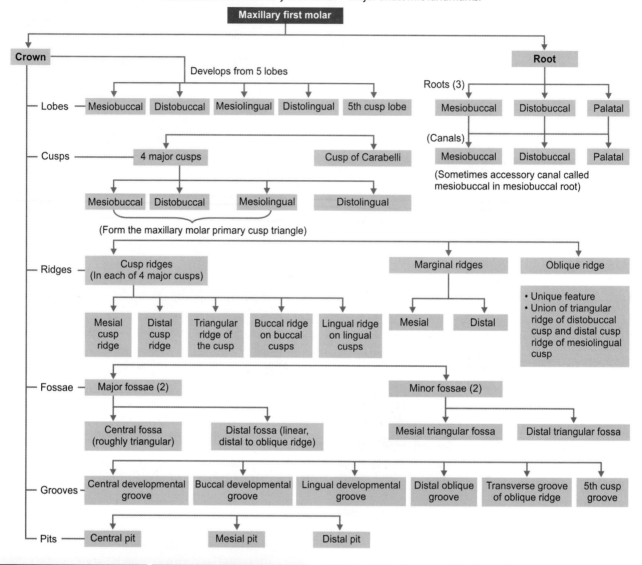

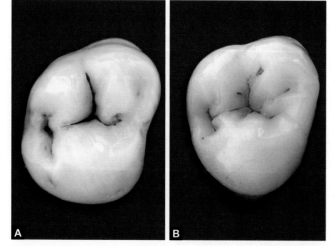

**Figs. 14.16A and B:** The maxillary second molars are of two forms: (A) 4 cusp or rhomboidal type; (B) 3 cusp type or heart-shaped type.

**Table 14.2:** Maxillary second molar—chronology and measurements.

| Chronology | |
| --- | --- |
| First evidence of calcification | 2½–3 years |
| Enamel completed | 7–8 years |
| Eruption | 12–13 years |
| **Measurements** *Dimensions suggested for carving technique (in mm)* | |
| Cervico-occlusal length of crown | 7.0 |
| Length of root | Buccal—11.0; lingual—12.0 |
| Mesiodistal diameter of crown | 9.0 |
| Mesiodistal diameter of crown at cervix | 7.0 |
| Buccolingual diameter of crown | 11.0 |
| Buccolingual diameter of crown at cervix | 10.0 |
| Curvature of cervical line—mesial | 1.0 |
| Curvature of cervical line—distal | 0.0 |

**Flowchart 14.2:** Maxillary first molar—summary.

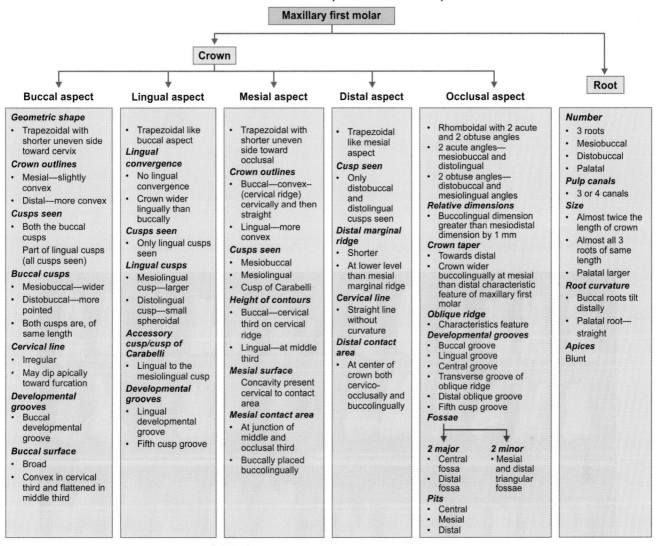

**DETAILED DESCRIPTION OF MAXILLARY SECOND MOLAR FROM ALL ASPECTS (FIGS. 14.17 TO 14.19)**

## Crown

### Buccal Aspect (Fig. 14.20)

**Geometric shape:** It is *trapezoidal* with shorter uneven side toward the cervical portion.

**Crown outlines:**

*Mesial outline:*
- The mesial outline is nearly a straight line extending mesio-occlusally up to the mesial contact area where it becomes convex.
- Its maximum convexity *(mesial contact area)* is at the junction of occlusal and middle third of crown.

*Distal outline:*
- The distal outline is convex from cervix to the point where it joins the occlusal outline.
- Its maximum convexity *(distal contact area)* is at the middle third of the crown.

*Occlusal outline:*
- The occlusal outline is formed by the cusp tips and ridges of the buccal cusps separated by the buccal groove
- The outline appears to tilt cervically in a distal direction.

*Cervical outline:* The cervical line on buccal surface is nearly straight mesiodistally.

**Buccal surface within the outlines:**
- Buccal surface is similar to that of maxillary permanent first molar. But the crown is shorter and narrower mesiodistally.

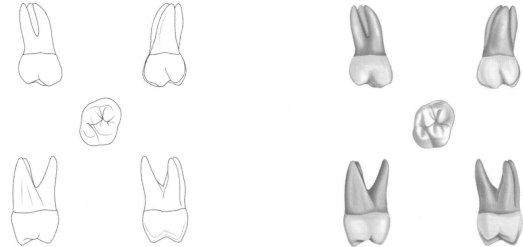

**Fig. 14.17:** Maxillary second molar—line drawings.

**Fig. 14.18:** Maxillary second molar—graphic illustrations.

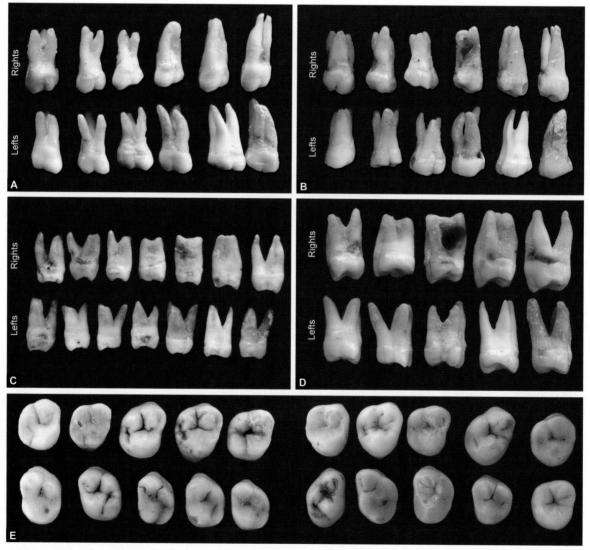

**Figs. 14.19A to E:** Maxillary second molar—typical specimen from all aspects: (A) Buccal aspect; (B) Lingual aspect; (C) Mesial aspect; (D) Distal aspect; (E) Occlusal aspect.

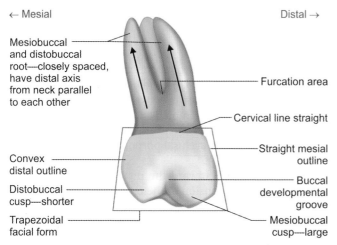

Fig. 14.20: Maxillary second molar—buccal aspect.

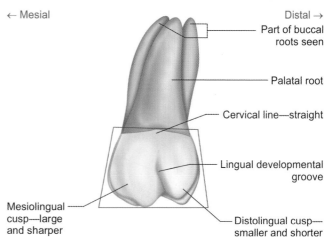

Fig. 14.21: Maxillary second molar—lingual aspect.

- The distobuccal cusp is much smaller and shorter than the mesiobuccal cusp. Thus, a part of distolingual cusp can be seen from the buccal aspect.
- The *buccal developmental groove* separates the two buccal cusps.

### Lingual Aspect (Fig. 14.21)

**Geometric shape:** *Trapezoidal* similar to buccal aspect.

**Crown outlines:**

*Mesial outline*
*Distal outline* } are similar to buccal aspect
*Cervical outline*

*Occlusal outline:* The occlusal outline is formed by the cusp tips and cusp ridges of sharper mesiolingual cusp and rounded distolingual cusp. The outline is interrupted by the lingual developmental groove.

**Lingual surface within the outlines:**
- The distolingual cusp is much smaller and shorter than the mesiolingual cusp.
- The lingual surface is smoothly convex except for the *lingual developmental groove* separating the two lingual cusps.
- There is no fifth cusp seen.

### Mesial Aspect (Fig. 14.22)

**Geometric shape:** The crown is trapezoidal with shorter uneven side toward the occlusal portion.

**Crown outlines:**

*Buccal outline:*
- The buccal outline is more convex in its cervical third and is less convex from there up to the mesiobuccal cusp tip.
- *Height of buccal contour* is in the cervical third of the crown. Buccal contour of all the molars exhibit maximum convexity at the cervical third—due to buccal cervical ridge.

*Lingual outline:*
- The lingual outline is convex from cervix to the mesiolingual cusp tip.

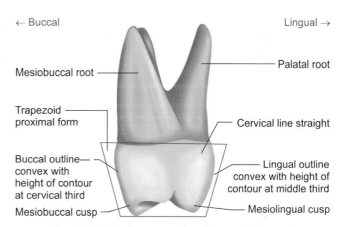

Fig. 14.22: Maxillary second molar—mesial aspect.

- *Height of lingual contour*—at the middle third.

*Occlusal outline:* The mesial marginal ridge forms a smooth concave arc merging with the mesial cusp ridges of mesiobuccal and mesiolingual cusps.

*Cervical outline:* The cervical line is almost a straight line.

**Mesial surface within the outlines:**
- The mesial surface is smoothly convex and the crown appears shorter than that of maxillary permanent first molar
- The mesiobuccal and mesiolingual cusps are almost of same length, although the mesiolingual cusp is larger.

### Distal Aspect (Fig. 14.23)

**Geometric shape:** *Trapezoidal* like that of mesial aspects.

**Crown outlines:**

*Buccal outline*
*Lingual outline* } are similar to mesial aspect
*Cervical outline*

*Occlusal outline:*
- The distal marginal ridge is at a lower level than mesial marginal ridge.

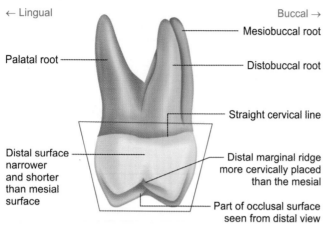

**Fig. 14.23:** Maxillary second molar—distal aspect.

- It is rather irregular and slopes cervically toward the smaller distobuccal cusp.

### Distal surface within the outlines:
- The distal surface is narrower and shorter than the mesial surface.
- As the distal marginal ridge is more cervically placed, some portion of occlusal surface can be seen. Some part of buccal surface and mesiobuccal cusp can also been seen from distal aspect.

## Occlusal Aspect (Fig. 14.24)

**Geometric shape:** In the four-cusp type—
- The occlusal aspect appears *more rhomboidal.*
- The mesiobuccal and distolingual line angles are—acute.
- The distobuccal and mesiolingual line angles are—obtuse.
  *In the three-cusp type:* The occlusal form is *heart shaped,* highlighting the primary cusp triangle of the maxillary molars. The distolingual cusp is very small.

**Relative dimensions:** The buccolingual dimension is more than the mesiodistal dimension, especially so in the four cusp

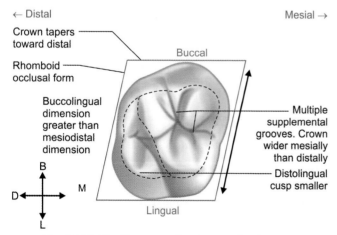

**Fig. 14.24:** Maxillary second molar—occlusal aspect.

type with rhomboid form. The distobuccal cusp is small and less well developed.

### Rhomboidal form:
- The tooth resembles maxillary permanent first molar.
- Mesiolingual cusp is the largest followed by the mesiobuccal cusp. The distobuccal cusp is less well-developed and its small size accentuates the rhomboid outline of occlusal aspect.
- The distolingual cusp is small and appears to be separated from the rest of the occlusal portion. The oblique ridge is less prominent.
- The crown tapers toward the distal surface. Thus, the buccolingual dimension of the crown is greater mesially than distally. Multiple supplemental grooves can be seen along with the developmental grooves.

### Heart-shaped form:
- This type of maxillary second molar resembles maxillary third molar.
- The mesiolingual cusp is as well developed as seen in the first maxillary molar.
- But the distolingual cusp is very small or absent making the crown appears heart shaped.

## Root

Morphology of the root can be described under the following headings:

| | |
|---|---|
| *Number:* | Three roots originating from a common root base |
| *Size:* | Roots are as long as those of maxillary first molar roots |
| *Form:* | • The buccal roots are more distally inclined than that of maxillary first molar, often reaching out of the distal extremity of the crown |
| | • The lingual root does not diverge much lingually and it is within the confines of the crown when seen from proximal aspects |
| | • The mesiobuccal and distobuccal roots are in close approximation and they have a parallel course |
| *Curvature:* | All three roots are inclined distally |
| *Apex:* | Apices of the root are sharper than that of maxillary first molar |

## Variations (Figs. 14.25A and B)
- Fused root
- Long or short root
- Supernumerary roots
- Crown with accentuated rhomboid outline and multiple small tubercles.

## Developmental Anomalies
- Dilaceration of roots
- Concrescence.

Flowchart 14.3 shows major anatomic landmarks of maxillary second molar and **Flowchart 14.4** summarizes the tooth anatomy.

**Box 14.2** shows the identification features of the tooth.

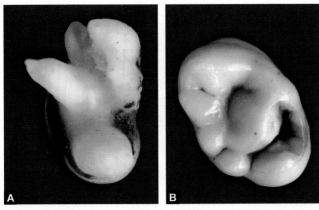

**Figs. 14.25A and B:** Maxillary second molar—variation: (A) Supernumerary root; (B) Accentuated rhomboid form with multiple small tubercles on the occlusal surface.

## PERMANENT MAXILLARY THIRD MOLAR

The third molars in both the dental arches are highly variable in their size and form than any other teeth. They are the most common teeth to be congenitally missing. In maxillary third molar, crown is smaller and shows resemblance to heart-

---

**Box 14.2: Maxillary second molar—identification features.**

- *Identification features of maxillary second molar:*
  - Crown is shorter with comparatively long roots. The root is trifurcated
  - There is no evidence of the fifth cusp development
  - Mesiolingual cusp is the largest
  - Distolingual cusp is small or absent
  - The oblique ridge is less prominent
  - The roots do not spread out much, tend to fuse and have a distal inclination
- *Side identification:*
  - The crown is wider mesially than distally
  - The distolingual cusp is small or absent
  - The roots are not wide apart and are inclined distally

---

**Flowchart 14.3:** Maxillary second molar—major anatomic landmarks.

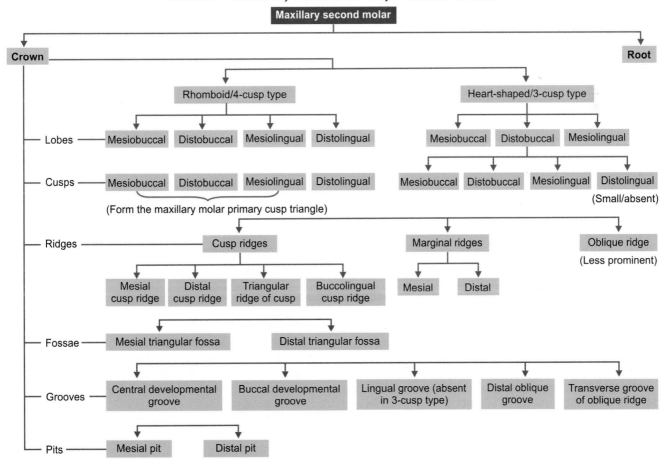

**Flowchart 14.4:** Maxillary second molar—summary.

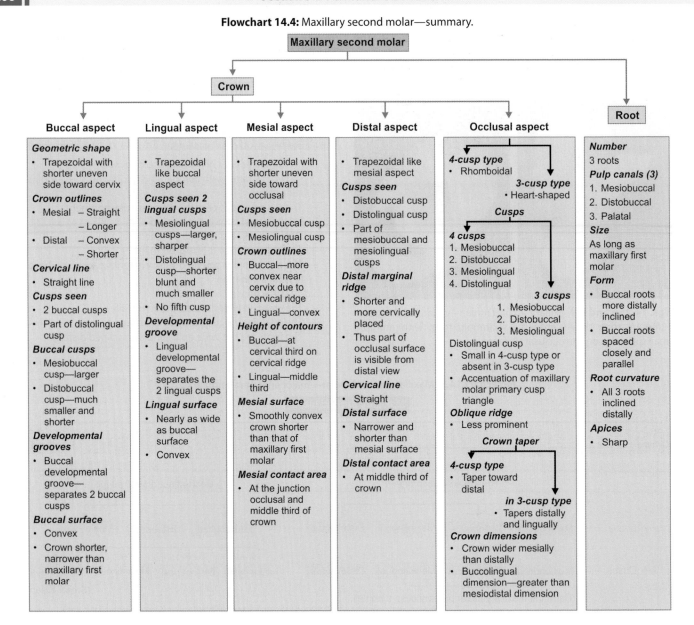

shaped type of permanent maxillary second molar when viewed occlusally (**Fig. 14.26**). The distolingual cusp is very small and poorly developed, or may even be completely absent. The tooth assists the second molar in function. The roots are shorter and have a strong tendency to fuse. Sometimes, the maxillary third molars appear as developmental anomalies with little or no resemblance to adjacent teeth. The maxillary third molar is directly compared with the maxillary second molar in its description.

The maxillary and mandibular third molars are the last teeth to erupt into oral cavity at around 17–21 years of age. Since they erupt late in life, they are also commonly referred to as the *wisdom teeth*. The chronology and measurements of the maxillary third molar are given in **Table 14.3**.

## DETAILED DESCRIPTION OF MAXILLARY THIRD MOLAR FROM ALL ASPECTS (FIGS. 14.27 TO 14.29)

### Crown

#### *Buccal Aspect (Fig. 14.30)*

- The mesiobuccal and distobuccal cusps are seen from buccal aspect. When compared to maxillary second molar, the crown is shorter in length and narrower in its mesiodistal width. The distobuccal cusp is much smaller than the mesiobuccal cusp.
- The cervical line is irregular without much curvature.
- Buccal developmental groove is seen separating the two buccal cusps.

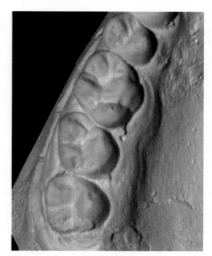

**Fig. 14.26:** Maxillary third molar resembles heart-shaped second molar occlusally.

**Table 14.3:** Maxillary third molar—chronology and measurements.

| Chronology | |
|---|---|
| First evidence of calcification | 7–9 years |
| Enamel completed | 12–16 years |
| Eruption | 17–21 years |
| Roots completed | 18–25 years |
| **Measurements** *Dimensions suggested for carving technique (in mm)* | |
| Cervico-occlusal length of crown | 6.5 |
| Length of root | 11.0 |
| Mesiodistal diameter of crown | 8.5 |
| Mesiodistal diameter of crown at cervix | 6.5 |
| Buccolingual diameter of crown | 10.0 |
| Buccolingual diameter of crown at cervix | 9.5 |
| Curvature of cervical line—mesial | 1.0 |
| Curvature of cervical line—distal | 0.0 |

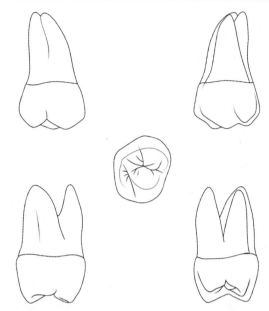

**Fig. 14.27:** Maxillary third molar—line drawings.

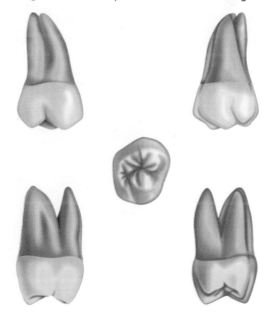

**Fig. 14.28:** Maxillary third molar—graphic illustrations.

## Lingual Aspect (Fig. 14.31)

- The mesiolingual cusp occupies most of the lingual aspect of the crown and thus, there is no lingual developmental groove.
- Sometimes, a small distolingual cusp may be present.
- The lingual surface is spheroidal.

## Mesial and Distal Aspects (Figs. 14.32 and 14.33)

- The distal surface is shorter and narrower than the mesial surface.
- The cervical line on proximal surfaces is rather straight.

## Occlusal Aspect (Fig. 14.34)

From the occlusal view, the tooth generally resembles the heart-shaped type of maxillary permanent second molar.

*Geometric shape:* The occlusal aspect has a heart-shaped outline formed by the three major cusps, namely mesiobuccal, distobuccal, and mesiolingual.

*Relative dimensions:*
- The buccolingual dimension is greater than mesiodistal dimension.
- The crown is larger buccally than lingually.

*Occlusal features:* The occlusal form can be irregular with small tubercles and multiple supplemental grooves. Sometimes, the tooth has four cusps and shows close resemblance to maxillary second molar.

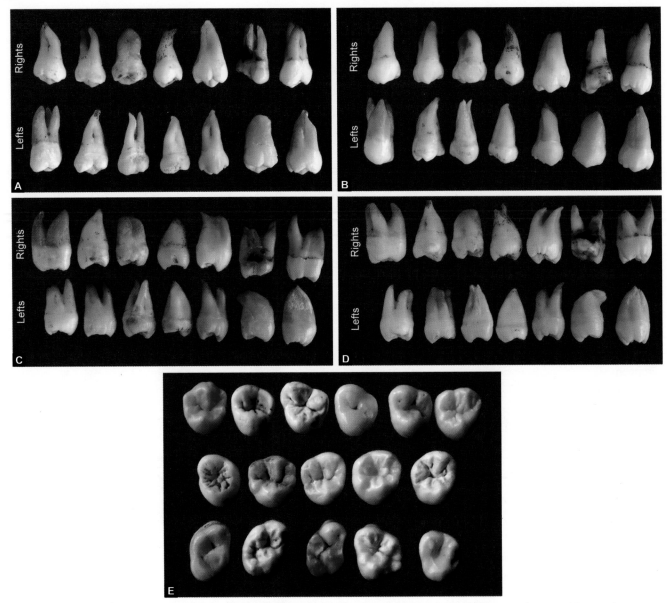

**Figs. 14.29A to E:** Maxillary third molar—typical specimen from all aspects: (A) Buccal aspect; (B) Lingual aspect; (C) Mesial aspect; (D) Distal aspect; (E) Occlusal aspect.

### Root

- Though maxillary third molars have three roots, they function like a single unit as they are often fused together. The fused roots may show division in apical end.
- The roots collectively bend in a distal direction.

### Variations (Fig. 14.35)

- Crown and root of the tooth can be well formed resembling maxillary second molar.
- Very long or very short roots.

- The crown form varies greatly and often sometimes appears like anomalies.

### Clinical Considerations

- Third molars are the most common teeth to be congenitally missing. They may be impacted in the jaw **(Fig. 14.36)**
- They often erupt buccally rather than in line with the dental arch due to shorter space.

**Flowchart 14.5** shows the major anatomic landmarks of maxillary third molar.

← Distal                                    Mesial →

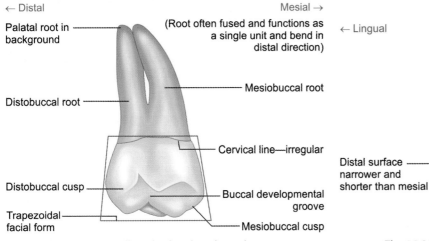

Palatal root in background

(Root often fused and functions as a single unit and bend in distal direction)

Distobuccal root

Mesiobuccal root

Cervical line—irregular

Distobuccal cusp

Buccal developmental groove

Trapezoidal facial form

Mesiobuccal cusp

**Fig. 14.30:** Maxillary third molar—buccal aspect.

← Lingual                                    Buccal →

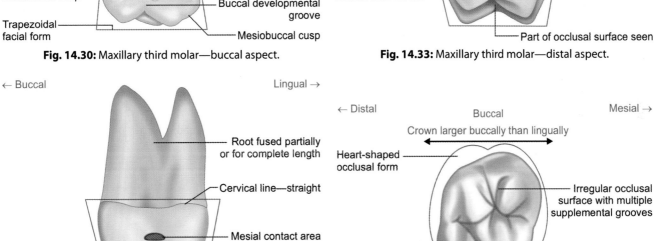

Distal surface narrower and shorter than mesial

Part of occlusal surface seen

**Fig. 14.33:** Maxillary third molar—distal aspect.

← Buccal                                    Lingual →

Root fused partially or for complete length

Cervical line—straight

Mesial contact area at center of crown

Mesiobuccal cusp

Mesiolingual cusp

Trapezoidal proximal form with longer uneven side toward cervix

**Fig. 14.31:** Maxillary third molar—mesial aspect.

← Distal          Buccal          Mesial →

Crown larger buccally than lingually

Heart-shaped occlusal form

Irregular occlusal surface with multiple supplemental grooves

Very small/absent distolingual cusp

Lingual

**Fig. 14.34:** Maxillary third molar—occlusal aspect.

← Mesial                                    Distal →

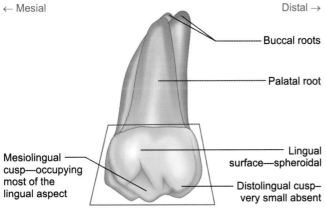

Buccal roots

Palatal root

Mesiolingual cusp—occupying most of the lingual aspect

Lingual surface—spheroidal

Distolingual cusp—very small absent

**Fig. 14.32:** Maxillary third molar—lingual aspect.

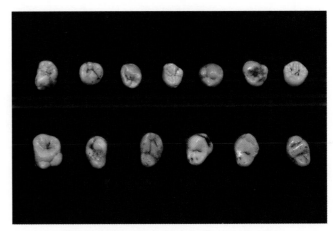

**Fig. 14.35:** Maxillary third molars—variations.

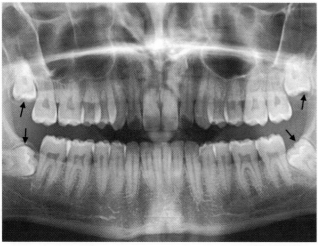

**Fig. 14.36:** The third molars are the most commonly impacted teeth.

Flowchart 14.6 summarizes the morphology of maxillary third molar.

Box 14.3 shows the identification features of maxillary third molar.

The differences between maxillary first, second and third molars (type traits) are given in Table 14.4.

| Box 14.3: Maxillary third molar—identification features. |
|---|
| *Identification features of maxillary third molar:* |
| • Smaller tooth with fused roots |
| • The crown has heart-shaped occlusal outline with a well-developed mesiolingual cusp forming most of the lingual portion |
| • Very small or no distolingual cusp |
| • Multiple supplemental grooves and several small tubercles giving an irregular occlusal form to the tooth |

**Flowchart 14.5:** Maxillary third molar—major anatomic landmarks.

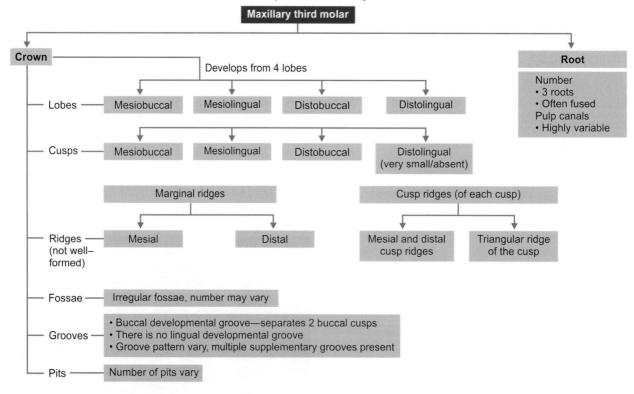

**Flowchart 14.6:** Maxillary third molar—summary.

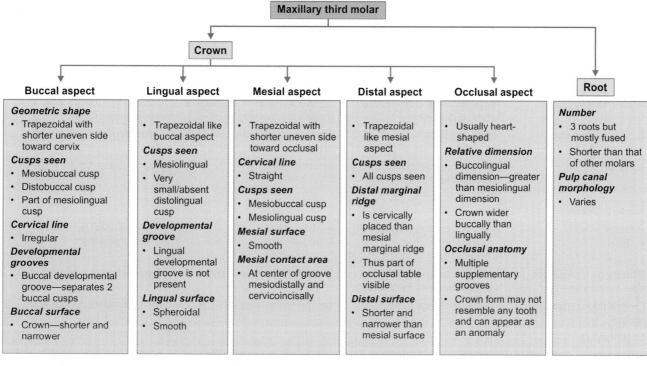

**Table 14.4:** Differences between maxillary first, second, and third molars (type traits).

| Characteristics | Maxillary first molar | | Maxillary second molar | | Maxillary third molar | |
|---|---|---|---|---|---|---|
| *Synonym* | 6-year molar | | 12-year molar | | Wisdom tooth | |
| *Tooth nomenclature* | Right | Left | Right | Left | Right | Left |
| Universal system | 3 | 14 | 2 | 15 | 1 | 16 |
| Zsigmondy/Palmer system | 6⌋ | ⌊6 | 7⌋ | ⌊7 | 8⌋ | ⌊8 |
| FDI system | 16 | 26 | 17 | 27 | 18 | 28 |
| ***Chronology*** | | | | | | |
| First evidence of calcification | At birth | | 2.5–3 years | | 7–9 years | |
| Eruption | 6 years | | 12–13 years | | 17–21 years | |
| Root completion | 9–10 years | | 14–16 years | | 18-25 years | |
| ***General features*** | | | | | | |
| Tooth size | Largest tooth in the arch | | Smaller than first molar | | Smallest molar | |
| Variation in form, eruption pattern, timing | Least variable | | Two crown forms: <br> 1. Rhomboidal (4 cusp type) <br> 2. Heart shaped like third molar (3 cusp type) | | • Most variable tooth in the arch <br> • May be congenitally missing (agenesis), impacted, <br> • Crown form may be irregular, looking like anomaly | |
| Developmental lobes | 5 lobes | | 4 lobes | | 3 or 4 lobes | |
| Number of cusps | 5 | | 4 | | 4 or 3 cusps | |
| ***Crown*** | | | | | | |
| *Buccal aspect*: | | | | | | |
| Crown width | Widest of three | | Moderate width | | Smallest of the three | |
| Height of buccal cusps | Mesiobuccal and distobuccal cusps of same height | | Distobuccal cusp slightly shorter than mesiobuccal cusp | | Distobuccal cusp much shorter than mesiobuccal cusp | |

*Contd...*

*Contd...*

| Characteristics | Maxillary first molar | Maxillary second molar | Maxillary third molar |
|---|---|---|---|
| Crown height | Crown height on distal slightly lesser than on mesial | Distal crown height much shorter than mesial | Distal crown height much more shorter than mesial |
| Distal crown tilt | Crown nearly upright on the root base | Crown shows slight distal tilt on root base due to shorter distobuccal cusp | More distal tilt on root base |
| Mesial and distal profiles | Mesial and distal crown outlines nearly equal sized | Distal crown outline shorter than mesial crown outline | Distal outline much shorter than mesial outline form |
| Occlusal surface slant | Nearly horizontal | Slants cervically from mesial to distal | Slants more cervically toward distal |
| Buccal pit | More pronounced, buccal groove often ends here in buccal pit (often site of caries) | Less marked | May be absent |
| *Proximal contacts:* <br> • Mesial <br> • Distal | • At junction of occlusal and middle third <br> • Middle third | • Middle third <br> • Middle third | • Middle third <br> • No distal contact |
| Visibility of distal surface from buccal view | Portion of distal surface visible, as the distal surface tapers buccally | Distal surface of crown not visible | Distal surface of crown not visible |
| Cervical ridge on buccal surface | Prominent cervical ridge | Less prominent cervical ridge | Least prominent cervical ridge |
| *Lingual aspect:* | | | |
| Crown width | Lingually crown is as wide or wider than buccal surface | Lingual width narrower than on buccal | Narrower on lingual than buccal |
| Lingual convergence | Least or no lingual convergence present | Slight lingual convergence | More lingual convergence |
| Number of cusps on lingual aspect | 2 lingual cusps + 1 accessory cusp (cusp of Carabelli) | 2 (in 4 cusp type/rhomboid shaped); 1 (in 3 cusp type/heart shaped 2nd molar) | Usually 1 (distolingual cusp absent) |
| Distolingual cusp | Never missing | Distolingual cusp is absent in 3 cusp type | Usually absent |
| Size of distolingual cusps | Distolingual cusp smaller than mesiolingual cusp | Distolingual cusp much smaller than mesiolingual cusp | Least in size or entirely absent |
| Accessory cusp (cusp of Carabelli) | • Cusp of Carabelli is additional cusp lingual to mesiolingual cusp <br> • Carabelli's trait may be expressed as a well-formed cusp, a tubercle, groove or a pit <br> • Carabelli's trait is the characteristic feature of maxillary first molar | Rarely present | Not present |
| Lingual developmental groove | Present between two lingual cusp, relatively long | Present in 4 cusp type/rhomboid form of second molar | Absent |
| *Proximal aspects:* | | | |
| Number of cusps visible from mesial aspect | Mesiobuccal, mesiolingual, and cusp of Carabelli | Mesiobuccal and mesiolingual | Mesiobuccal and mesiolingual |
| Buccolingual width | Crown is narrower buccolingually on distal than mesial side | Crown is more narrower buccolingually on distal side | Crown is much narrower buccolingually on distal side |
| Contact areas | Mesial contact area narrower than distal | Mesial and distal contact areas are equally broader | • Broad mesial contact <br> • No distal contact |

*Contd...*

*Contd...*

| Characteristics | Maxillary first molar | Maxillary second molar | Maxillary third molar |
|---|---|---|---|
| Height of contour | | | |
| Buccal | At cervical third (prominent cervical ridge) | Cervical third | Cervical third |
| Lingual | Middle third (when cusp is large, lingual crest of contour more occlusally) | Middle third | Middle third |
| Distal surface area | Shorter | Shorter and narrower | Shorter and narrower |
| *Occlusal aspect*: | | | |
| • Geometric shape | Rhomboidal | Rhomboidal/Heart shaped | Heart shaped |
| • Cusp of Carabelli | Present | Absent | Absent |
| • Oblique ridge | Prominent | Less prominent | Varied |
| • Distolingual cusp size | Relatively large | Smaller | Smallest/absent |

(FDI: Federation Dentaire Internationale)

## BIBLIOGRAPHY

1. Ash MM, Nelson SJ. Wheeler's Dental Anatomy, Physiology and Occlusion, 8th edition. Saunders: St Louis; 2003.
2. Khraisat A, Alsoleihat F, Subramani K, et al. Hypocone reduction and Carabelli's traits in contemporary Jordanians and the association between Carabelli's trait and the dimensions of the maxillary first permanent molar. Coll Antropol. 2011;35(1):73-8.
3. Townsend GC, Brown T. The Carabelli's trait in Australian aboriginal dentition. Arch Oral Biol. 1981;26:809-14.

## MULTIPLE CHOICE QUESTIONS

1. Nonfunctional cusp of maxillary permanent first molar is:
   a. Mesiobuccal cusp
   b. Distobuccal cusp
   c. Mesiolingual cusp
   d. Cusp of Carabelli
2. How many cusps are seen in maxillary permanent first molar?
   a. Four
   b. Five
   c. Two
   d. Three
3. Tripod design of maxillary permanent first molar is best suited to resist:
   a. Oblique occlusal forces
   b. Horizontal force
   c. Vertical force
   d. Transverse force
4. The geometrical shape of buccal aspect of maxillary permanent first molar is:
   a. Trapezoidal
   b. Triangular
   c. Octagonal
   d. Hexagonal
5. Mesial contact area of maxillary permanent first molar is located at:
   a. Occlusal third of the crown
   b. At the junction of occlusal and middle third of the crown
   c. Cervical third of the crown
   d. None of the above
6. The cervical line on the buccal surface of maxillary permanent first molar is:
   a. Regular
   b. In occlusal direction
   c. In apical direction and irregular
   d. None of the above
7. Which is the largest cusp of maxillary permanent first molar?
   a. Mesiobuccal cusp
   b. Distobuccal cusp
   c. Mesiolingual cusp
   d. Distolingual cusp
8. Which cusp is sharper in maxillary permanent first molar?
   a. Mesiobuccal cusp
   b. Distobuccal cusp
   c. Mesiolingual cusp
   d. Distolingual cusp
9. Groove separating mesiobuccal cusp from distobuccal cusp of maxillary permanent first molar is:
   a. Mesiobuccal developmental groove
   b. Distobuccal developmental groove
   c. Buccal developmental groove
   d. Transverse developmental groove
10. Groove separating mesiolingual cusp from distolingual cusp of maxillary permanent first molar is:
   a. Mesiobuccal developmental groove
   b. Distobuccal developmental groove
   c. Lingual developmental groove
   d. Transverse developmental groove

**Answers**

1. d    2. b    3. a    4. a    5. b    6. c    7. c    8. b
9. c    10. c

# 15
**CHAPTER**

# The Permanent Mandibular Molars

## INTRODUCTION

The mandibular molars along with their maxillary counterparts are the most efficient grinding teeth in the dental arches. The three mandibular molars resemble each other in morphology and their size decreases from first to third molars. The mandibular molars have larger crowns and two well-developed roots which are suitably spaced to impart maximum anchorage in the alveolar bone. In mandibular molars, the mesiodistal dimension of the crown is larger than the buccolingual dimension by about 1 mm. It can be remembered that the maxillary molars are wider buccolingually than they are mesiodistally.

## PERMANENT MANDIBULAR FIRST MOLAR

Mandibular and maxillary first molars are among the first permanent teeth to erupt into oral cavity along with the mandibular central incisors at around 6 years of age **(Fig. 15.1)**. The mandibular first molar is the largest tooth in the mandibular arch. It has five cusps: two buccal, two lingual,

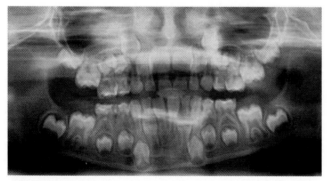

**Fig. 15.1:** Mandibular and maxillary first molars are the first permanent teeth to erupt into oral cavity with mandibular central incisors at 6 years of age (6 years molars).

**Table 15.1:** Mandibular first molar—chronology and measurements.

| Chronology | |
|---|---|
| First evidence of calcification | At birth |
| Enamel completed | 2½–3 years |
| Eruption | 6–7 years |
| Roots completed | 9–10 years |
| **Measurements** *Dimensions suggested for carving technique (in mm)* | |
| Cervico-occlusal length of crown | 7.5 |
| Length of root | 14.0 |
| Mesiodistal diameter of crown | 11.0 |
| Mesiodistal diameter of crown at cervix | 9.0 |
| Buccolingual diameter of crown | 10.5 |
| Buccolingual diameter of crown at cervix | 9.0 |
| Curvature of cervical line—mesial | 1.0 |
| Curvature of cervical line—distal | 0.0 |

and a distal cusp; and two roots—mesial and distal. The chronology and measurements of the mandibular first molar are given in **Table 15.1**.

## DETAILED DESCRIPTION OF MANDIBULAR FIRST MOLAR FROM ALL ASPECTS (FIGS. 15.2 TO 15.4)

### Crown

#### Buccal Aspect (Fig. 15.5)

***Geometric shape:*** The buccal aspect is *trapezoidal* with its shorter uneven side toward the cervical portion.

***Crown outlines:***

*Mesial outline:*
- It is convex except near the cervical line where it is concave.
- Its maximum convexity *(mesial contact area)* is at the junction of occlusal and middle thirds.

*Distal outline:* This outline begins as a straight line near cervix and soon becomes convex forming the *distal contact area* at the middle third of crown.

*Occlusal outline:* It is formed by the cusp ridges of the two buccal cusps and a small distal cusp. The outline is interrupted by two developmental grooves separating the three cusps.

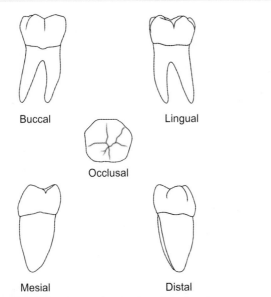

**Fig. 15.2:** Mandibular first molar—line drawing.

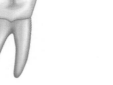

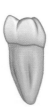

**Fig. 15.3:** Mandibular first molar—graphic illustrations.

*Cervical outline:* The cervical line on buccal surface is curved apically and often shows a sharp dip pointing toward the bifurcation area.

**Buccal surface within the outlines:**
- All the five cusps are visible from buccal aspect.
- The lingual cusps are seen in the background as they are at higher level than the buccal cusps.
- Most of the buccal surface is formed by the two buccal cusps and the distal cusp (mesial portion).
- The mesiobuccal cusp is wider than the distobuccal cusp, which is relatively sharper of the two.
- The mesial and distal cusp ridges of the two buccal cusps are relatively flat and meet at more obtuse angles.
- The two buccal cusps are separated by the *mesiobuccal developmental groove* which runs for half the distance of buccal surface to end in the buccal pit. It is placed slightly mesial to the root bifurcation.
- The distobuccal and distal cusps are separated by the *distobuccal developmental groove* which approaches the distobuccal line angle of the crown. Occasionally, this groove may be absent.
- The buccal surface is convex in the occlusal third except for the interruption of buccal grooves and it is more convex in the cervical third forming the buccal cervical ridge.
- There is a linear concavity in the middle third of the crown extending in a mesiodistal direction, just above the cervical ridge of buccal surface.

## Lingual Aspect (Fig. 15.6)

**Geometric shape:** It is *trapezoidal* like the buccal aspect.

**Crown outlines:** The lingual aspect has four outlines:
- Mesial outline
- Distal outline
} are similar to buccal aspect

- Occlusal outline: It is formed by sharp cusp tips of the lingual cusps and their cusp ridges. The outline is interrupted by the lingual developmental groove in its midway.
- Cervical outline: The cervical line on lingual surface is irregular and may bend apically toward the root bifurcation.

**Lingual surface within the outlines:**
- From lingual aspect, only lingual cusps and small part of distal cusp are seen.
- The crown tapers lingually making the lingual surface narrower than the buccal surface and a part of distal cusp are also visible. Thus, a part of mesial and distal surfaces of the crown can be seen from lingual aspect.
- The two lingual cusps are almost of same width and are sharper and longer than the buccal cusps.
- The mesiolingual cusp tip is at a higher level than the distolingual cusp.
- The distal cusp tip is at a much lower level.
- The *lingual developmental groove* separating the two lingual cusps runs for a shorter distance on the lingual surface and is in line with the bifurcation of the root.
- The lingual surface is smoothly convex in the occlusal portion, and becomes flat in the cervical third.
- There is a shallow concavity in the center of the lingual surface at middle third.

## Mesial Aspect (Fig. 15.7)

**Geometric shape:** The proximal aspect is *rhomboidal* like that of all the mandibular posteriors.

**Crown outlines:**

*Buccal outline:*
- It is more convex in the cervical third at the buccal cervical ridge and from there, it is slightly convex up to the flattened mesiobuccal cusp tip

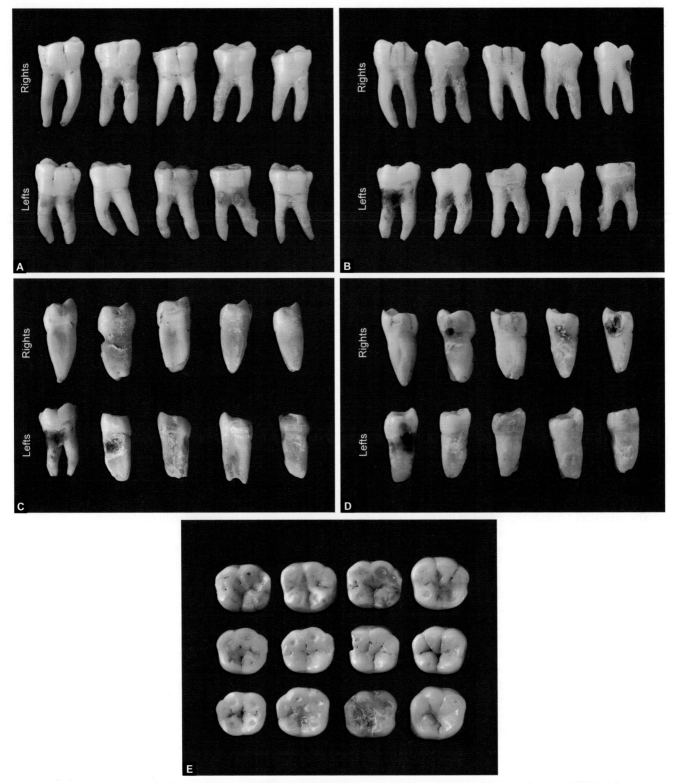

**Figs. 15.4A to E:** Mandibular first molar—typical specimen from all aspects: (A) Buccal aspect; (B) Lingual aspect; (C) Mesial aspect; (D) Distal aspect; (E) Occlusal aspect.

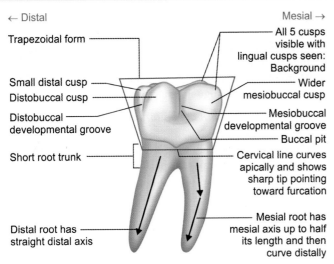

**Fig. 15.5:** Mandibular first molar—buccal aspect.

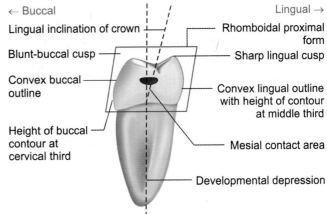

**Fig. 15.7:** Mandibular first molar—mesial aspect.

- The *height of buccal contour* is in the cervical third of the crown.

*Lingual outline:*
- This outline is evenly convex from cervix to the mesiolingual cusp tip.
- The *height of lingual contour* is at the middle third.

*Occlusal outline:*
- It shows a sharp mesiolingual cusp tip at a higher level than the flattened mesiobuccal cusp tip.
- The mesial marginal ridge merges smoothly with the mesial ridge of mesiolingual and mesiobuccal cusps and forms a concave outline.

*Cervical outline:* The cervical line on mesial surface may be straight or slightly curved occlusally and is at a higher level lingually than buccally.

***Mesial surface within the outlines:***
- Only two cusps namely, mesiodistal and mesiolingual cusps can be seen from this aspect.

- The crown shows a lingual inclination on its root base when seen from proximal view. However, the buccal and lingual cusp tips are within the confines of the root base.
- The mesial surface is smoothly convex except for the shallow concavity just below the contact area, which joins the central depression on mesial surface of the mesial root.
- The *mesial contact area* is at the junction of occlusal and middle third of the crown cervico-occlusally and in the center of the crown buccolingually below the mesial marginal ridge.

### Distal Aspect (Fig. 15.8)

***Geometric shape:*** It is *rhomboid* similar to the mesial aspect.

***Crown outlines:***

*Buccal outline* ⎱
*Lingual outline* ⎰ are similar to buccal aspect

*Occlusal outline:*
- The distal marginal ridge is shorter and is at a lower level than the mesial marginal ridge.

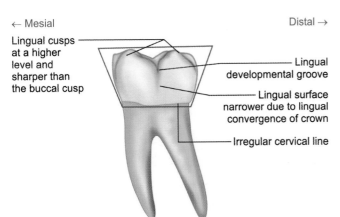

**Fig. 15.6:** Mandibular first molar—lingual aspect.

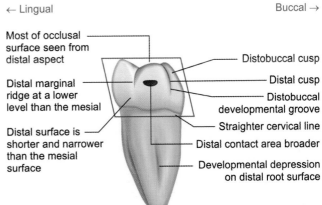

**Fig. 15.8:** Mandibular first molar—distal aspect.

- It is placed lingual to the center of the crown buccolingually.

*Cervical outline:* The cervical line on the distal surface is rather straight without occlusal curvature.

### Distal surface within the outlines:

- The distal surface is shorter and narrower than the mesial surface. Most of the buccal surface and some portion of lingual surface can be seen from this aspect as the crown tapers distally.
- The distolingual and the distal cusps are in the direct line of view. Most of the distobuccal cusp is also seen along with the distobuccal developmental groove.
- Most of the occlusal surface along with the mesial marginal ridge is visible from this aspect as the crown is placed with a distal inclination on the root base and distal marginal ridge is at a lower level.
- The distal surface is smoothly convex.
- The *distal contact area* is on the distal contour of the distal cusp and is placed more buccally and at a higher level than the mesial contact area. The distal contact area is broader than the mesial as the tooth contacts with the second molar tooth distally.

### Occlusal Aspect (Figs. 15.9A and B)

*Geometric shape:* The occlusal aspect of first molar is roughly *hexagonal with unequal sides.* When the distal cusp is very small, the occlusal aspect looks quadrilateral which is the basic form of all mandibular molars.

*Boundaries of occlusal surface:* The occlusal surface is bounded by the cusp ridges of all the five cusps and the marginal ridges.

### Relative dimensions:

- The mesiodistal measurement of the crown is greater than the buccolingual measurement.
- The crown is bulkier mesially than distally as the crown tapers in a distal direction toward the small distal cusp.

*Lingual convergence:*
- Furthermore, the mesial and distal surfaces converge lingually making the lingual surface of the crown narrower than the buccal surface.
- More of buccal surface can be seen from occlusal aspect and very little of lingual surface.

### Occlusal surface within the boundaries:

*Cusps and cusp ridges:*
- From the developmental point of view, the mandibular molars have four major cusps; distal cusp is a minor cusp, although it is often functional. Whereas, the maxillary molars have three major cusps.
- Among the five cusps of mandibular first molars, mesiobuccal (largest) > mesiolingual > distolingual > distobuccal > distal.
- The cusp ridges of the buccal cusps and distal cusp are usually flattened by occlusal wear. The lingual cusps are sharp with well-defined cusp ridges.
- Each cusp has a triangular ridge along with two inclined planes on either side of the triangular ridge. As expected, the triangular ridges of the lingual cusps are well defined.

*Fossae and marginal ridges:*
- *Fossae*
  - There is one major fossa namely *central fossa* and two minor fossae *mesial and distal triangular fossae.*
  - The *central fossa* is a circular large depression in the center of the occlusal surface.
  - It is bounded buccally by the distal slope of mesiobuccal cusp, the mesial and distal slopes of the distobuccal cusp and the mesial slope of distal cusp. Lingually, it is limited by the distal slope of mesiolingual and the mesial slope of distolingual cusp.
  - The *mesial and distal triangular fossae* have the mesial and distal marginal ridges as their base; and the mesial and distal pits as apex respectively.

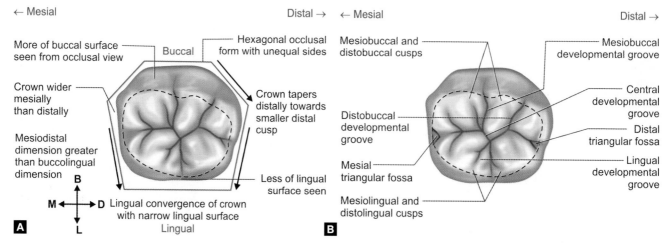

**Figs. 15.9A and B:** Mandibular first molar—occlusal aspect.

- *Marginal ridges:* The distal marginal ridge is shorter and at a lower level than the well-developed mesial marginal ridge.

*Grooves and pits:*

- There are four developmental grooves and some supplemental grooves are seen on the occlusal surface.
- There are three pits. The *central pit* is at the center of the central fossa. The *mesial and distal pits* are in the mesial and distal triangular fossae, respectively.
- The *central developmental groove* originates at the central pit and runs in the opposite directions. Its mesial course from the central pit is relatively smooth and terminates in the mesial triangular fossa. Again from the central pit, the central groove takes a rather irregular course in a distal direction and ends in the distal triangular fossa.
- The *mesiobuccal developmental groove* joins the central developmental groove just mesial to the central pit and runs buccally separating the mesiobuccal and distobuccal cusps and ends on the buccal surface in the buccal pit.
- The *distobuccal developmental groove* joins the central groove, distal to the central pit and runs distobuccally between the distobuccal and distal cusps to end on the buccal surface.
- The *lingual developmental groove* takes a lingual course from the central pit and extends onto the lingual surface separating the two lingual cusps.
- Several supplemental grooves can be seen originating from the developmental grooves.

## Root

Morphology of the root can be described under the following headings:

| | |
|---|---|
| *Number:* | Two well-developed roots—mesial and distal |
| *Size:* | Roots are nearly twice as long as the crown. Both the roots are of same length |
| *Form:* | • The mandibular first molar has a short root trunk and the bifurcation is more near to the cervical line (3–4 mm). There are developmental depressions on the buccal and lingual surfaces of the root trunk extending from the bifurcation point up to the cervical lines |
| | • The mesial root has a straight vertical axis up to half its length, and its apical half is curved distally |
| | • The distal root slants distally from the root base without much curvature |
| *Developmental depressions:* | • There are developmental depressions on mesial and distal surfaces of both the roots extending for the entire length of roots |
| | • The developmental depressions help to provide increased anchorage to the roots in the alveolar bone |
| *Cross-section of roots:* | Cross-sections of both roots show that roots are thinner in the center due to developmental depressions and broader buccally and lingually |
| *Apex:* | Mesial root has a blunt apex and distal root has a relatively sharp apex |

## Variations (Figs. 15.10A and B)

- The mesial root may be bifurcated at the apical third.
- There can be an extra cusp on the occlusal surface called cusp intermedium.

## Developmental Anomalies

- Dilacerations
- Concrescence
- Taurodontism.

## Clinical Considerations

- The mandibular first molars are most commonly affected by dental caries as they erupt early in life and have multiple grooves.

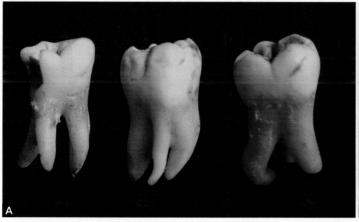 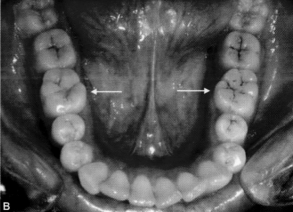

**Figs. 15.10A and B:** Mandibular first molar—variations: (A) Bifurcated mesial root; (B) Supernumerary cusp or six-cusped molar (cusp intermedium).

- The mandibular first molars occlude with the maxillary first molar and they together form an important key of occlusion.
- The maxillary and mandibular first molars erupt (about 6–7 years) when all the primary teeth are still intact and functioning. Thus they provide broader occlusal table assisting the primary molars in mastication of more complex food for growing children.

**Flowcharts 15.1 and 15.2** summarize the anatomy of mandibular first molar.

**Box 15.1** shows the tooth's identification features.

## PERMANENT MANDIBULAR SECOND MOLAR

The permanent mandibular second molar is smaller than the mandibular first molar from all aspects. It has four well-developed cusps, but there is no distal cusp. The tooth has two roots, mesial and distal, which may be as long as that

> **Box 15.1: Mandibular first molar—identification features.**
>
> - *Identification features of mandibular first molar*:
>   - The mandibular first molars have five cusps and two well-formed roots
>   - The distal cusp is the smallest cusp and helps to identify the tooth and its side
> - *Side identification*:
>   - Smallest cusp, i.e. the distal cusp helps in identifying the side
>   - Roots often show distal curvature

of mandibular first molar, though they are not as broad buccolingually. Both the roots have a marked distal inclination and are closely spaced.

The chronology and measurements of the mandibular second molar are given in **Table 15.2**.

**Flowchart 15.1:** Mandibular first molar—major anatomic landmarks.

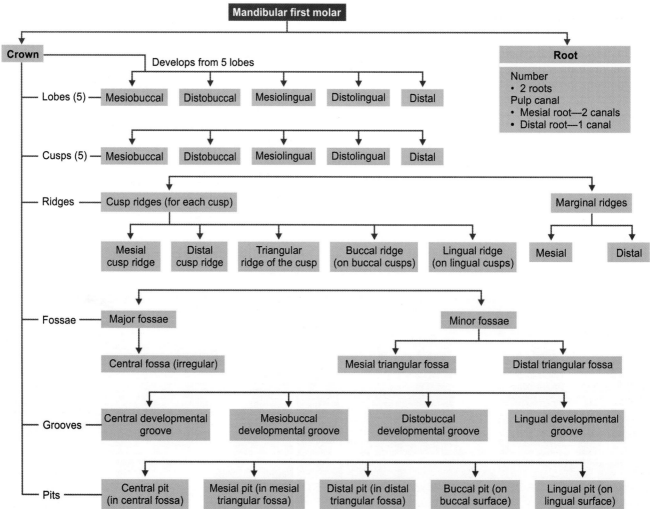

**Flowchart 15.2:** Mandibular first molar—summary.

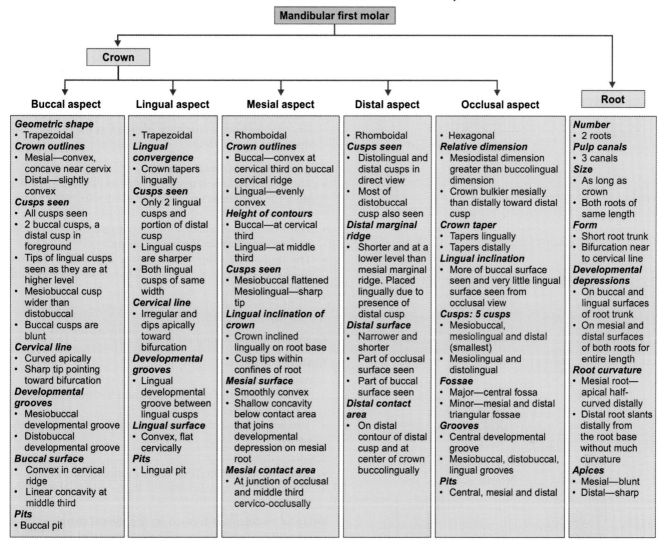

| Buccal aspect | Lingual aspect | Mesial aspect | Distal aspect | Occlusal aspect | Root |
|---|---|---|---|---|---|
| **Geometric shape**<br>• Trapezoidal<br>**Crown outlines**<br>• Mesial—convex, concave near cervix<br>• Distal—slightly convex<br>**Cusps seen**<br>• All cusps seen<br>• 2 buccal cusps, a distal cusp in foreground<br>• Tips of lingual cusps seen as they are at higher level<br>• Mesiobuccal cusp wider than distobuccal<br>• Buccal cusps are blunt<br>**Cervical line**<br>• Curved apically<br>• Sharp tip pointing toward bifurcation<br>**Developmental grooves**<br>• Mesiobuccal developmental groove<br>• Distobuccal developmental groove<br>**Buccal surface**<br>• Convex in cervical ridge<br>• Linear concavity at middle third<br>**Pits**<br>• Buccal pit | • Trapezoidal<br>**Lingual convergence**<br>• Crown tapers lingually<br>**Cusps seen**<br>• Only 2 lingual cusps and portion of distal cusp<br>• Lingual cusps are sharper<br>• Both lingual cusps of same width<br>**Cervical line**<br>• Irregular and dips apically toward bifurcation<br>**Developmental grooves**<br>• Lingual developmental groove between lingual cusps<br>**Lingual surface**<br>• Convex, flat cervically<br>**Pits**<br>• Lingual pit | • Rhomboidal<br>**Crown outlines**<br>• Buccal—convex at cervical third on buccal cervical ridge<br>• Lingual—evenly convex<br>**Height of contours**<br>• Buccal—at cervical third<br>• Lingual—at middle third<br>**Cusps seen**<br>• Mesiobuccal flattened Mesiolingual—sharp tip<br>**Lingual inclination of crown**<br>• Crown inclined lingually on root base<br>• Cusp tips within confines of root<br>**Mesial surface**<br>• Smoothly convex<br>• Shallow concavity below contact area that joins developmental depression on mesial root<br>**Mesial contact area**<br>• At junction of occlusal and middle third cervico-occlusally | • Rhomboidal<br>**Cusps seen**<br>• Distolingual and distal cusps in direct view<br>• Most of distobuccal cusp also seen<br>**Distal marginal ridge**<br>• Shorter and at a lower level than mesial marginal ridge. Placed lingually due to presence of distal cusp<br>**Distal surface**<br>• Narrower and shorter<br>• Part of occlusal surface seen<br>• Part of buccal surface seen<br>**Distal contact area**<br>• On distal contour of distal cusp and at center of crown buccolingually | • Hexagonal<br>**Relative dimension**<br>• Mesiodistal dimension greater than buccolingual dimension<br>• Crown bulkier mesially than distally toward distal cusp<br>**Crown taper**<br>• Tapers lingually<br>• Tapers distally<br>**Lingual inclination**<br>• More of buccal surface seen and very little lingual surface seen from occlusal view<br>**Cusps: 5 cusps**<br>• Mesiobuccal, mesiolingual and distal (smallest)<br>• Mesiolingual and distolingual<br>**Fossae**<br>• Major—central fossa<br>• Minor—mesial and distal triangular fossae<br>**Grooves**<br>• Central developmental groove<br>• Mesiobuccal, distobuccal, lingual grooves<br>**Pits**<br>• Central, mesial and distal | **Number**<br>• 2 roots<br>**Pulp canals**<br>• 3 canals<br>**Size**<br>• As long as crown<br>• Both roots of same length<br>**Form**<br>• Short root trunk<br>• Bifurcation near to cervical line<br>**Developmental depressions**<br>• On buccal and lingual surfaces of root trunk<br>• On mesial and distal surfaces of both roots for entire length<br>**Root curvature**<br>• Mesial root—apical half-curved distally<br>• Distal root slants distally from the root base without much curvature<br>**Apices**<br>• Mesial—blunt<br>• Distal—sharp |

**Table 15.2:** Mandibular second molar—chronology and measurements.

| Chronology | |
|---|---|
| First evidence of calcification | 2½–3 years |
| Enamel completed | 7–8 years |
| Eruption | 11–13 years |
| Roots completed | 14–15 years |
| **Measurements**<br>*Dimensions suggested for carving technique (in mm)* | |
| Cervico-occlusal length of crown | 7.0 |
| Length of root | 13.0 |
| Mesiodistal diameter of crown | 10.5 |
| Mesiodistal diameter of crown at cervix | 8.0 |
| Buccolingual diameter of crown | 10.0 |
| Buccolingual diameter of crown at cervix | 9.0 |
| Curvature of cervical line—mesial | 1.0 |
| Curvature of cervical line—distal | 0.0 |

## DETAILED DESCRIPTION OF MANDIBULAR SECOND MOLAR FROM ALL ASPECTS (FIGS. 15.11 TO 15.13)

### Crown

*Buccal Aspect (Fig. 15.14)*

***Geometric shape:*** Trapezoidal

***Crown outlines:***

*Mesial and distal outlines:* These outlines are usually convex with their maximum convexity at the center of middle third of the crown.

*Occlusal outline:*
• It is formed by the flattened cusp ridges of two buccal cusps.
• It is divided by the buccal developmental groove.
• The lingual cusps may be seen from buccal view.

*Cervical outline:* The cervical outline on buccal surface of the tooth may be a straight line or may tip apically near the bifurcation.

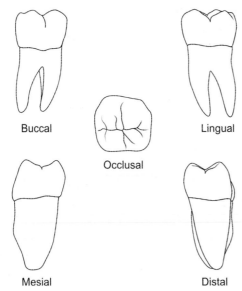

**Fig. 15.11:** Mandibular second molar—line drawing.

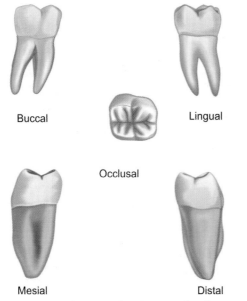

**Fig. 15.12:** Mandibular second molar—graphic illustrations.

### Buccal surface within the outlines:
- The crown appears shorter and narrower than that of mandibular first molar.
- The mesiobuccal and distobuccal cusps are equal in their width and are separated by a short buccal developmental groove which ends within the occlusal third of the crown.
- The buccal aspect has only one developmental groove as there is no distal cusp. The buccal cervical ridge may not be as pronounced as in the mandibular first molar.

### Lingual Aspect (Fig. 15.15)

***Geometric shape:*** *Trapezoidal* like that of the buccal aspect.

***Crown outlines:***
- Mesial outline
- Distal outline ⎱ are similar to that of buccal aspect
- Cervical outline ⎰
- *Occlusal outline:* It is formed by the cusp ridges of two lingual cusps and is separated by the lingual developmental groove. The buccal cusps are not seen as the lingual cusp tips are at a higher level.

### Lingual surface within the outlines:
- The lingual surface is nearly as wide as the buccal surface since the tooth does not converge much toward the lingual aspect.
- The mesiolingual and distolingual cusps are of equal width and are sharper than the buccal cusps.
- The *lingual developmental groove* separating the two lingual cusps runs for a short distance onto the lingual surface.

### Mesial Aspect (Fig. 15.16)

***Geometric shape:*** Rhomboidal

***Crown outlines:***

*Buccal outline:*
- It is convex in the cervical third and becomes flat for the rest of its course.
- The *height of buccal contour* is in the cervical third of the crown.

*Lingual outline:*
- It is convex from cervix up to the mesiolingual cusp tip.
- The *height of lingual contour* is in the middle third of the crown.

*Occlusal outline:* It is formed by the mesial marginal ridge along with the mesial ridges of mesiobuccal and mesiolingual cusps.

*Cervical outline:* The cervical line on the mesial surface is rather straight and regular.

### Mesial surface within the outlines:
- The mesial aspect is similar to that of mandibular first molar.
- Only mesiobuccal and mesiolingual cusps are seen from the mesial aspect.
- The crown shows a lingual inclination on the root base.
- The mesial surface is convex for most of its part and may be flattened near the cervical line, below the contact area.
- *Mesial contact area:* It is at the center of the mesial surface both cervico-occlusally and buccolingually.

### Distal Aspect (Fig. 15.17)

***Geometric shape:*** It is *rhomboidal* like the mesial aspect.

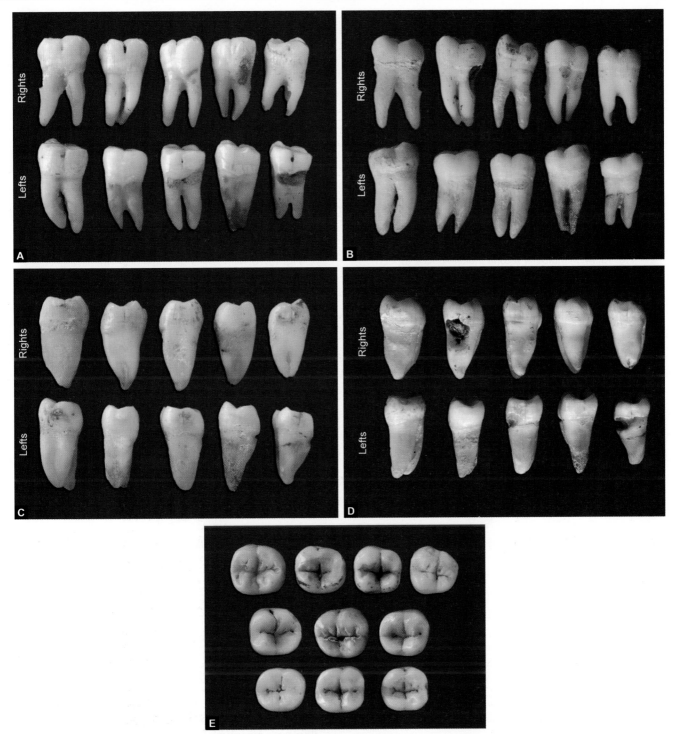

**Figs. 15.13A to E:** Mandibular second molar—typical specimen from all aspects: (A) Buccal aspect; (B) Lingual aspect; (C) Mesial aspect; (D) Distal aspect; (E) Occlusal aspect.

← Distal  Mesial →

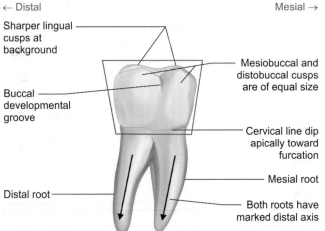

**Fig. 15.14:** Mandibular second molar—buccal aspect.

Labels (Fig. 15.14):
- Sharper lingual cusps at background
- Buccal developmental groove
- Distal root
- Mesiobuccal and distobuccal cusps are of equal size
- Cervical line dip apically toward furcation
- Mesial root
- Both roots have marked distal axis

← Buccal  Lingual →

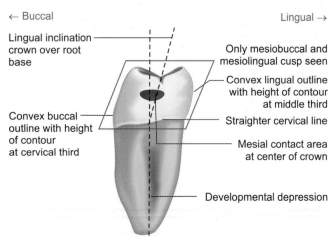

**Fig. 15.16:** Mandibular second molar—mesial aspect.

Labels (Fig. 15.16):
- Lingual inclination crown over root base
- Convex buccal outline with height of contour at cervical third
- Only mesiobuccal and mesiolingual cusp seen
- Convex lingual outline with height of contour at middle third
- Straighter cervical line
- Mesial contact area at center of crown
- Developmental depression

← Mesial  Distal →

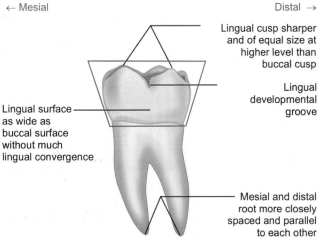

**Fig. 15.15:** Mandibular second molar—lingual aspect.

Labels (Fig. 15.15):
- Lingual surface as wide as buccal surface without much lingual convergence
- Lingual cusp sharper and of equal size at higher level than buccal cusp
- Lingual developmental groove
- Mesial and distal root more closely spaced and parallel to each other

← Lingual  Buccal →

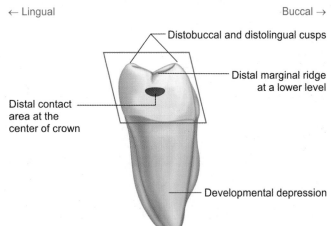

**Fig. 15.17:** Mandibular second molar—distal aspect.

Labels (Fig. 15.17):
- Distal contact area at the center of crown
- Distobuccal and distolingual cusps
- Distal marginal ridge at a lower level
- Developmental depression

***Crown outlines:***
- Buccal outline
- Lingual outline
- Cervical outline

} are similar to that of mesial aspect

- *Occlusal outline:* The distal marginal ridge is at a lower level than the mesial marginal ridge. Some of occlusal surface can be seen from distal aspect.

***Distal surface within the outlines:***
- The distobuccal and distolingual cusps are seen and there is no distal cusp.
- Some part of occlusal surface can be seen from this aspect as the distal marginal ridge is at a lower level.
- The *distal contact area*: It is at the center of the distal surface both cervico-occlusally and buccolingually. Generally, the contact area both mesially and distally is at the same level in case of molars.

## Occlusal Aspect (Figs. 15.18A and B)

***Geometric shape:*** The occlusal aspect of the second molar is rectangular, with the opposing sides nearly equal in length. All the four angles are nearly equal and form right angles.

***Relative dimensions:***
- The mesiodistal dimension is greater than the buccolingual dimension.
- From occlusal view, it can be appreciated that the tooth is as wide lingually as it is buccally. This is because the tooth does not taper much lingually.
- It can also be noted that the distal outline of the crown is more rounded than the mesial outline. Viewed occlusally, the crown is squarish and broader mesially and is more rounded distally.
- There is often a prominence seen cervically near the mesiobuccal line angle.

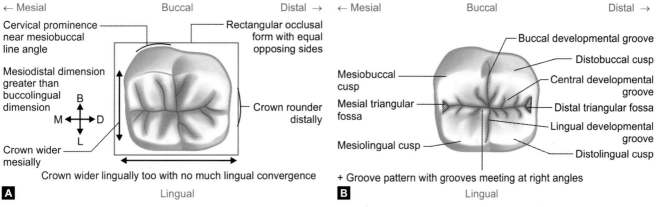

**Figs. 15.18A and B:** Mandibular second molar—occlusal aspect.

*Occlusal surface within the boundaries:*

*Cusps and cusp ridges:*
- The mandibular second molar has four cusps.
- The mesiobuccal and distobuccal cusps are almost equal in size, although the cervical portion of the tooth near mesiobuccal cusp may be more bulky.
- The mesiolingual and distolingual cusps are equally well developed. In general, the lingual cusp ridges are well defined than the more flattened buccal cusp ridges.
- The triangular ridges of all the cusps converge toward the center of the occlusal surface.

*Fossae and marginal ridges:*
- There are two fossae: *mesial and distal triangular fossae.*
- The mesial and distal triangular fossae are nearly equal in size and may have supplemental grooves.
- The *mesial and distal marginal ridges* are well developed and form the base of respective triangular fossa.

*Grooves and pits:*
- There are three pits: *central, mesial, and distal pits.*
- The *groove pattern* forms a typical plus mark "+" or a cross in the center of occlusal aspect, dividing the occlusal portion into four nearly equal parts.
- The *central developmental groove* runs across the occlusal surface from mesial pit to the distal pit.
- The *buccal and lingual grooves* meet the central groove at right angles at the central pit and they run onto the buccal and lingual surfaces of the crown, respectively.
- There is no distobuccal groove.

## Root

Morphology of the root can be described under the following headings:

| | |
|---|---|
| *Number:* | Two roots like mandibular first molar: the mesial and the distal |
| *Size:* | The roots are usually a little shorter than that of mandibular first molar |
| *Form:* | • The mesial and distal roots are closely spaced and they are nearly parallel to each |

other. Both the roots have their axes distally inclined
- The roots may be fused for all or part of their length
- The roots are not as broad buccolingually as those of mandibular first molar

| | |
|---|---|
| *Developmental depressions:* | • The mesial and distal roots have developmental depressions on their mesial and distal surfaces |
| | • The depressions are often seen extending for only apical half of the roots |
| *Curvature:* | Apical ends of the roots in some cases show a mesial curvature |
| *Apex:* | Pointed |

## Variations

The mesial and distal roots can vary in their length and development.

## Developmental Anomalies

- Dilaceration
- Concrescence
- Taurodontism.

Mandibular second molar anatomy is summarized in **Flowcharts 15.3 and 15.4**.

**Box 15.2** shows identification features of the tooth.

## PERMANENT MANDIBULAR THIRD MOLAR

The mandibular third molars exhibit considerable variation in their size, form, and position. Their occlusal anatomy in particular is highly variable from having four cusps like mandibular second molar, five cusps like mandibular first molar, to more than five cusps appearing like small tubercles **(Fig. 15.19)**. When their variation in size is considered, the crowns of mandibular third molars tend to be oversized rather than undersized. Whereas the maxillary third molars tend to be smaller when they are not normal sized.

**Flowchart 15.3:** Mandibular second molar—major anatomic landmarks.

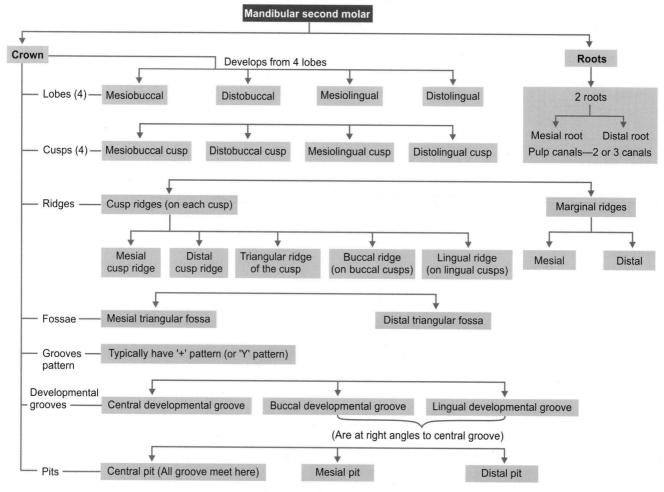

Box 15.2: Mandibular second molar—identification features.

- *Identification features of mandibular second molar:*
  – The mandibular second molar has four cusps and two roots
  – The occlusal aspect has a plus "+" or cross-shaped groove pattern, dividing the occlusal surface into four nearly equal parts
  – Both the roots are distally inclined and extend parallelly and are close to each other
  – Viewed occlusally, there is a cervical prominence seen at mesiobuccal line angle of the crown
- *Side identification:*
  – Viewed from occlusal aspect, the crown is wider mesially than distally
  – Often, there is a prominence cervically near mesiobuccal line angle when viewed from occlusal aspect
  – The roots are inclined distally

The two roots present are shorter, often malformed, and have a tendency to fuse. The roots are more distally inclined than those of first and second mandibular molars. In general,

the mandibular third molars resemble mandibular second molars whom they assist in function. The mandibular third molars are the most common teeth to be impacted, either partially or completely. They can be congenitally absent often bilaterally.

The chronology and measurements of the mandibular third molar are given in **Table 15.3**.

## DETAILED DESCRIPTION OF MANDIBULAR THIRD MOLAR FROM ALL ASPECTS (FIGS. 15.20 TO 15.22)

### Crown

#### *Buccal Aspect (Fig. 15.23)*

- *Geometric shape:* Buccal and lingual aspects of the tooth appear trapezoidal.
- The crown is a little smaller or of same size as that of mandibular second molar.
- The two buccal cusps are seen from buccal aspect, and they are separated by the *buccal developmental groove.*

**Flowchart 15.4:** Mandibular second molar—summary.

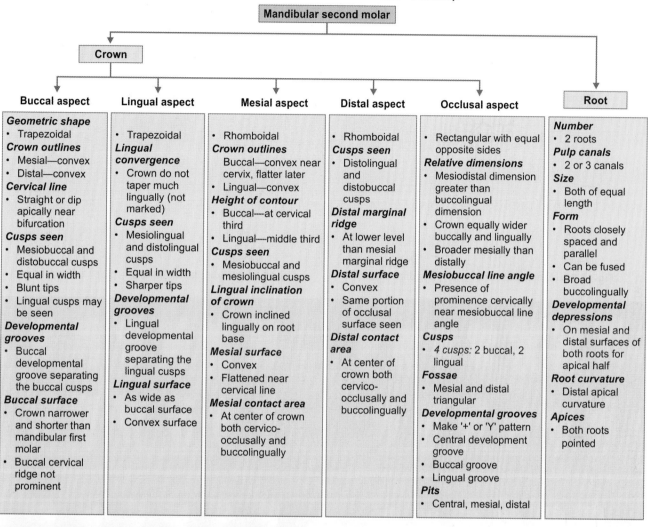

**Mandibular second molar**

**Crown**

### Buccal aspect

*Geometric shape*
- Trapezoidal

*Crown outlines*
- Mesial—convex
- Distal—convex

*Cervical line*
- Straight or dip apically near bifurcation

*Cusps seen*
- Mesiobuccal and distobuccal cusps
- Equal in width
- Blunt tips
- Lingual cusps may be seen

*Developmental grooves*
- Buccal developmental groove separating the buccal cusps

*Buccal surface*
- Crown narrower and shorter than mandibular first molar
- Buccal cervical ridge not prominent

### Lingual aspect

- Trapezoidal

*Lingual convergence*
- Crown do not taper much lingually (not marked)

*Cusps seen*
- Mesiolingual and distolingual cusps
- Equal in width
- Sharper tips

*Developmental grooves*
- Lingual developmental groove separating the lingual cusps

*Lingual surface*
- As wide as buccal surface
- Convex surface

### Mesial aspect

- Rhomboidal

*Crown outlines*
- Buccal—convex near cervix, flatter later
- Lingual—convex

*Height of contour*
- Buccal—at cervical third
- Lingual—middle third

*Cusps seen*
- Mesiobuccal and mesiolingual cusps

*Lingual inclination of crown*
- Crown inclined lingually on root base

*Mesial surface*
- Convex
- Flattened near cervical line

*Mesial contact area*
- At center of crown both cervico-occlusally and buccolingually

### Distal aspect

- Rhomboidal

*Cusps seen*
- Distolingual and distobuccal cusps

*Distal marginal ridge*
- At lower level than mesial marginal ridge

*Distal surface*
- Convex
- Same portion of occlusal surface seen

*Distal contact area*
- At center of crown both cervico-occlusally and buccolingually

### Occlusal aspect

- Rectangular with equal opposite sides

*Relative dimensions*
- Mesiodistal dimension greater than buccolingual dimension
- Crown equally wider buccally and lingually
- Broader mesially than distally

*Mesiobuccal line angle*
- Presence of prominence cervically near mesiobuccal line angle

*Cusps*
- 4 cusps: 2 buccal, 2 lingual

*Fossae*
- Mesial and distal triangular

*Developmental grooves*
- Make '+' or 'Y' pattern
- Central development groove
- Buccal groove
- Lingual groove

*Pits*
- Central, mesial, distal

### Root

*Number*
- 2 roots

*Pulp canals*
- 2 or 3 canals

*Size*
- Both of equal length

*Form*
- Roots closely spaced and parallel
- Can be fused
- Broad buccolingually

*Developmental depressions*
- On mesial and distal surfaces of both roots for apical half

*Root curvature*
- Distal apical curvature

*Apices*
- Both roots pointed

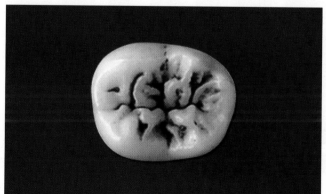

**Fig. 15.19:** Occlusal anatomy of mandibular third molar is highly variable from having 4–5 cusps or many small tubercles.

- Mesial and distal outlines are convex with their maximum convexity at a level occlusal to the center of the crown cervico-occlusally.
- The cervical line may be straight or irregular.

**Table 15.3:** Mandibular third molar—chronology and measurements.

| Chronology | |
|---|---|
| First evidence of calcification | 8–10 years |
| Enamel completed | 12–16 years |
| Eruption | 17–21 years |
| Roots completed | 18–25 years |
| **Measurements** *Dimensions suggested for carving technique (in mm)* | |
| Cervico-occlusal length of crown | 7.0 |
| Length of root | 11.0 |
| Mesiodistal diameter of crown | 10.0 |
| Mesiodistal diameter of crown at cervix | 7.5 |
| Buccolingual diameter of crown | 9.5 |
| Buccolingual diameter of crown at cervix | 9.0 |
| Curvature of cervical line—mesial | 1.0 |
| Curvature of cervical line—distal | 0.0 |

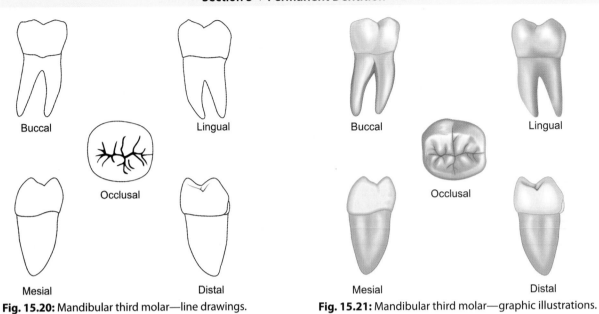

**Fig. 15.20:** Mandibular third molar—line drawings.

Buccal

Lingual

Occlusal

Mesial

Distal

**Fig. 15.21:** Mandibular third molar—graphic illustrations.

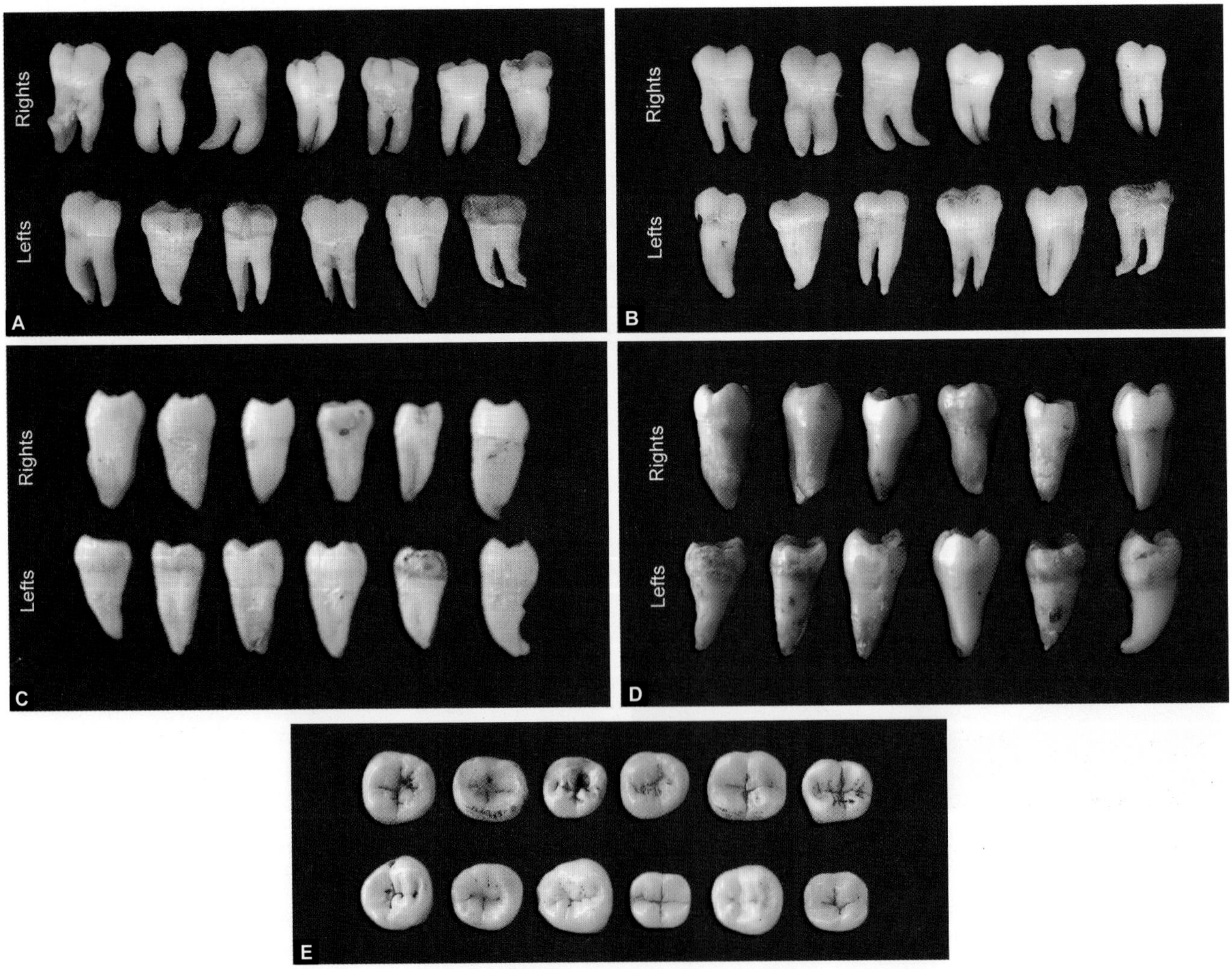

Buccal

Lingual

Occlusal

Mesial

Distal

Rights

Lefts

A

Rights

Lefts

B

Rights

Lefts

C

Rights

Lefts

D

E

**Figs. 15.22A to E:** Mandibular third molar—typical specimen from all aspects: (A) Buccal aspect; (B) Lingual aspect; (C) Mesial aspect; (D) Distal aspect; (E) Occlusal aspect.

### Lingual Aspect (Fig. 15.24)

- It is similar to buccal aspect in general.
- The two lingual cusps are seen from this aspect and are separated by the *lingual developmental groove*.

### Mesial Aspect (Fig. 15.25)

- *Geometric shape:* Rhomboidal
- The mesiobuccal and mesiolingual cusps are seen from this aspect whose mesial slopes merge with the mesial marginal ridge.
- The *height of buccal contour* is at cervical third and that of *lingual contour* is at the middle third of the crown.
- The *mesial contact area* is broad, centered buccolingually, and a little occlusal to the center of the tooth cervico-occlusally.

### Distal Aspect (Fig. 15.26)

- *Geometric shape:* Rhomboidal

- The distobuccal and distolingual cusp tips are usually at a lower level than the mesiobuccal and mesiolingual cusp tips.
- Distal marginal ridge is at a lower level than the mesial marginal ridge.
- Thus the cusps along with most of the portion of occlusal surface can be seen from the distal aspect.
- The third molars have only one contact area—mesial, as they are the last teeth in the dental arches.

### Occlusal Aspect (Fig. 15.27)

**Geometric shape:** It is quadrilateral similar to that of mandibular second molar.

**Relative dimensions:** The mesiodistal dimension is greater than the buccolingual dimension. Crown tends to be smaller distally than mesially.

**Occlusal anatomy:**

- Usually the mandibular third molars have an occlusal design similar to that of mandibular second molar with four cusps

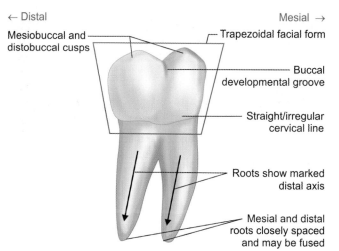

← Distal        Mesial →

Mesiobuccal and distobuccal cusps

Trapezoidal facial form

Buccal developmental groove

Straight/irregular cervical line

Roots show marked distal axis

Mesial and distal roots closely spaced and may be fused

**Fig. 15.23:** Mandibular third molar—features on buccal aspect.

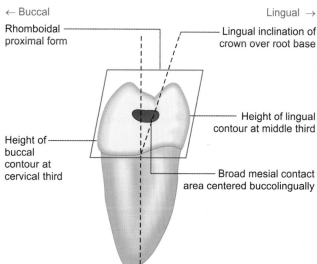

← Buccal        Lingual →

Rhomboidal proximal form

Lingual inclination of crown over root base

Height of lingual contour at middle third

Height of buccal contour at cervical third

Broad mesial contact area centered buccolingually

**Fig. 15.25:** Mandibular third molar—features on mesial aspect.

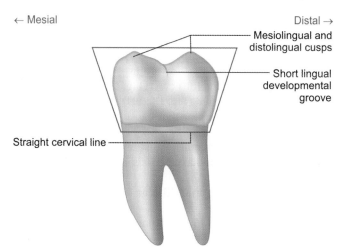

← Mesial        Distal →

Mesiolingual and distolingual cusps

Short lingual developmental groove

Straight cervical line

**Fig. 15.24:** Mandibular third molar—features on lingual aspect.

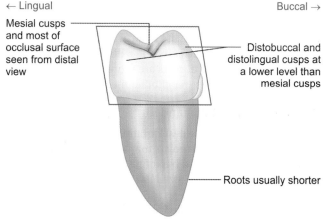

← Lingual        Buccal →

Mesial cusps and most of occlusal surface seen from distal view

Distobuccal and distolingual cusps at a lower level than mesial cusps

Roots usually shorter

**Fig. 15.26:** Mandibular third molar—features on distal aspect.

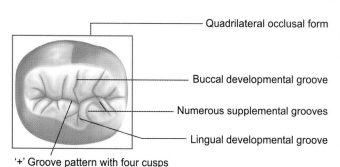

Fig. 15.27: Mandibular third molar—features on occlusal aspect.

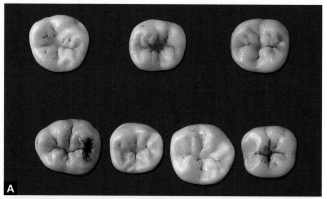

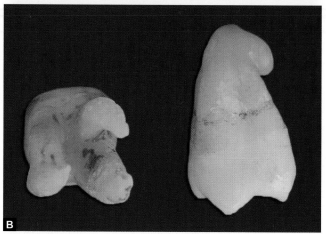

Figs. 15.28A and B: Mandibular third molar—variations.

and "+" shaped groove pattern. They may also show "*Y*" *groove pattern*.

- Some third molars may also resemble mandibular first molars carrying five cusps. There are yet others which may appear like anomalies with more than five cusps or several small tubercles roughened by multiple grooves.
- When they are well formed and resemble mandibular second molars, the occlusal surface is divided into four parts by central, buccal, and lingual developmental grooves.

## Root

Morphology of the root can be described under the following headings:

| | |
|---|---|
| *Number:* | Two roots which may be fused |
| *Size:* | • The roots are generally small, poorly developed and shorter than that of mandibular second molar. |
| | • Even when the crown is oversized, the roots tend to be shorter |
| *Form:* | • The mesial and distal roots may be separated or fused for all or part of their length |
| | • The roots are inclined distally to a greater extent than seen in the mandibular second molars |
| | • Both the roots taper more rapidly from cervix to their apical ends |
| | • May be curved in a distal direction |
| *Apex:* | Apices of roots are more pointed than those of other mandibular molars |

## Variations (Figs. 15.28A and B)

- Third molars show greatest variation in form.
- The mandibular third molars may resemble second molar or sometimes the mandibular first molar.
- The crowns can be oversized having five or more than five cusps.
- The roots can be bifurcated at their apical ends.
- The roots may be very short.

## Developmental Anomalies

- Dilaceration
- Concrescence.

## Clinical Considerations (Figs. 15.29A to D)

- The mandibular third molars are the most commonly impacted teeth, either partially or completely, often due to lack of space in the jaw **(Fig. 15.29A)**.
- When the tooth is partially erupted, the surrounding mucosa may get inflamed which is called as *pericoronitis* **(Fig. 15.29B)**. This condition can be quite painful and may cause difficulty in opening the mouth.
- Impacted third molars are often associated with cyst development (dentigerous cyst) **(Fig. 15.29C)**.
- When partially erupted **(Fig. 15.29D)**, food impaction and inaccessibility to cleaning may cause caries of the tooth or its adjacent tooth.
- The impacted tooth may also cause resorption of the roots of mandibular second molar when it is in close approximation with the latter tooth.
- The maxillary and mandibular third molars can be congenitally absent.

**Flowcharts 15.5 and 15.6** summarize the mandibular third molar anatomy.

**Box 15.3** shows identification features of the tooth.

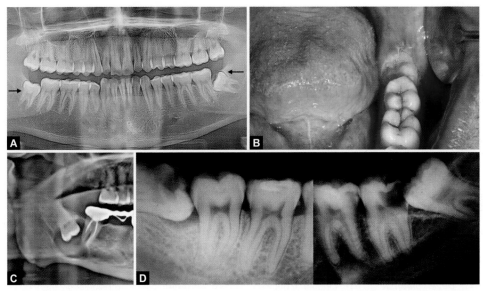

**Figs. 15.29A to D:** (A) Impacted mandibular third molars; (B) Pericoronitis of partially erupted mandibular third molar; (C) Dentigerous cyst developing around an unerupted mandibular third molar; (D) Caries in the partially impacted mandibular third molar or its adjacent tooth.

**Flowchart 15.5:** Mandibular third molar—major anatomic landmarks.

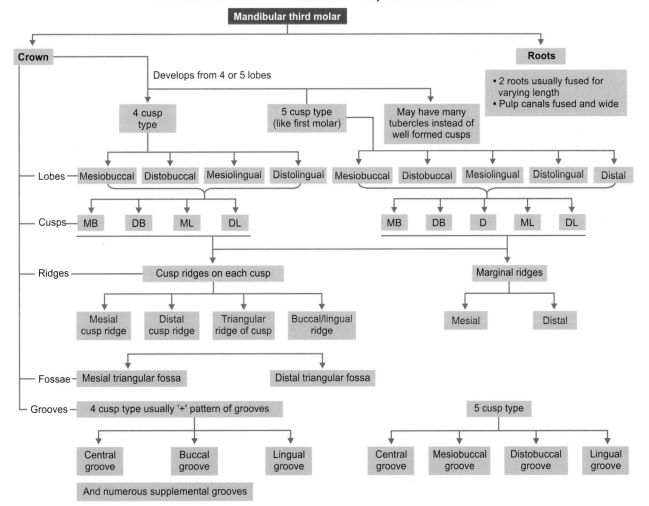

Flowchart 15.6: Mandibular third molar—summary.

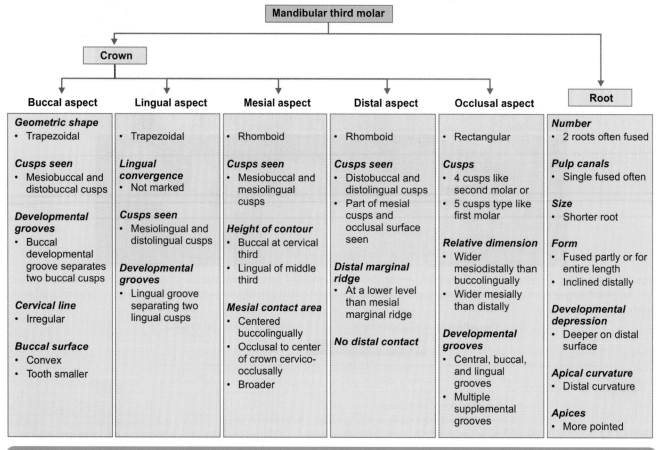

**Mandibular third molar**

**Crown**

**Buccal aspect**

*Geometric shape*
- Trapezoidal

*Cusps seen*
- Mesiobuccal and distobuccal cusps

*Developmental grooves*
- Buccal developmental groove separates two buccal cusps

*Cervical line*
- Irregular

*Buccal surface*
- Convex
- Tooth smaller

**Lingual aspect**
- Trapezoidal

*Lingual convergence*
- Not marked

*Cusps seen*
- Mesiolingual and distolingual cusps

*Developmental grooves*
- Lingual groove separating two lingual cusps

**Mesial aspect**
- Rhomboid

*Cusps seen*
- Mesiobuccal and mesiolingual cusps

*Height of contour*
- Buccal at cervical third
- Lingual of middle third

*Mesial contact area*
- Centered buccolingually
- Occlusal to center of crown cervico-occlusally
- Broader

**Distal aspect**
- Rhomboid

*Cusps seen*
- Distobuccal and distolingual cusps
- Part of mesial cusps and occlusal surface seen

*Distal marginal ridge*
- At a lower level than mesial marginal ridge

*No distal contact*

**Occlusal aspect**
- Rectangular

*Cusps*
- 4 cusps like second molar or
- 5 cusps type like first molar

*Relative dimension*
- Wider mesiodistally than buccolingually
- Wider mesially than distally

*Developmental grooves*
- Central, buccal, and lingual grooves
- Multiple supplemental grooves

**Root**

*Number*
- 2 roots often fused

*Pulp canals*
- Single fused often

*Size*
- Shorter root

*Form*
- Fused partly or for entire length
- Inclined distally

*Developmental depression*
- Deeper on distal surface

*Apical curvature*
- Distal curvature

*Apices*
- More pointed

**Box 15.3: Mandibular third molar—identification features.**

*Identification features of mandibular third molar:*
- Usually, the mandibular third molars are similar to mandibular second molars, but a little smaller in size
- The occlusal surface shows more number of supplemental grooves
- The roots are shorter and more pointed and have an extreme distal tilt
- They often have fused roots

The Differences between maxillary and mandibular molars (arch traits) are given in **Table 15.4** and Differences between mandibular first, second, and third molars (type traits) are given in **Table 15.5**.

**Table 15.4: Differences between maxillary and mandibular molars (arch traits).**

| Characteristics | Maxillary molars | Mandibular molars |
|---|---|---|
| **Tooth nomenclature** | | |
| Universal system | Right 1, 2, 3; left 14, 15, 16 | Right 30, 31, 32; left 17, 18, 19 |
| Zsigmondy/Palmer system | Right 6̲, 7̲, 8̲; Left 6̲, 7̲, 8̲ | Right 6̅, 7̅, 8̅; Left 6̅, 7̅, 8̅ |
| FDI system | Right 16, 17, 18; left 26, 27, 28 | Right 46, 47, 48; left 36, 37, 38 |
| **General features:** | | |
| Development | 4 to 5 lobes<br>One lobe for each cusp | 4 to 5 lobes<br>One lobe for each cusp |
| Number of cusps | • In general, 3 large cusps and 1 small cusp—the distolingual cusp<br>• 3 large cusps make the maxillary molar primary cusp triangle(they are mesiobuccal, mesiolingual, and distobuccal cusps) | • In general, 4 large cusps—2 buccal, 2 lingual<br>• First molar has 5 cusps; the additional small cusp is the distal cusp<br>• No cusp of Carabelli |

*Contd...*

*Contd...*

| Characteristics | Maxillary molars | Mandibular molars |
|---|---|---|
| | • An accessory cusp is present only in first molar—cusp of Carabelli | |
| Size of the cusps | 2 buccal cusps are unequal—mesiobuccal cusp is larger than distobuccal cusp<br>2 lingual cusp are unequal, distolingual is the smallest of all cusps | 2 main buccal cusps—mesiobuccal and distobuccal are equal in size<br>2 lingual cusps are of equal size |
| Crown dimensions | Buccolingual diameter is greater than the mesiodistal diameter | Mesiodistal diameter is larger than buccolingual |
| Oblique ridge | Oblique ridge on occlusal surface is a characteristic feature of maxillary molars | No oblique ridge |
| **Crown** | | |
| *Buccal aspect:* | | |
| Geometric form | Trapezoid | Trapezoid |
| Crown width | Mesiodistal width is greater than cervicoincisal crown height | Mesiodistal width is much greater than crown height |
| Buccal cusps | Sharper | Blunt and often attrited |
| Lingual cusp visibility | Only a part of lingual cusps is visible from buccal view | All the cusps are visible from buccal view due to blunt buccal cusps |
| Visibility of distal surface | Distal surface is visible because of crown form | Not visible from this view |
| Developmental grooves on buccal surface | One buccal groove separating the buccal cusps | Two buccal grooves—on first molar (and third molar)<br>One buccal groove—second and third molars |
| *Contact areas* | | |
| Mesial distal | • At or near the junction of occlusal and middle third<br>• At middle third | • At or near the junction of occlusal and middle third<br>• At middle third |
| Buccal surface | Relatively vertical | Buccal surface bends lingually from middle third |
| *Lingual aspect:* | | |
| Geometric form | Trapezoid | Trapezoid |
| Lingual convergence | • First molar—no lingual taper<br>• Less lingual convergence in second and third molars | Marked lingual tapering of crown, especially in first molar |
| Visibility of proximal surfaces from lingual view | Portion of mesial surface visible from this view | Portion of both mesial and distal surfaces visible from this view |
| *Proximal aspect:* | | |
| Geometric form | Trapezoid | Rhomboid |
| Lingual crown tilt | Crown upright over root base | Crown tilted lingually over the root base (a feature common to all the mandibular teeth) |
| Buccal cervical ridge | Less prominent | More prominent, especially on first molar |
| Proximal surfaces | Distal surface narrower than mesial | Distal surface narrower than mesial |
| *Occlusal aspect:* | | |
| Geometric form | Rhomboid—with 2 acute and 2 obtuse angles | Quadrilateral |
| Crown dimension | Buccolingual diameter greater than mesiodistal | Mesiodistal diameter greater than buccolingual |
| Lingual convergence | • No marked lingual convergence<br>• Crown converges toward buccal in first molar | Marked lingual convergence in all molars |
| Mesiodistal width | Mesiodistal width at lingual is greater than that at buccal in first molar | Mesiodistal dimension greater buccally than lingually |
| Crown taper | Crown tapers from mesial toward distal aspect | Crown tapers from mesial toward distal aspect |
| Buccolingual width | Greater mesially than distally | Greater mesially than distally |

*Contd...*

*Contd...*

| Characteristics | Maxillary molars | Mandibular molars |
|---|---|---|
| Number of cusps | • First molar—5 cusp<br>• Second and third molars—4 cusps | • First molar—5 cusps<br>• Second molar—4 cusps<br>• Third molar—4 or 5 cusps |
| Accessory cusp | Cusp of Carabelli on first molar | No accessory cusp |
| Largest cusp | Mesiopalatal cusp | Mesiobuccal cusp |
| Size of lingual cusps | Unequal in size | Equal in size |
| Centric holding cusps | Lingual cusps | Buccal cusps |
| Primary cusp triangle | • Developmentally only 3 major cusps (2 buccal and mesiolingual cusps) are considered as primary<br>• They make a triangular arrangement | No primary cusp triangle present |
| Third molars | When not of normal size, tends to be smaller | When not of normal size, tends to be larger |
| Third molars resemblance | Third molars resemble second molar | Third molars resemble first or second molar |
| Distolingual cusp size | Decreases from first molar to third molar in which it may be absent completely | No significant decrease in size |
| Oblique ridge | • Ridge running obliquely on occlusal surface<br>• Formed by union of distal ridge of mesiopalatal cusp and triangular ridge of distobuccal cusp<br>• Most prominent on first molar and barely visible on third molar | No oblique ridge |
| Fossae | Four fossae:<br>• 2 major fossae—central and distal<br>• 2 minor fossae—mesial and distal triangular fossae | Three fossae:<br>• One major central fossa<br>• Two minor—mesial and distal triangular fossae |
| Groove pattern | No "Y" or "+" pattern | "Y" or "+" pattern |
| **Root** | | |
| Number | • Roots—2 buccal and 1 palatal<br>• Tripod arrangement—gives good anchorage in alveolar bone | 2 roots—1 mesial and 1 distal |
| Size | Palatal root—strongest and longest | Two roots are equal in size and length |
| Root trunk | Long | Short, nearer to cervical line especially in second molar |

(FDI: Federation Dentaire Internationale)

**Table 15.5: Differences between mandibular first, second, and third molars (type traits).**

| Characteristics | Mandibular first molar | | Mandibular second molar | | Mandibular third molar | |
|---|---|---|---|---|---|---|
| *Synonym* | 6-year molar | | 12-year molar | | Wisdom tooth | |
| ***Tooth nomenclature*** | Right | Left | Right | Left | Right | Left |
| Universal system | 30 | 19 | 31 | 18 | 32 | 17 |
| Zsigmondy/Palmer system | 6⌐ | ⌐6 | 7⌐ | ⌐7 | 8⌐ | ⌐8 |
| FDI system | 46 | 36 | 47 | 37 | 48 | 38 |
| ***Chronology*** | | | | | | |
| First evidence of calcification | At birth | | 2.5–3 years | | 8–10 years | |
| Eruption | 6–7 years | | 11–13 years | | 17–21 years | |
| Root completion | 9–10 years | | 14–15 years | | 18–25 years | |
| Development | 5 lobes | | 4 lobes | | 4 and 5 lobes | |
| Tooth size | Largest tooth in mandibular arch | | Smaller than first molar | | Smallest of mandibular molars | |
| Number of cusps | Five: 2 buccal; 2 lingual; 1 distal | | Four: 2 buccal; 2 lingual | | Four: 2 buccal; 2 lingual | |

*Contd...*

*Contd...*

| Characteristics | Mandibular first molar | Mandibular second molar | Mandibular third molar |
|---|---|---|---|
| Variations | Least variable | Less variable | • Highly variable<br>• Can be 4 or 5 cusps (like first molar)<br>• Small or large<br>• May be congenitally missing<br>• Impaction common |
| *Buccal aspect:* | | | |
| Number of cusps on buccal aspect | *Three:* Mesiobuccal, distobuccal, and distal cusps | *Two:* Mesiobuccal and distobuccal | *Two:* Mesiobuccal and distobuccal |
| Size of buccal cusps | Mesiobuccal cusp is the largest | Both the buccal cusps nearly same size | Both the buccal cusps nearly same size |
| Mesiodistal crown width | Greatest mesiodistal width among all permanent teeth | Mesiodistal width less than first molar | Mesiodistal width less |
| Mesiodistal width at cervix | Crown narrower at cervix | Crown appear broader at cervix due to absence of distal cusp | Broader at cervix |
| Relative crown dimensions | Mesiodistal crown width is much greater than cervico-occlusal height | Mesiodistal crown width is slightly greater than cervico-occlusal height | Mesiodistal crown width may be equal to or greater than cervico-occlusal height |
| Crown height | • Crown appears shorter due to its greater mesiodistal width<br>• Crown is shorter at distal than mesial side | • Crown appears longer<br>• Its length is nearly same; both mesially and distally | Crown height varies |
| Developmental groove on buccal surface | Two developmental grooves—mesiobuccal and distobuccal, long groove | • One buccal development groove—relatively shorter<br>• Also distobuccal developmental groove | Varies:<br>• One buccal developmental groove (in 4 cusp type)<br>• Two buccal developmental groove (in 5 cusp type) |
| Buccal pit | • Commonly present, caries can occur<br>• Mesiobuccal developmental groove terminates in this pit | Less common | Varies |
| Visibility of lingual cusps | Since buccal cusps are blunt, the lingual cusp are visible from buccal view | The lingual cusp are visible | The lingual cusp are visible |
| *Proximal contact areas:*<br>• Mesial<br>• Distal | • At junction occlusal and middle third<br>• At middle third | • At middle third<br>• At middle third | • Middle third<br>• No distal contact |
| Crown taper to cervical | Mesial and distal outlines taper noticeably from contact areas to cervical line | Less tapering mesial and distal crown outlines | May or may not taper to cervical |
| Distal crown tilt | Crown appears to be tilted to distal on root base due to shorter crown height distally | Not much distal tilt | May or may not show distal crown tilt |
| Occlusal surface tilt | Occlusal surface slopes cervically from mesial to distal direction | Occlusal surface is horizontal | May be horizontal or slanting |
| *Lingual aspect:* | | | |
| Lingual convergence | Marked lingual convergence | No much tapering toward lingual | Can vary |
| Lingual surface | Narrower than the buccal surface since crown tapers toward lingual | Nearly of same width as buccal surface | Narrower or of same width |

*Contd...*

*Contd...*

| Characteristics | Mandibular first molar | Mandibular second molar | Mandibular third molar |
|---|---|---|---|
| Visibility of buccal profile | Buccal profile and portion of proximal surfaces visible from lingual aspect | Not visible | May or may not be visible |
| Lingual cusps | Longer and more pointed than the buccal cusps | Longer and more pointed than the buccal cusps | Variable |
| Cusp visibility | Lingual cusp and a part of distal cusp visible | Only lingual cusps visible | Only lingual cusps (like third molar—4 cusp type) |
| Developmental groove on lingual surface | Lingual groove separates mesiolingual and distolingual cusps | Lingual groove shorter | Shorter or not present |
| Lingual pit | Often present lingual groove terminates here | May be present | Usually absent |
| *Proximal aspects:* | | | |
| Crown height | Shorter on distal aspect than mesial | Crown height nearly same on mesial and distal aspect | Variable |
| Lingual crown inclination over root base | Crown more tilted lingually | Moderately tilted lingually | Less tilt lingually |
| Contact areas | Mesial contact area is smaller than distal, as tooth contacts with a premolar on mesial side | Both contact areas are broader as the tooth contacts with molar on both sides | • Broad mesial contact<br>• No distal contact |
| *Height of contours:* | | | |
| • Buccal contour<br>• Lingual contour | • At cervical third<br>• At middle third | • At cervical third<br>• At middle third | • At cervical third<br>• At middle third |
| Buccal cervical ridge | More prominent | Less prominent | Least prominent |
| Occlusal surface visibility | Greater occlusal surface visible from distal view | Some portion of occlusal surface visible from distal view | Can vary |
| Cusps seen from distal aspect | Distal, distobuccal, and distolingual cusps | Distobuccal and distolingual cusps | Distobuccal and distolingual cusps |
| *Occlusal aspect:* | | | |
| Occlusal form | Hexagonal with unequal size | Rectangular with opposing sides equal | Varies |
| Relative crown dimensions | Mesiodistal dimension much greater than buccolingual dimension | Mesiodistal dimension slightly greater than buccolingual dimension | Varies |
| Lingual convergence | More pronounced taper | Less taper | Less taper |
| Mesiodistal crown width | Greater on buccal side than on lingual | Nearly equal on buccal and lingual | Nearly equal on buccal and lingual or greater on buccal |
| Crown taper to distal | Marked tapering toward distal | Less taper | Varies |
| Buccolingual width | Greater mesially than distally | Nearly equal both on mesial and distal | Varies |
| Cervical bulge | Not present | Prominent cervical bulge at mesiobuccal line angle | Not present |
| Occlusal table | Broadest of all teeth in the arch | Smaller than first molar | Smaller/bigger |
| *Marginal ridges:* | | | |
| • Mesial<br>• Distal | • Straight and converge lingually<br>• Distal shorter, not well developed | • Curved and do not converge to lingual<br>• Mesial and distal marginal ridge of same length | • More curved<br>• Equal or vary |
| Distal cusp | Present | Not present | • Absent (in 4 cusp type)<br>• Present (in 5 cusp type) |
| Groove pattern | Main developmental grooves form "Y" pattern | Main developmental grooves form "+" pattern | "+" pattern or "Y" pattern |

*Contd...*

Contd...

| Characteristics | Mandibular first molar | Mandibular second molar | Mandibular third molar |
|---|---|---|---|
| **Root** | | | |
| Number | *Two:* Mesial and distal | *Two:* Mesial and distal | Two or fused to one root |
| Size | Broader buccolingually | Narrower than first molar | Much narrower |
| Length | Mesial and distal roots of same length | Shorter than that of first molar | Much shorter |
| Spacing between roots | Spread wide apart | Closely spaced/sometimes partly fused | Very close/fused |
| Vertical axis of roots | • Mesial root straight for half length, then curved distally; • Distal root slants distally for whole length | • Both nearly parallel • Both roots have more distal inclination | Straight or curved distally |
| Developmental depression on root | Extend longitudinally on both roots for entire length | Extend for only apical half of root length | Less marked depression/absent |
| Variations | Less likely | Less likely | More commonly vary—supernumerary root, crooked root |

(FDI: Federation Dentaire Internationale)

## BIBLIOGRAPHY

1. Ash MM, Nelson SJ (Eds). Wheeler's Dental Anatomy, Physiology and Occlusion, 8th edition. Saunders: St Louis; 2003.
2. Brand RW, Isselhard DE (Eds). Anatomy of Orofacial Structures, 5th edition. CV Mosby: St Louis; 1994.
3. Sicher H, DuBrul EL (Eds). Oral Anatomy, 7th edition. CV Mosby: St Louis; 1975.
4. Woelfel JB, Scheid RC (Eds). Dental Anatomy: Its relevance to dentistry, 5th edition. Williams and Wilkins: Baltimore; 1997.

## MULTIPLE CHOICE QUESTIONS

1. In mandibular arch, the size of the molar teeth:
   a. Increases from first molar to third molar
   b. Decreases from first molar to third molar
   c. Remains same for all three molars
   d. None of the above
2. Mandibular molar crowns are:
   a. Wider mesiodistally than buccolingually
   b. Wider buccolingually than mesiodistally
   c. Equal in mesiodistal and buccolingual dimensions
   d. None of the above
3. The largest tooth of mandibular arch in permanent dentition is:
   a. Mandibular second premolar
   b. Mandibular first molar
   c. Mandibular second molar
   d. Mandibular third molar
4. Mandibular first molar has:
   a. 3 cusps
   b. 4 cusps
   c. 5 cusps
   d. 6 cusps
5. Mandibular first molar has:
   a. 2 roots; buccal and lingual
   b. 2 roots; mesial and distal
   c. 3 roots; 2 buccal and lingual
   d. 3 roots; 2 mesial and distal
6. Buccal and lingual aspects of mandibular first molar are:
   a. Triangular
   b. Rhomboidal
   c. Trapezoidal with shorter uneven side toward the cervix
   d. Trapezoidal with shorter uneven side toward the occlusal portion
7. Buccal surface of the mandibular first molar has:
   a. No developmental groove
   b. One developmental groove
   c. Two developmental grooves
   d. Three developmental grooves
8. In permanent mandibular first molars, the cusps visible from buccal view are:
   a. Two buccal cusps only
   b. Two buccal cusps and the distal cusp
   c. Two buccal cusps and two lingual cusps
   d. All five cusps can be seen
9. The cusps present in permanent mandibular first molar are:
   a. Mesiobuccal, distobuccal, mesiolingual, distolingual, and distal
   b. Mesiobuccal, middle distal, mesiolingual, and distolingual
   c. Mesiobuccal, distobuccal, mesiolingual, distolingual, and cusp of Carabelli
   d. None of the above
10. The 2 buccal cusps of mandibular first molar are separated by:
   a. The central developmental groove
   b. The oblique developmental groove
   c. The mesiobuccal developmental groove
   d. The distobuccal developmental groove

**Answers**

| 1. b | 2. a | 3. b | 4. c | 5. b | 6. c | 7. c | 8. d |
| 9. a | 10. c | | | | | | |

# 16
**CHAPTER**

# Pulp Morphology

## INTRODUCTION

Dental pulp is the only soft tissue component of the tooth; the other three components of tooth being the hard mineralized tissues namely, enamel, dentin, and cementum. The dental pulp harbors neurovascular bundles and lymphatic channels. Various functions have been attributed to the pulp including formative, nutritive, sensory, and defensive. Although its initial function is to form dentin during the developmental period of tooth, the dental pulp remains active throughout life and responds to various stimuli such as caries, trauma, and restorative procedures by forming secondary and reparative dentin as may be required to maintain vitality of the pulp.

Knowledge of pulp morphology is essential for sound clinical practice. For instance, it is important to avoid exposing the pulp while removing caries and restoring the tooth. When the pulp is diseased or a tooth is nonvital the entire pulp tissue is removed and the pulp cavity is filled

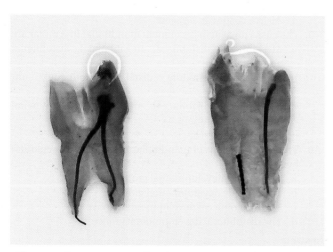

**Fig. 16.1:** Transparent tooth model of failed root canal therapy. Note broken file in the right specimen.

using an inert material such as gutta-percha (root canal treatment). Thorough understanding of pulp morphology is a prerequisite for performing successful root canal treatment. False assumptions about the root canal anatomy of teeth may lead to misdiagnosis, missed canals, and breakage of root canal instruments during root canal treatment **(Fig. 16.1)**.

Several methods have been used to examine root canal system including in vitro methods such as sectioning of teeth, clearing and staining of teeth (transparent tooth model), radiographs, and more advanced microcomputed tomography imaging.

## THE TERMINOLOGY

The terminology related to the pulp morphology is explained before proceeding further toward describing the pulp anatomy of each tooth in detail **(Figs. 16.2A and B)**.

### Pulp Cavity

The dental pulp occupies the central cavity within the tooth, the *pulp cavity*. The pulp cavity is encased by rigid dentinal walls all around except at the apical foramen through which the blood vessels and nerves enter and leave the pulp. At the apical foramen the pulp becomes continuous with the periodontal ligament.

For descriptive purposes, the pulp cavity is divided into a coronal portion—the *pulp chamber* and a radicular portion—the *root canal(s)*. All teeth have single pulp chamber while the number of root canals vary accordingly to the tooth type and class. The pulp cavity confines to the external form of the tooth in basic shape. The pulp chamber follows the external shape of the crown while the root canals take the basic shape of roots.

### Pulp Chamber

As mentioned above, the pulp chamber is that portion of the pulp present within the crown portion of the tooth. The pulp chamber closely follows the external crown morphology especially in a younger tooth.

All teeth have a single pulp chamber that has a roof and four walls. Extension of the roof of the pulp chamber directly under a cusp or developmental lobe is called as the *Pulp Horn* or *Cornua*. Pulp horns are at a higher level in primary teeth.

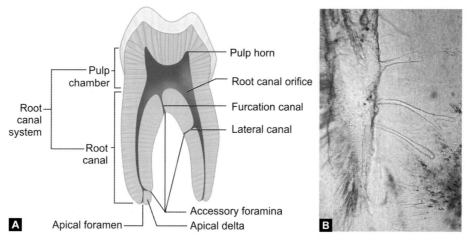

**Figs. 16.2A and B:** (A) Mesiodistal section of a mandibular molar; (B) Photomicrograph of a ground section of tooth showing apical delta.

In permanent teeth pulp horns are especially prominent under buccal cusp of premolars and mesiobuccal cusp of molar teeth. During cavity preparation and restoration of teeth, it is important to avoid the pulp horns to prevent exposure of pulp tissue. The walls of the pulp chamber derive their names from the corresponding walls of the tooth surface, e.g. buccal wall or lingual wall of the pulp chamber.

In anterior teeth, the pulp chamber gradually merges into the single root canal and the division becomes indistinct. In multirooted teeth, the pulp chamber opens into two or more root canals. The entrance (orifices) to the root canals is located on the floor of the pulp chamber, usually below the center of the cusp tips.

## Root Canals

Both the terms *root canal* and *pulp canal* are accepted; the term root canal is commonly used though the term *root canal system* is appropriate for multirooted teeth.

The root canal is the portion of the pulp from the canal orifice to the apical foramen. Each root has at least one root canal, many have two (e.g. mandibular molars have two root canals in their mesial root). When roots are fused, the tooth still maintains the usual number of root canals.

Small *accessory canals* can be found at the apical third of the root and furcation areas of multirooted teeth in varying frequencies. The term *"lateral canals"* is often used for the small canals that lead from main canal to the lateral aspect of the root. Both accessory and lateral canals develop due to a break in Hertwig's epithelial root sheath or when the sheath grows around existing blood vessels during root formation.

The apical foramen and lateral or accessory canals form channels of communication between the main body of the root canal and the periodontal ligament space. Thus they can act as route of extension of inflammation from one tissue to the other. Infection in pulp can produce changes in the periodontal tissue and more rarely the vice versa.

Apical delta refers to the branching pattern of small accessory canals and minor foramina seen at the apex of some tooth roots. The pattern is said to be reminiscent of a river delta when sectioned and viewed using a microscope **(Fig. 16.2B)**.

### Classification of Root Canals

Root canal morphology is quite complex. The root canal configurations have been classified by various researchers (Weine, Vertucci, etc.) according to the number of canals, intracanal branching, fusion, and exit from the canal. Weine's classification is considered here.

### *Weine's classification of root canals (Fig. 16.3A):*
- *Type* I: Single canal from pulp chamber to apex.
- *Type II:* Two canals leaving from the chamber and merging to form a single canal short of the apex.

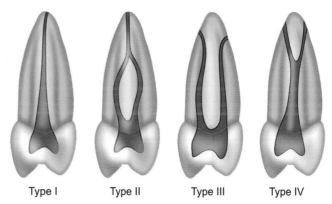

Type I          Type II          Type III          Type IV

**Fig. 16.3A:** Weine's classification of root canal configurations: Type I: Single canal from pulp chamber to apex; Type II: Two canals leaving the chamber and merging to form a single canal short of the apex; Type III: Two separate and distinct canals from chamber to apex; Type IV: One canal leaving the chamber and dividing into two separate and distinct canals.

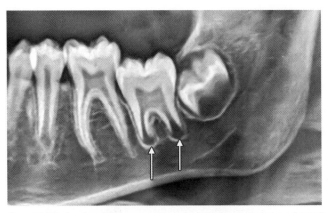

**Fig. 16.3B:** In developing tooth, apical foramen is large, funnel shaped, and centrally located (arrows). It becomes small and eccentrically placed after root completion.

- *Type III:* Two separate and distinct canals from chambers to apex.
- *Type IV:* One canal leaving the chamber and dividing into two separate and distinct canals.

### Apical Foramen and Accessory Foramina

The apical foramen is the opening at each root tip, or apex, through which nerve fibers and blood vessels pass from the alveolar region to the pulp cavity. Accessory canals communicate through accessory foramina. In the young, developing tooth, the apical foramen is large, funnel shaped, and centrally located **(Fig. 16.3B)**. The wide foramen is filled with periodontal tissue that is later replaced by dentin and cementum.

As the root completes its development, the apical foramen becomes smaller in diameter and more eccentric in position. After root completion, the apical foramen is seldom located at the very end, i.e. anatomic apex. It may be located on mesial, distal, labial or lingual surfaces of root usually slightly eccentrically.

Knowledge of the age at which calcification and closure of root apex occurs is essential for endodontic practice, especially when treating pulp involved teeth of children and adolescents. In general, the root apex is completely formed about 2–3 years after eruption of the tooth (refer **Tables 3.1 and 3.2** in Chapter 3).

### AGE-RELATED CHANGES IN PULP MORPHOLOGY

The size and shape of the pulp cavity are influenced by age. The dental pulp gets smaller with age, because of secondary dentin deposition that occurs throughout life. In addition, tertiary or reparative dentin that is formed in response to various stimuli such as caries, trauma, etc. also contributes to decreasing size of the pulp. In a young person, the pulp horns are long, pulp chambers are large, root canals are wide, and apical foramina are widely open. With advancing age, pulp horns recede, pulp chambers become smaller in height and

root canals become narrower **(Figs. 16.4A and B)**. The floor of the pulp chamber is nearly flat in young teeth, later becomes convex. The incidence of pulp stones or calcifications also increases with age. They appear as radiopacities in pulp cavity on a radiograph **(Fig. 16.5)**.

### CLINICAL APPLICATIONS

A thorough understanding of root canal anatomy with all the variations and complexities is essential for the clinicians to successfully localize, disinfect, and seal root canal system.

**Figures 16.6A and B** give ideal access opening for maxillary and mandibular teeth.

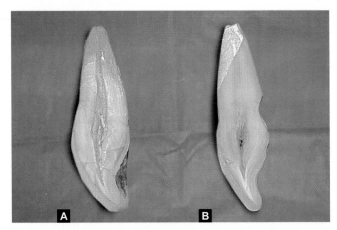

**Figs. 16.4A and B:** Longitudinal sections of maxillary central incisor from (A) young and (B) old individuals to show shrinkage of pulp size with age due to secondary dentin formation.

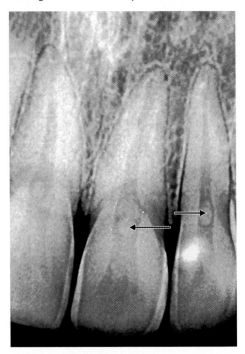

**Fig. 16.5:** Pulp stones.

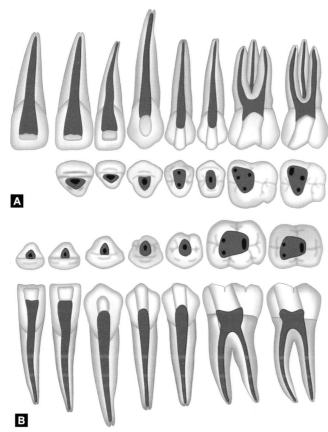

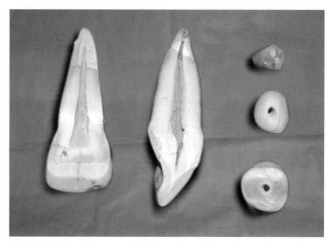

**Fig. 16.7:** Maxillary central incisor. Sections of natural specimen: Mesiodistal, labiolingual, cross-section of root at cervical, mid-root, and apex.

**Figs. 16.6A and B:** Ideal design of access opening for maxillary and mandibular permanent teeth.

## DETAILED DESCRIPTION OF PULP ANATOMY OF PERMANENT TEETH

### Maxillary Teeth

#### *Permanent Maxillary Central Incisor (Fig. 16.7)*

***Pulp chamber:***
- Viewed proximally (labiolingual section), the pulp chamber of maxillary central incisor is wider at cervix and tapers toward the incisal ridge.
- Viewed labially (mesiodistal section), the pulp chamber follows the crown outline and may show three pulp horns that correspond to the developmental mamelons in a young tooth. The pulp chamber is wider in the mesiodistal section than in the labiolingual section, with widest dimension incisally.
- The division between root canal and pulp chamber is indistinct.

***Root canal:***
- The maxillary central incisor has one root with one root canal.
- The root canal is conical in shape, broader labiolingually, and centrally located.
- The root canal tapers gradually toward the apical foramen, where it may curve slightly either distally or labially.

***Cross-section:***
- In a young tooth, cross-section of the root at cervix shows a roughly triangular outline with the base of the triangle at the labial aspect of the root.
- The cross-section of the root canal becomes oval or round at mid-root level and round at the apex.

***Access opening:*** Inverted triangular-shaped access cavity is cut with its base at the cingulum to give a straight line access.

#### *Permanent Maxillary Lateral Incisor (Fig. 16.8)*

***Pulp chamber:***
- Pulp chamber of maxillary permanent lateral incisor is similar but smaller than that of maxillary permanent central incisor.
- It is broad mesiodistally, with its broadest part incisally.
- The division between root canal and pulp chamber is indistinct.

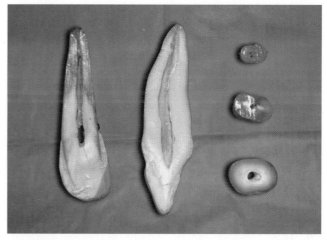

**Fig. 16.8:** Maxillary lateral incisor. Sections of natural specimen: Mesiodistal, labiolingual, cross-section of root at cervical, mid-root, and apex.

*Root canal:* The root canal is conical like that of central incisor but is of smaller diameter.

*Cross-section:* In cross-section, the canal is ovoid labiolingually at cervical level and mid-root level. It becomes round at the apical third.

*Access opening:* The access cavity is similar to that of central incisor but is smaller and more ovoid.

### Permanent Maxillary Canine (Fig. 16.9)

*Pulp chamber:*
- The pulp chamber of maxillary permanent canine is the largest among all anterior teeth. The pulp chamber is broader labiolingually than is mesiodistally.
- Viewed proximally (on labiolingual section), the pulp chamber is wider cervically and single pulp horn extends toward the single cusp.
- On mesiodistal section, the pulp chamber is narrow resembling a flame.
- The division between the pulp chamber and root canal is indistinct.

*Root canal:*
- The single root canal of maxillary permanent canine is larger and longer than that of maxillary incisors.
- It is wider labiolingually than in mesiodistal dimension.
- The pulp canal may show sudden narrowing at middle third of root and from this level it tapers gradually to apical foramen. Abrupt constriction of root canal should be borne in mind during root canal treatment to avoid over instrumentation.

*Cross-section:* Cross-section of the root canal at cervix and mid-root level is oval with greater diameter labiolingually and may become round at apex.

*Access opening:* Oval-shaped access cavity is cut that reflects the shape of the root canal.

### Permanent Maxillary First Premolar (Fig. 16.10)

*Pulp chamber:*
- Viewed proximally (buccolingual section), the pulp chambers of maxillary first premolar is broad with two pulp horns pointing toward the buccal and lingual cusps. The buccal pulp horn is more prominent than the lingual or palatal pulp horn in young teeth.
- The floor of the pulp chamber is located in coronal third of root below cervical line. It is convex, generally has two canal orifices, one buccal and one lingual.
- Viewed from buccal aspect, the mesiodistal dimension of pulp chamber is much narrower. The pulp horns are superimposed on one another and appear blunted. The pulp chamber cannot be differentiated from root canal from this view.

*Root canals:*
- The maxillary first premolar generally has two roots (85%), although fused or partially fused roots are not uncommon. When roots are fused a groove may be seen that divides the root into buccal or lingual portions. Regardless of whether maxillary first premolars have one or two roots, they usually have two root canals that exit by separate apical foramina. A single root and single root canal is present in less than 10% of the cases. A small number (5%) of maxillary first premolars may have three roots and three root canals.
- The two canals take the shape of their respective roots and get tapered toward apex.

*Cross-section:*
- Cross-section at cervical level shows a typical kidney-shaped appearance with indentation on mesial aspect that is formed by mesial developmental groove and depression.
- The root canal is also kidney-shaped or oval at cervical level.
- At mid-root level two round or oval-shaped canals can be seen
- The root canals are round and small at apex.

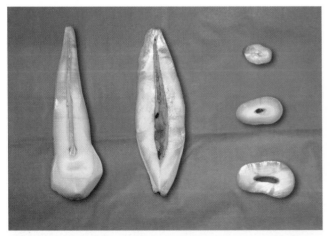

**Fig. 16.9:** Maxillary canine. Sections of natural specimen: Mesiodistal, buccolingual, cross-section of root at cervical, mid-root, and apex.

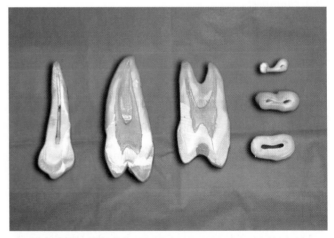

**Fig. 16.10:** Maxillary first premolar. Sections of natural specimen: Mesiodistal, buccolingual, cross-section of root at cervical, mid-root, and apex.

*Access cavity:* An oval-shaped access cavity is cut on occlusal surface between the cusp tips to gain access to buccal and lingual canals.

### Permanent Maxillary Second Premolar (Fig. 16.11)

*Pulp chambers:*
- The pulp chamber of maxillary second premolar is wider buccolingually than mesiodistally.
- It shows two pulp horns similar to maxillary first premolar.
- The pulp chamber extends apically well below the cervical margin.

*Pulp canals:* The maxillary second premolar generally has single root and single root canal (90% cases). The tooth can sometimes have two root canals.

*Cross-section:* The cervical cross-section of the root shows flattened oval canal. The root canal is slightly oval at mid-root level and becomes round at apical third.

*Access cavity:* The access cavity preparation is oval similar to the first premolars.

### Permanent Maxillary First Molar (Fig. 16.12)

*Pulp chamber:*
- The pulp chamber of maxillary first molar is the largest in the maxillary arch. It is rhomboidal in shape; its buccolingual dimension is wider than the mesiodistal dimension.
- The roof of the pulp chamber projects to form four pulp horns one to each of the major cusps. The mesiobuccal pulp horn is longest, more nearer to tooth surface than other pulp horns.
- The floor of the pulp chamber lies below the cervical margin. Generally, three openings of root canal can be located at three angles of the floor.

*Root canals:*
- The maxillary first molar generally has three roots and respective three canals namely the mesiobuccal,

distobuccal, and palatal. Sometimes, a fourth canal can be found in the mesiobuccal root.
- The distobuccal canal is narrower than the mesiobuccal root canal. The palatal root canal is the widest and the longest of the three root canals.

*Cross-section:*
- The cervical cross-section of the root shows rhomboidal shaped pulp cavity with three canal orifices.
- Cross-section at mid-root level shows larger round-shaped palatal canal, small oval-shaped distobuccal canal, and oval elongated or kidney-shaped mesiobuccal canal.

*Access cavity:*
- The access opening is triangular, with rounded corner extending toward mesiobuccal cusp tip, mesial marginal ridge, and oblique ridge.
- When accessory canal MB-2 is present, the access preparation is modified into a rhomboid-shaped cavity.

### Permanent Maxillary Second Molar (Fig. 16.13)

*Pulp chamber:*
- The pulp chamber of maxillary second molar is similar to that of maxillary first molar but is smaller.
- Mesiodistal dimension is much narrower than buccolingual. Thus, pulp chamber is more rhomboidal and the mesiobuccal and distobuccal canals are more closely placed.
- The floor of the pulp is apical to the cervical line.

*Root canal:*
- Three roots of maxillary second molar are less divergent than those of maxillary first molar. Thus, the canal orifices are closely placed on the pulpal floor.
- The mesiobuccal and distobuccal roots may be fused. Then only two root canals may be present, the buccal and palatal.

*Cross-section:* The cervical cross-section shows rhomboidal pulp floor with three/two canal orifices.

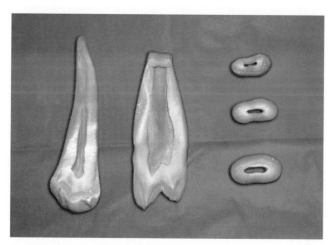

**Fig. 16.11:** Maxillary second premolar. Sections of natural specimen: Mesiodistal, buccolingual, cross-section of root at cervical, mid-root, and apex.

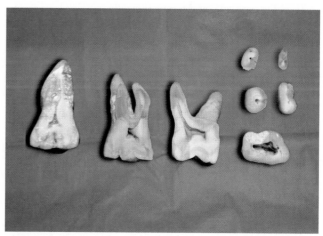

**Fig. 16.12:** Maxillary first molar. Sections of natural specimen: Mesiodistal, buccolingual, cross-section of root at cervical, mid-root, and apex.

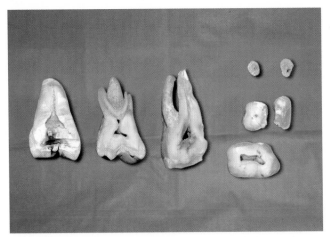

**Fig. 16.13:** Maxillary second molar sections of natural specimen: Mesiodistal, buccolingual, cross-section of root at cervical, mid-root, and apex.

*Access cavity:* The access opening for maxillary second molar is same as that of maxillary first molars.

### Permanent Maxillary Third Molar (Fig. 16.14)

The maxillary third molar has the most variable anatomy among the maxillary teeth. It is smaller than the other molars. The roots are short and often fused. Anatomy of pulp chamber and root canals of the maxillary third molars vary and cannot be generalized. Often they have three roots and three canals.

### Mandibular Teeth

### Permanent Mandibular Central Incisor (Fig. 16.15)

*Pulp chamber:*
- Being the smallest tooth in permanent dentition, the pulp chamber of mandibular central incisor is small and narrower mesiodistally than labiolingually. It is constricted at cervical margin.
- Viewed proximally (labiolingual section), the pulp chamber is wider cervically and tapers incisally.
- The division between pulp chamber and root canal is indistinct.

*Pulp canal:* The mandibular central incisor generally has a single root with single root canal. Some teeth may show two root canals. However, they fuse at apex and exit by a single foramen.

*Cross-section:* Cervical cross-section shows a labiolingually oval pulp cavity. The canal becomes round at apex.

*Access cavity:* The access opening is long and oval incisogingivally.

### Permanent Mandibular Lateral Incisor (Fig. 16.16)

*Pulp chamber:*
- In contrast to maxillary incisor, the tooth and pulp cavity of mandibular lateral incisor is larger than that of mandibular central incisor.

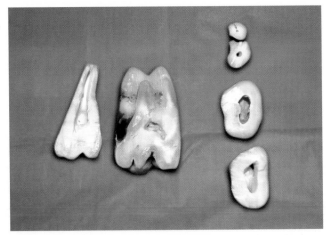

**Fig. 16.14:** Maxillary third molar. Sections of natural specimen: Mesiodistal, buccolingual, cross-section of root at cervical, mid-root, and apex.

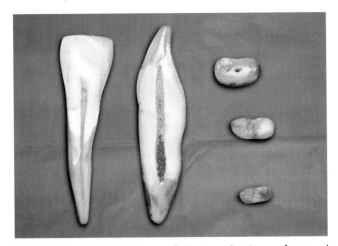

**Fig. 16.15:** Mandibular central incisor. Sections of natural specimen: Mesiodistal, labiolingual, cross-section of root at cervical, mid-root, and apex.

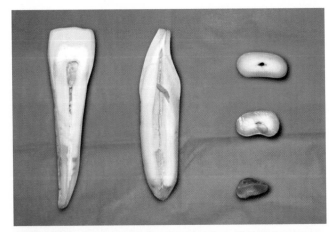

**Fig. 16.16:** Mandibular lateral incisor. Sections of natural specimen: Mesiodistal, labiolingual, cross-section of root at cervical, mid-root, and apex.

- The pulp chamber is similar in shape to that of mandibular central incisor but is larger.

**Pulp canals:**
- The mandibular lateral incisor has one root and one canal.
- Two root canals occur more frequently than seen in mandibular central incisor. When present, the two canals exit by separate foramina.

**Cross-section:** The cervical cross-section of the pulp is oval and round at mid-root and apex.

**Access cavity:** Access opening is oval, similar to that of mandibular central incisor.

### Permanent Mandibular Canine (Fig. 16.17)

**Pulp chamber:**
- The pulp chamber of mandibular permanent canine is similar to that of maxillary canine but is smaller in dimension.
- The pulp chamber is narrower mesiodistally than labiolingually. It has single pulp horn that extends toward the cusp tip.
- Pulp chamber and root canal are not well demarcated.

**Root canal:**
- The mandibular canine usually has single root and single root canal.
- A common variation is to exhibit bifurcated root with two root canals that exit by two separate foramina.

**Cross-section:** Cervical cross-section shows oval-shaped pulp canal. It becomes small and round apex.

**Access cavity:** Access opening is oval shaped, similar to that of maxillary canine.

### Permanent Mandibular First Premolar (Fig. 16.18)

**Pulp chamber:**
- The pulp chamber is wider buccolingually than mesiodistally. Unlike other premolars, it has only one pulp horn under well-developed buccal cusp. Small lingual pulp horn may be visible in a young tooth, but soon becomes indistinct with age. This gives the pulp chamber a resemblance to that of mandibular canine.
- Lingual inclination of the crown over root base is also reflected in the pulp chamber form.
- The division between pulp chamber and root canal is indistinct.

**Root canal:**
- The mandibular first premolar has one root with one root canal.
- The root canal becomes constricted toward the middle third of the root.
- In 25% of the cases, the main root canal may divide into two canals at apex.

**Cross-section:** The root canal is slightly oval at cervical and mid-root level and becomes small and round at apex.

**Access cavity:** An oval access opening gives access to the pulp canal. Lingual tilt of the crown has to be borne in mind to prevent preparations.

### Permanent Mandibular Second Premolar (Fig. 16.19)

**Pulp chamber:** The pulp chamber of mandibular second premolar is similar to that of mandibular first premolar; however, the tooth has a prominent lingual horn under well-formed lingual cusp(s) in addition to buccal pulp horn.

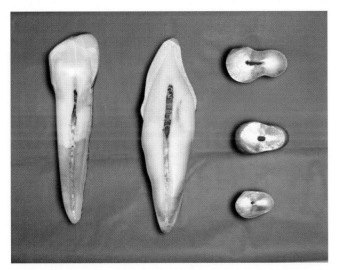

**Fig. 16.17:** Mandibular canine. Sections of natural specimen: Mesiodistal, labiolingual, cross-section of root at cervical, mid-root, and apex.

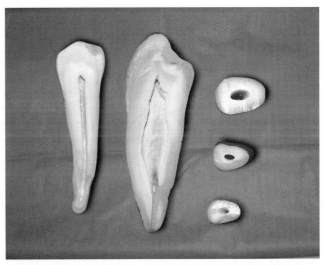

**Fig. 16.18:** Mandibular first premolar. Sections of natural specimen: Mesiodistal, buccolingual, cross-section of root at cervical, mid-root, and apex.

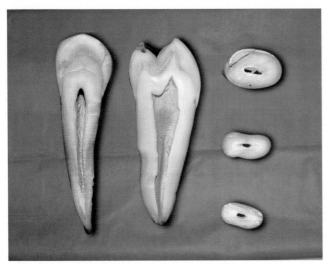

**Fig. 16.19:** Mandibular second premolar. Sections of natural specimen: Mesiodistal, buccolingual, cross-section of root at cervical, mid-root, and apex.

*Root canal:*
- The mandibular second premolar root is wider buccolingually than the mandibular first premolar and it often shows a distal curvature.
- The root canal is wider buccolingually, becomes constricted at mid-root level and then gets tapered toward apex.

*Cross-section:* The cervical cross-section shows oval-shaped pulp cavity buccolingually. It is round at mid-root level and apex.

*Access cavity:* It is similar to that of mandibular first molar, oval-shaped opening is needed.

### Permanent Mandibular First Molar (Fig. 16.20)

*Pulp chamber:*
- The pulp chamber of mandibular first molar is wider mesiodistally than buccolingually.
- The pulp chamber is rectangular when viewed from buccal and lingual aspects.
- It has four pulp horns under four major cusps—the mesiobuccal, distobuccal, mesiolingual, and distolingual.
- The lingual horns are longer and at a higher level than the buccal pulp horns.
- The floor of the pulp chamber is broad and is at or below cervical margin.

*Root canals:*
- The mandibular first molar has two roots and three root canals. The mesial root has two canals—the mesiobuccal and the mesiolingual.
- The distal root canal is more oval and wider buccolingually than the mesial roots.
- Rarely, the mandibular first molar can have three roots. The distal root sometimes may shows two canals.

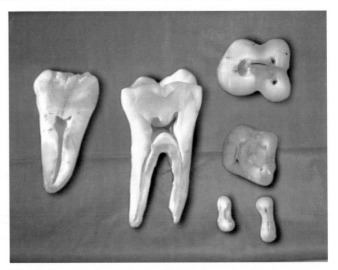

**Fig. 16.20:** Mandibular first molar. Sections of natural specimen: Mesiodistal, buccolingual, cross-section of root at cervical, mid-root, and apex.

*Cross-section:*
- The cross-section of the tooth at cervix is quadrilateral in shape with mesial wall of pulp wider than the distal.
- At mid-root level, the distal root canal is long and oval shaped. The mesial root canal is slightly oval.

*Access cavity:*
- The access opening is trapezoidal with round corners, wider toward mesial surface of the crown.
- The access cavity is made rectangular if a second distal canal is present.

### Permanent Mandibular Second Molar (Fig. 16.21)

*Pulp chamber:* The pulp chamber of mandibular second molar closely resembles that of the mandibular first molar.

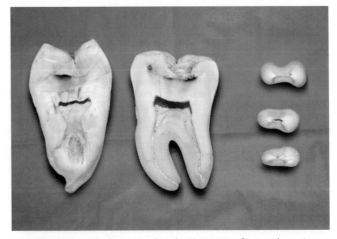

**Fig. 16.21:** Mandibular second molar. Sections of natural specimen: Mesiodistal, buccolingual, cross-section of root at cervical, mid-root, and apex.

*Root canal:*
- The tooth has two roots and three canals similar to mandibular first molars.
- A common variation seen is the presence of only two canals—the mesial and distal.

*Cross-section:* Cervical cross-section is quadrilateral with small canal orifices closely placed. The root canals at mid-root level are oval in shape.

### Permanent Mandibular Third Molar (Fig. 16.22)

- The mandibular third molar pulp morphology varies greatly. The pulp cavity resembles that of mandibular second molar but the roots are short, often fused and curved.
- The tooth may have one to four roots and one to six canals. C-shaped canals can be seen due to fusion of roots.

## BIBLIOGRAPHY

1. Barker BC, Parsons KC, Mills PR, et al. Anatomy of root canals. I. Permanent incisors, canines and premolars. Aust Dent. 1973;18(5):320-7.
2. Barker BC, Parsons KC, Mills PR, et al. Anatomy of root canals. II. Permanent maxillary molar. Aust Dent J. 1974;19(1):46-50.
3. Barker BC, Parsons KC, Mills PR, et al. Anatomy of root canals. III. Permanent mandibular molar. Aust Dent J. 1974;19(6):408-13.
4. Okumura T. Anatomy of the root canals. J Am Dent Assoc. 1927;14:632.
5. Vertucci FJ, Williams RG. Furcation in the human mandibular 1st molars. Oral Surg. 1974;38:308.
6. Vertucci FJ, Seelig A, Gillis R. Root canal morphology of the human maxillary second premolar. Oral Surg. 1974;38(3):456-64.
7. Vertucci FJ, Gegauff A. Root canal morphology of the human maxillary first premolar. Oral Surg. 1979;99(2):194-8.

## MULTIPLE CHOICE QUESTIONS

1. As age advances, the dental pulp gets _____
   a. Becomes larger with age
   b. Remains unchanged
   c. Becomes smaller with age
   d. None of the above
2. The hard mineralized components of tooth are the following, except:
   a. Dental pulp
   b. Enamel
   c. Dentin
   d. Cementum
3. The functions of pulp include:
   a. Formative
   b. Nutritive
   c. Sensory and defensive
   d. All of the above
4. According to Weine's classification of root canal system, Type II is _____
   a. Single canal from pulp chamber to apex
   b. Two canals leaving from the chambers and merging to form a single canal short of the apex
   c. Two separate and distinct canals from chamber to the apex

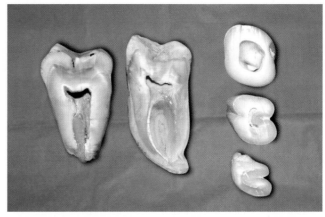

**Fig. 16.22:** Mandibular third molar. Sections of natural specimen: Mesiodistal, buccolingual, cross-section of root at cervical, mid-root, and apex.

   d. One canal leaving the chamber and dividing into two separate and distinct canals
5. The pulp cavity is encased by rigid dentin walls all around, except:
   a. At the center of the root
   b. At the cervix of the root
   c. At apical foramen through which the blood vessels enters and leaves the pulp
   d. None of the above
6. The coronal portion of the pulp cavity is termed as:
   a. Pulp chamber
   b. Root canal
   c. Both of the above
   d. None of the above
7. The radicular portion of the pulp cavity is termed as:
   a. Pulp chamber
   b. Root canal
   c. Both of the above
   d. None of the above
8. Which of the following statements is correct?
   I All teeth have single pulp chambers
   II Number of root canals differs from tooth to tooth
   a. Statement I and II are incorrect
   b. Statement I and II are correct
   c. Only statement I is correct
   d. Only statement II is correct
9. The extension of the roof of the pulp chamber directly under a cusp or developmental lobe is called as the:
   a. Pulp chambers
   b. Pulpal extension
   c. Pulp stones
   d. Pulp horns
10. During cavity preparation and restorations of tooth, it is important to avoid the pulp horns to prevent:
    a. Exposure of the pulp tissue
    b. Morphology of the tooth crown
    c. Superinfection of the tooth
    d. All of the above

**Answers**

1. c    2. a    3. d    4. b    5. c    6. a    7. b    8. b
9. d    10. a

# 6 SECTION

# Dento-osseous Structures: Temporomandibular Joint

## Section Outline

# 17
## CHAPTER

# Dento-osseous Structures: Blood Supply, Lymphatics and Innervation

## INTRODUCTION

Maxilla and mandible are the osseous structures that support the teeth by their alveolar processes. They form the *viscerocranium or splanchnocranium or face* of the skull. The cranial vault and the cranial base form the *neurocranium* of the skull. The anatomy of the dento-osseous structures along with blood supply, lymphatic drainage, and innervations are discussed in this chapter.

The skull or craniofacial complex is divided into neurocranium and viscerocranium or face (**Fig. 17.1**):
- Neurocranium made up of:
  - The cranial vault (calvarium)
  - The cranial base.

- Viscerocranium (face) made up of:
  - The nasomaxillary complex
  - The mandible.

## SKULL AND JAWS AT BIRTH

The skull at birth is far different from that of the adult skull. There are differences in shape and proportion of the face and cranium and the degree of development and fusion of the individual bones. At birth, the infant skull consists of 45 bony elements, separated by cartilage or connective tissue. This number is reduced to 22 bones in the adult life after the completion of ossification of skull. Some bones, which are single bones in adulthood, appear as separate constituent parts at birth; for example, frontal, occipital, and mandible bones. Other skull bones are widely separated from their neighboring bones at birth by loose connective tissue. Open spaces between the adjacent flat bones of skull are called "*fontanelle*" (**Fig. 17.2**), which allows significant growth of brain and also provides the cranium sufficient flexibility to pass through the birth canal during parturition.

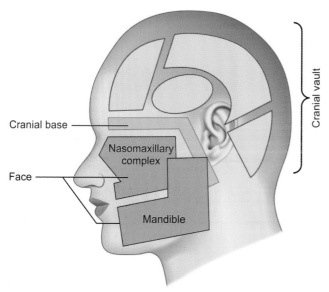

**Fig. 17.1:** The skull is divided into neurocranium and viscerocranium (face).

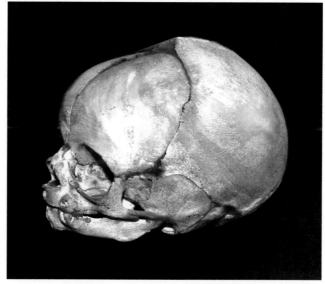

**Fig. 17.2:** Fetal skull showing fontanelle.

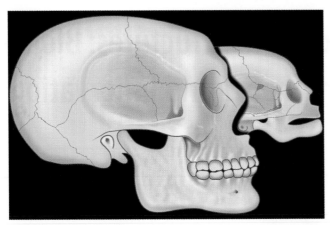

**Fig. 17.3:** Relative sizes of face and cranium at birth and adult life.

The relative sizes of face and cranium at birth and in adult life is noticeably different. The cranium grows rapidly in prenatal period, accommodating the rapidly developing brain. In contrast, the face appears small in vertical dimension because the nasomaxillary complex and mandible with their alveolar bones are relatively small at birth (**Fig. 17.3**).

## DEVELOPMENT OF SKULL OR CRANIOFACIAL COMPLEX

The neurocranium, especially the cranial base develops from endochondral ossification, where primary cartilage is converted into bone.

The facial bones, i.e. bones of viscerocranium are formed by intramembranous ossification, where bone is directly formed from undifferentiated mesenchymal tissue with no cartilaginous precursor. The membranous bones may later develop secondary cartilages to provide rapid growth for example, condylar cartilage of the mandible.

Cranium and facial skeleton (maxilla and mandible) grow at different rates. Growth of the cranium being intimately associated with growth of brain follows the neural growth curve, where most of the growth occurs in first few years of life. Growth of the facial skeleton, on the other hand, follows general somatic growth curve.

## BONES OF NEUROCRANIUM

The neurocranium is the portion which functions to support, house, and protect the brain. It consists of the cranial vault and the cranial base.

The cranial vault covers the upper and outer surface of the brain. It consists of a number of flat bones, which are formed by intramembranous ossification. They include the following:
- Frontal bone
- Temporal bone (paired)
- Parietal bone (paired)
- Occipital bone.

Adaptive growth occurs at the coronal, sagittal, parietal, temporal, and occipital sutures to accommodate the rapidly expanding brain.

As the brain expands, the separate bones of the cranial vault are displaced in an outward direction. This intramembranous sutural growth replaces the fontanelles that are present at birth.

The cranial base develops from endochondral ossification. It is formed by the following three bones:
1. Ethmoid bone
2. Sphenoid bone
3. Occipital bone.

## VISCEROCRANIUM OR FACE

The facial skeleton gives us our appearance and functions of both respiration and digestion. The maxilla or the upper jaw is joined to the other bones of the cranium and is not movable. The mandible or lower jaw on the other hand is a separate bone and is movable. The maxilla and mandible are discussed further in detail.

### Maxilla

The maxilla consists of two bones—the right and the left maxillae that are sutured together at the midline. The maxillae join to form the whole of the upper jaw, the roof of the mouth—hard palate, floor, and the lateral wall of nasal cavity and orbital floors.

Each maxilla is an irregular bone that consists of the following parts (**Fig. 17.4**):
- A body
- Four processes:
  1. Zygomatic process

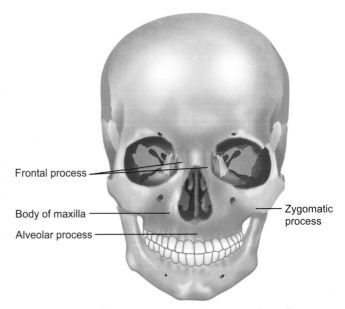

**Fig. 17.4:** Skull illustration showing parts of maxilla.

2. Frontal process
3. Palatine process
4. Alveolar process.

The maxilla joins other cranial and facial bones including frontal, nasal, ethmoidal, and malar bones by way of sutures.

### Body of the Maxilla

The body of the maxilla is hollow and contains maxillary air sinus space which is also called the *antrum of Highmore* (**Fig. 17.5**). The body of the maxilla has the following four surfaces:
1. Anterior (facial)
2. Posterior (infratemporal)
3. Orbital

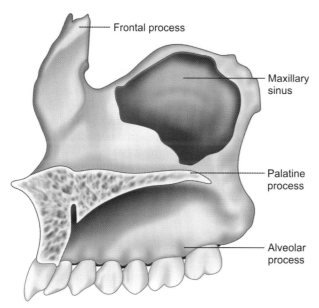

**Fig. 17.5:** Body of the maxilla houses maxillary sinus.

4. Nasal.

There are several important landmarks on the body of the maxilla (**Fig. 17.6**):

• The *infraorbital foramen* through which the infraorbital nerve and vessels pass is on the anterior surface of the body just above the canine fossa.
• The alveolar ridge over the root of the canine tooth is pronounced and is called the *canine eminence.*
• The shallow concavity anterior to the canine eminence, overlying the root of maxillary lateral incisor, is known as the *incisive fossa.*
• A deeper concavity that lies posterior to the canine eminence, over the roots of maxillary premolars, is named the *canine fossa*
• The inferior portion of the infratemporal surface that overhangs the root of the third molar is more prominent and is called the *maxillary tuberosity.*
• The nasal surface forms the lateral wall of the nasal fossa.
• The orbital surface of the maxillary body is smooth and forms most of the orbital floor.
• The junction of the orbital surface and the anterior surface forms the *infraorbital margin.*

### Process of Each Maxilla

*Zygomatic process*: The zygomatic process extends laterally to articulate with the zygomatic bone. It is a pyramidal projection where anterior, infratemporal, and orbital surfaces of the maxillary bone converge. This process along with the zygomatic bone and zygomatic process of temporal bone, form the zygomatic arch. Zygomatic arch serves as the origin of masseter muscle.

*Frontal (frontonasal) process:* Frontal process of maxilla extends posterosuperiorly between the nasal and lacrimal bones. It articulates superiorly with the frontal bone, anteriorly

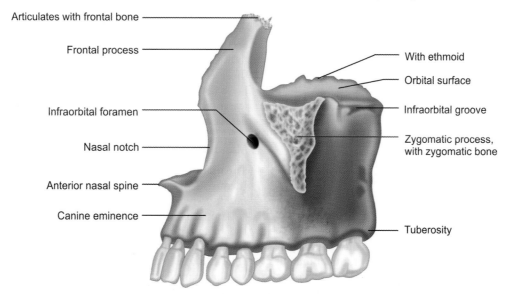

**Fig. 17.6:** Body of the maxilla.

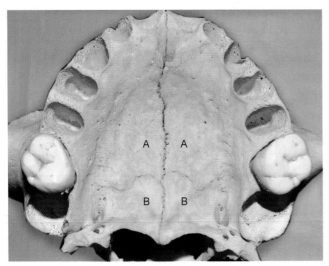

**Fig. 17.7:** Palatine process of maxilla (A) along with the horizontal plates of palatine bones (B) form the hard palate.

with the nasal bone, and posteriorly with the lacrimal bone. It also forms the lateral wall of the nose.

***Palatine process (Fig. 17.7):*** The right and left palatine processes of maxillae extend horizontally from the medial surface of respective maxilla and join in the midline at the median palatine suture. The inferior surface of the palatine process forms the anterior two-thirds of the hard palate. The inferior surface of the palatine processes is rough and pitted for palatine mucous glands and exhibits numerous small foramina. The smoother superior surface of palatine processes forms the floor of the nasal cavity.

The palatine process of each maxilla articulates posteriorly with the horizontal plates of the palatine bones at the *transverse palatine suture.* The horizontal plates of palatine bones form the posterior one-third of the hard palate. The posterior border of the horizontal palatine plates is concave and in the midline forms a sharp ridge called the *posterior nasal spine.*

The palatine process of maxilla blends smoothly with the palatal portion of the maxillary alveolar process. *Incisive fossa or canal* lies in the midline just posterior to the central incisors. Two lateral incisive canals are seen in the incisive fossa which transmits the *greater palatine artery* and the *nasopalatine nerves.*

The mucosa over the median palatine suture in the mouth is a smooth ridge called *midpalatine raphe.* In a person born with cleft palate, a part or all of the palatine process of maxilla are absent. Sometimes, the bony margins are raised in the midline to form palatine torus.

***Alveolar process:*** The alveolar process extends inferiorly from the bodies of the maxillae, surround the roots of maxillary teeth, and give them osseous support within bony sockets. The alveolar process merges smoothly with the palatine process medially and with the zygomatic process laterally.

The maxilla contains 8 permanent teeth or 5 primary teeth on each side. The shape of the alveolus or socket varies and corresponds exactly with the shape of the root of the tooth that each socket surrounds. For instance, sockets for incisors are single, that of canine is deepest and those for molars are widest and subdivided into two or three by septa.

The form of the alveolus is related to the functional demands put upon the teeth. When a tooth is lost, the alveolus that supports the missing tooth undergoes resorption. If all the teeth are lost, the alveolar process eventually gets completely resorbed.

The alveolar process of the jaw has a buccal or labial surface and lingual surfaces. The alveolar process is composed of two parallel plates of dense compact or cortical bone—*the outer and inner cortical plates.* Spongy or cancellous bone of varying thickness lies between the outer and inner cortical plates. The individual sockets are separated by plates of bone termed *the interdental septa.* In multirooted teeth, the roots are divided by *inter-radicular septa* (**Fig. 17.8A**).

The floor of the socket is called the *fundus* and its rim is called *alveolar crest.* The alveolar bone proper which forms the inner wall of the socket is perforated by many openings that carry nerve and blood vessels into periodontal ligament, and thus is also called the *cribriform plate.*

The alveolar bone proper also contains *bundle bone* into which the bundles of principal fibers of periodontal ligament are anchored and they continue into the bone as *Sharpey's fibers.* Radiographically, it is also referred as the *lamina dura* (**Fig. 17.8B**).

### Maxillary Sinus

The maxillary sinus is the largest paranasal air sinus and is situated in the body of the maxilla. It is shaped as a four-sided pyramid, the base of which faces medially toward the nasal cavity and apex is pointed laterally toward the zygomatic bone (**Fig. 17.9A**).

The roots of the posterior teeth, especially the first and second molars and sometimes premolars, are closely related to the floor of the maxillary sinus (**Fig. 17.9B**). The alveoli of these teeth are separated from the sinus floor by only a thin layer of bone. Thus care must be taken when extracting the fractured roots in this region to avoid creating an oroantral fistula.

### Mandible

The mandible is the largest and strongest bone of the skull. It consists of horizontal component—the horseshoe-shaped *body* and two vertical component—the *rami.*

The rami join the body posteriorly at an oblique angle at the angle of the mandible. The body of the mandible carries the mandibular teeth and their associated alveolar process (**Fig. 17.10**).

The mandible is attached to the cranial bone only by ligaments and muscles. It articulates with the cranium through the *temporomandibular joint (TMJ).* The mandible is the only

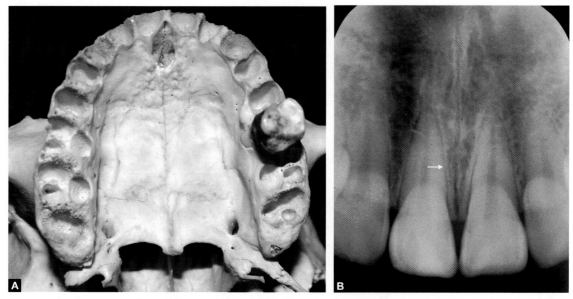

**Figs. 17.8A and B:** (A) Alveoli of maxillary teeth; (B) Lamina dura.

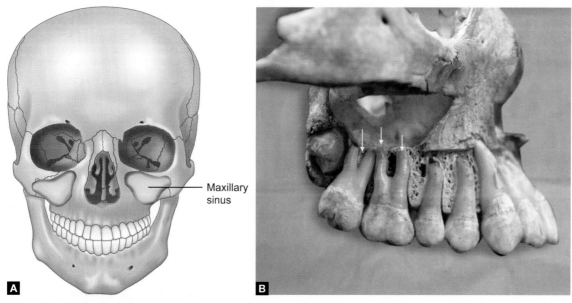

Maxillary sinus

**Figs. 17.9A and B:** (A) Maxillary sinus is shaped as a four-sided pyramid; (B) Maxillary first and second molars roots are closely related to floor and maxillary sinus.

bone in the skull that moves. All the muscles of mastication have their insertion into the mandible.

### Mandibular Body

The mandibular body has two surfaces—internal and external, and two borders—superior and inferior.

***External surface of mandibular body (Fig. 17.11):*** Prenatally, the mandibular body develops as two lateral halves **(Fig. 17.12)**. They join at midline during the first year after birth.

The line of fusion appears as a median ridge on external surface of the body called *symphysis.* Inferiorly, this ridge or symphysis forms a prominent triangular surface with base toward the lower border called the *mental protuberance.* The *mental tubercles* and the mental protuberance together form the human *chin,* a unique feature that is absent in other mammals. Posterior to the symphysis and above the mental protuberance, there is a shallow depression just below the alveolar border of central and lateral incisor called incisive fossa.

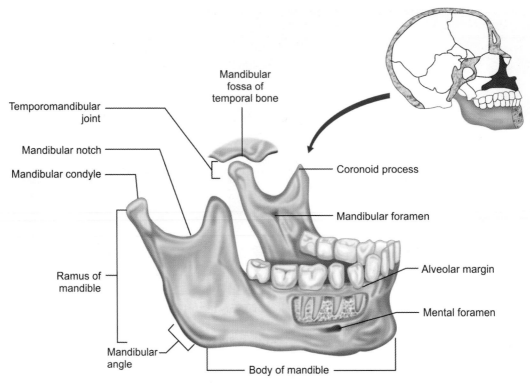

**Fig. 17.10:** Mandible has a horseshoe-shaped body and two rami. It articulates with cranium through temporomandibular joint.

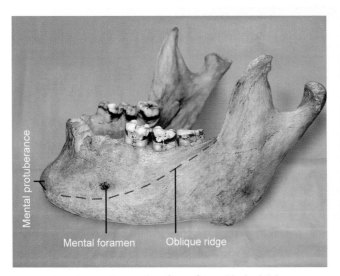

**Fig. 17.11:** External surface of mandibular body.

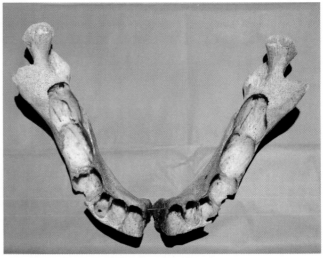

**Fig. 17.12:** Prenatally mandible develops as two lateral halves which join later at midline after birth.

Alveolar process over the root of the canine is prominent and forms the *canine eminence of mandible.* The *oblique ridge* extends obliquely from the mental tubercles where it is faint, ascends backwards sloping below the mental foramen, becoming more prominent near molar area as it continues into the anterior border of the ramus.

*Mental foramen,* through which the mental branches of inferior alveolar nerve and artery pass, is an important landmark on the external surface of mandible. It is positioned between the apices of premolars or directly below the apex of second premolar.

***Internal surface of mandibular body (Fig. 17.13):*** On the rear side of the mandible along the midline, there are two small eminences called the *superior and inferior genial spines or tubercles.* They give attachment to *geniohyoid and genioglossus*

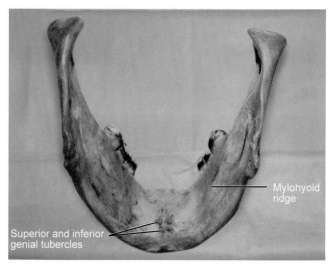

**Fig. 17.13:** Internal surface of mandibular body.

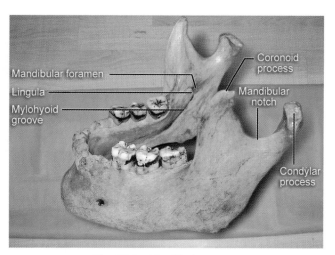

**Fig. 17.15:** Mandibular ramus.

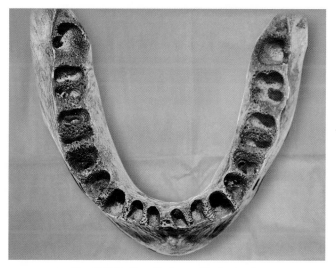

**Fig. 17.14:** Alveoli of mandibular teeth.

muscles, respectively. The *digastric fossae* are two depressions on the inferior surface of the mandible near midline, into which the *anterior belly of digastric muscles* are inserted.

The *mylohyoid line or ridge* arises near genial tubercles and passes obliquely to end on the anterior surface of the ramus. The *mylohyoid muscle* that forms the floor of the mouth takes origin from the mylohyoid ridge. The mylohyoid ridge separates two shallow fossae—the *sublingual fossa* above against which the *sublingual salivary gland* rests and the *submandibular fossa* below against which the *submandibular salivary gland* rests.

The alveoli of mandibular teeth are shown in **Figure 17.14**.

### Mandibular Ramus (Fig. 17.15)

The mandibular ramus is a quadrilateral bone with two processes along its superior border—the *coronoid and condylar processes.*

The coronoid process provides attachments to the *temporalis muscle* at its anterior border.

The head of the condyle fits into the mandibular fossa of the temporal bone to form a movable synovial joint—*the temporomandibular joint.* The concavity between the coronoid and condylar process is called the *mandibular notch or sigmoid notch.* The lateral surface of the ramus provides attachment for *masseter muscle.*

The medial surface of the ramus presents an irregular *mandibular foramen* that leads into the *mandibular canal* curving downward and inferior alveolar nerve and vessels pass through the mandibular canal. A triangular bony process, *lingula,* is seen overlapping the mandibular foramen anterosuperiorly. It gives attachment to the *sphenomandibular ligament.*

The *mylohyoid groove* may be seen running forward from behind the lingula, along which the mylohyoid nerve and vessels pass.

### BLOOD SUPPLY (FIG. 17.16)

### Blood Supply to Maxillary Teeth and Periodontium (Table 17.1 and Flowchart 17.1)

Maxillary artery is a branch of *external carotid artery* which in turn is a branch of *common carotid artery.* Maxillary artery gives off first branch posterosuperior alveolar artery, which supplies maxillary molars, alveolar bone, and supporting soft tissue structures. Maxillary artery gives of infraorbital artery, which in turn gives of two branches, anterosuperior alveolar artery and middle superior alveolar artery.

Middle superior alveolar artery runs downward between the sinus mucosa and bone and then supplies the maxillary premolar teeth and their supporting structures.

Anterosuperior alveolar artery arises from the infraorbital artery just before this vessel leaves the foramen and it runs

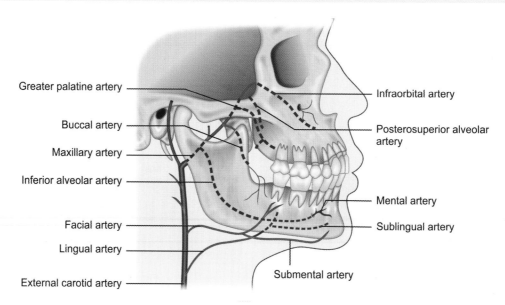

**Fig. 17.16:** Arterial supply of dento-osseous structures.

**Table 17.1:** Blood supply to maxillary teeth and periodontium.

| Structures | Blood supply |
|---|---|
| • Maxillary posterior teeth<br>• Alveolar bone of maxillary posteriors<br>• Membrane of sinus | Posterosuperior alveolar artery |
| • Gingiva of posterior teeth<br>• Alveolar mucosa of posterior teeth<br>• Cheek | Branches of posterosuperior alveolar artery |
| • Maxillary premolar teeth<br>• Alveolar bone of premolars<br>• Gingiva of premolars | Middle superior alveolar artery |
| • Maxillary anterior teeth and their supporting structures | Anterosuperior alveolar artery |

**Table 17.2:** Blood supply to mandibular teeth and periodontium.

| Structures | Blood supply |
|---|---|
| Anterior labial gingiva | Mental artery<br>Perforating branch of incisive artery |
| Posterior buccal gingiva | Buccal artery |
| Lingual gingiva (anterior and posterior) | Lingual artery and perforating branches of inferior alveolar artery |
| Tissue of chin | Mental artery |
| Individual tooth roots | Dental branches |
| • Individual septa<br>• Alveolar mucosa, periodontal membrane | Branches of dental artery |

down in the anterior aspect of the maxilla to supply the maxillary anterior teeth and their supporting structures such as alveolar mucosa, gingiva, and interdental septa.

**Flowchart 17.1:** Branches of maxillary artery.

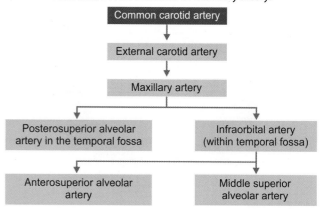

## Blood Supply to Mandibular Teeth and Periodontium (Table 17.2 and Fig. 17.16)

The blood supply to jaw bones and teeth is derived from the maxillary artery which is a branch of external carotid artery.

Maxillary artery gives off mylohyoid branch as it crosses the infratemporal fossa and then it traverses to give off inferior alveolar artery which enters the mandibular foramen in the ramus of the mandible.

Inferior alveolar artery gives off mental branch and incisive branch. Mental artery passes through mental foramen to supply anterior labial gingiva and tissues of the chin while the incisive branch enters incisive foramen to supply labial gingiva anteriorly. The anastomosis of mental artery and incisive artery serves as a good collateral blood supply for the mandible and teeth.

Third part of inferior alveolar artery is dental branches to the individual teeth, which serves the blood supply to the

**Table 17.3:** Blood supply to palate, lips, cheek, and tongue.

| Structures | Blood supply |
|---|---|
| Palate | • Greater palatine artery<br>• Lesser palatine artery |
| Tongue | Lingual artery |
| Cheek | Buccal branch of maxillary artery |
| Upper lip | Superior labial branch of facial artery |
| Lower lip | Inferior labial branch of facial artery |

individual tooth root and other branches that enter adjacent periodontal membrane and terminate in the gingiva. Numerous anastomosis of these arteries supplies the alveolar mucosa.

## BLOOD SUPPLY TO PALATE, CHEEK, TONGUE, AND LIPS (TABLE 17.3)

### Palate

The palate derives its blood supply from the greater and lesser palatine branches of maxillary artery. The greater palatine artery enters the palate through the greater palatine foramen and runs forward along with its nerve and vein in a groove at the junction of the palatine and alveolar process.

### Cheeks

The cheek derives its blood supply from the buccal branch of maxillary artery.

### Tongue

The tongue and floor of the mouth derives its blood supply from lingual artery.

### Lips

The lips (upper and lower lips) derive blood supply from superior and inferior labial branches of facial artery, where upper lip gets blood supply from superior labial branches of facial artery whereas lower lip obtains its blood supply from inferior labial branches of the facial artery.

## VENOUS DRAINAGE OF ORODENTAL TISSUES (FIG. 17.17)

The facial vein is the main vein for the venous drainage of orodental tissues. It begins at the medial corner of the eye by the confluence of supraorbital and supratrochlear veins and passes across the face behind the facial artery. It joins with the anterior branch of the retromandibular vein to form the common facial vein below the mandible.

### Teeth and Periodontium

Small veins from the teeth and alveolar mucosa pass into larger vein of each tooth surrounding the root apex or into the veins of interdental septa.

### Mandible

In the mandible, inferior alveolar vein is the prime vein for the venous drainage. Anteriorly, inferior alveolar vein drains through the mental foramen to join the facial vein while in the posterior region, it drains through mandibular foramen to join the pterygoid plexus of veins in the infratemporal fossa.

### Maxilla

Anteriorly, venous drainage in maxilla is from facial vein and posteriorly into the pterygoid plexus.

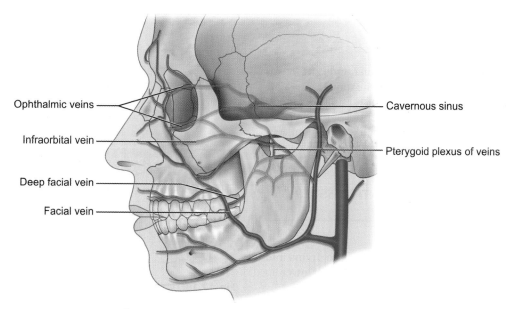

**Fig. 17.17:** Venous drainage of dento-osseous structures.

**Flowchart 17.2:** Venous drainage of palate.

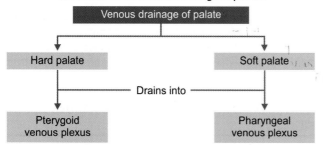

**Flowchart 17.3:** Venous drainage of lips.

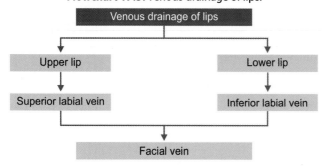

**Flowchart 17.4:** Venous drainage of tongue.

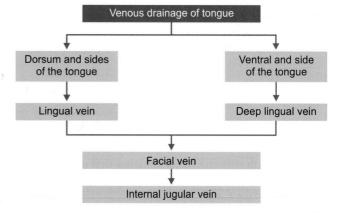

**Table 17.4:** Lymphatic drainage of orodental tissues.

| Orodental tissues | Lymphatic drainage |
|---|---|
| Lower part of the face | Submandibular lymph nodes |
| Medial part of lower lip | Submental group of lymph nodes |
| Posterior teeth | Submandibular lymph nodes |
| Anterior teeth | Submental group of lymph nodes |
| Labial or buccal gingiva of mandibular and maxillary teeth | Submandibular lymph nodes |
| Labial gingiva of mandibular anterior teeth | Submental group of lymph nodes |
| Lingual and palatal gingiva of teeth | Jugulodigastric lymph nodes |
| Hard palate | Jugulodigastric lymph nodes |
| Soft palate | Pharyngeal group of lymph nodes |

## Palate

The veins of the palate are rather diffuse and variable. However, those of the hard palate generally pass into the pterygoid venous plexus, those of the soft palate into the pharyngeal venous plexus (**Flowchart 17.2**).

## Lips

Venous drainage of the lips is mainly from the facial vein. Venous blood from upper lip drains into superior labial vein, whereas venous blood from lower lip drains into inferior labial veins (**Flowchart 17.3**).

## Tongue

Venous drainage of tongue is quite peculiar and is from two different routes for two different part of the tongue. The part of the tongue from dorsum surface and sides of the tongue drains into lingual vein, those of the ventral surface drains from the deep lingual veins. Venous blood from lingual vein drains into facial vein and later into internal jugular veins (**Flowchart 17.4**).

## LYMPHATIC DRAINAGE OF ORODENTAL TISSUES (TABLE 17.4 AND FIG. 17.18)

### Lower Part of the Face

Lymphatic drainage of the lower part of the face drains into submandibular lymph nodes and medial portion of lower lip into submental lymph nodes.

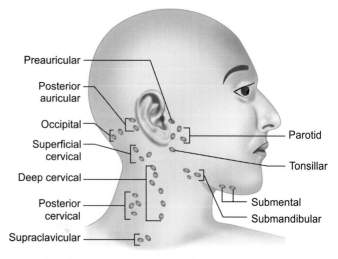

**Fig. 17.18:** Lymphatic drainage of dento-osseous structures.

## Maxillary and Mandibular Teeth

- The lymph vessels from the anterior teeth usually drain into the submental lymph nodes.
- The lymph vessels from the mandibular anterior teeth drain into the submental group of lymph nodes.
- The lymph vessels from the labial and buccal gingiva of the maxillary and mandibular teeth unite to drain into the submandibular lymph nodes.
- The lymph vessels from the labial gingival of mandibular anterior teeth drain into the submental group of lymph nodes.
- The lymph vessels from the lingual and palatal gingival drains into the jugulodigastric group of nodes, either directly or indirectly through the submandibular lymph nodes.

## Lymphatic Drainage of Palate

- The lymph vessels from most part of palate especially the hard palate drains into the jugulodigastric group of lymph nodes.
- The lymph vessels from soft palate drain into the pharyngeal lymph nodes.

## NERVE SUPPLY TO ORODENTAL TISSUES (FIG. 17.19)

There are different types of nerve fibers that supply the orodental tissues.

### Sensory Fibers or Afferent Fibers

These fibers convey impulses from peripheral organs to the central nervous system. They supply the skin of the entire face, the mucous membrane of the oral cavity and nasal cavity, the pharynx, and the base of the tongue and the teeth and their supporting structures (i.e. periodontal ligament, the alveolar process, and gingiva).

### Motor Fibers or Efferent Fibers

These fibers convey impulses from the central nervous system to the peripheral organs.

They supply the four pairs of muscles of mastication and several other muscles in the region of the mouth (mylohyoid, anterior belly of the digastric, tensor veli palatine, and the tensor tympani).

### Secretory Fibers

These are specialized fibers which upon stimulation increases secretory activity of a salivary gland.

## TRIGEMINAL NERVE (FIFTH CRANIAL NERVE)

Trigeminal nerve is the fifth cranial nerve and is the largest of all the sensory nerves of the face and scalp. It originates in the large semilunar or trigeminal ganglion within the above carotid canal medial to the foramen ovale on the internal surface of the temporal bone.

The trigeminal nerve gives off following three branches **(Flowchart 17.5):**
1. Ophthalmic nerve
2. Maxillary nerve
3. Mandibular nerve.

### Ophthalmic Nerve

The ophthalmic nerve comes out from skull via superior orbital fissure. This nerve gives of following three main branches:
1. Lacrimal
2. Frontal:
   - Supraorbital
   - Infraorbital
3. Nasociliary.

This nerve along with its branches supplies sensory innervations to the eyeball, the upper eye lid, the skin of the nose, the skin of the forehead, the skin of the scalp, part of nasal mucosa, and maxillary sinus and lacrimal glands. This nerve does not supply to any part of the oral cavity.

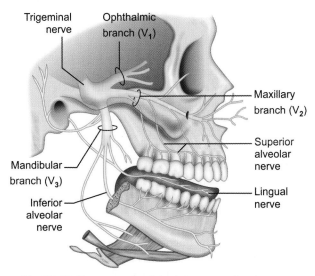

**Fig. 17.19:** Nerve supply of dento-osseous structures.

**Flowchart 17.5:** Divisions of trigeminal nerve.

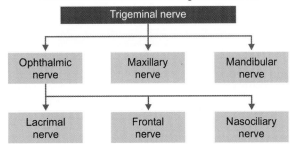

## Maxillary Nerve (Flowchart 17.6)

The maxillary nerve is the second division of trigeminal nerve and it exits from the skull through foramen rotundum.

The maxillary nerve has following four principle branches:
1. Pterygopalatine nerve:
   - Nasopalatine nerve
   - Palatine nerve
2. Posterosuperior alveolar nerve
3. Infraorbital nerve:
   - Middle superior alveolar nerve
   - Anterosuperior alveolar nerve
   - Anastomoses of infraorbital nerve
4. Zygomatic nerve.

### Pterygopalatine Branch of Maxillary Nerve

Pterygopalatine branch of maxillary nerve is the closest nerve as compared to other divisions of maxillary nerve; it gives off nasopalatine and palatine nerves.

*Nasopalatine nerve:* Nasopalatine nerve exits the palate through the incisive foramen to supply palatal and labial gingival of maxillary and mandibular molar and premolar teeth.

*Palatine nerve:* Palatine nerve gives off following three branches:

*1. Anterior palatine nerve:* This nerve enters the oral cavity through greater palatine foramen and runs anteriorly to supply the anterior part of mucosa of hard palate and palatal gingival of premolar and molar teeth.

*2. Middle palatine nerve:* This nerve enters the oral cavity through lesser palatine foramen to supply mucosa of soft palate and tonsils.

*3. Posterior palatine nerve:* This nerve like middle palatine nerve enters the lesser palatine foramen to supply the tonsils and the mucosa of the soft palate.

### Posterosuperior Alveolar Nerve

Posterosuperior alveolar nerve is the first terminal branch of maxillary nerve which enters via alveolar canal to supply following structures:
- The pulp of the maxillary molar teeth through the apical foramen except mesiobuccal root of the maxillary first molar
- Maxillary teeth and their supporting hard and soft tissue structures
- The mucosa of the maxillary sinus and cheek.

### Infraorbital Nerve

Infraorbital nerve enters the infraorbital canal and comes out through the infraorbital foramen onto the face. The infraorbital nerve gives off following three branches:

*1. Middle superior alveolar nerve:* It originates from infraorbital nerve in the infraorbital groove. It travels down through the lateral wall of the maxillary sinus and supplies the pulp of the maxillary premolars through the apical foramen and pulp in the mesiobuccal root of the maxillary first permanent molar; the mucosa of the maxillary sinus; supporting soft and hard tissue structures of premolar teeth.

*2. Anterosuperior alveolar nerve:* It originates from infraorbital nerve in the infraorbital canal and supplies maxillary anterior teeth and their supporting hard and soft tissue structures.

*3. Anastomoses of infraorbital nerve:* Anastomoses of infraorbital nerve supplies mucosa of the upper lip, mucosa of the lower eyelid, and mucosa of side of the neck.

### Zygomatic Nerve

Zygomatic nerve enters orbit via the inferior orbital fissure and then divides into zygomatic temporal and zygomaticofacial nerves. This nerve supplies the bone of temporal region and the orbit.

## Mandibular Nerve (Flowchart 17.7)

Mandibular division of trigeminal nerve exits from skull through the foramen ovale. This nerve is a mixed nerve; it has motor as well as sensory fibers. The motor fibers supply muscles and sensory fibers supply the teeth, soft and hard tissues.

### Motor Fibers

The motor fibers of mandibular division of trigeminal nerve have following nerves:
- Temporal nerve supplies to temporalis muscle
- Medial pterygoid nerve supplies to medial pterygoid muscle
- Lateral pterygoid nerve supplies to lateral pterygoid muscle
- Masseter nerve supplies to masseter muscle.

### Sensory Fibers

Sensory fibers of mandibular division of trigeminal nerve have following nerves:
- *Long buccal nerve:* It supplies to buccinator muscle hence this nerve is also called as buccinator nerve.
- *Lingual nerve:* The lingual nerve lies roughly about 2 mm below the foramen ovale and runs downward between the medial pterygoid muscle and ramus to the posterior part of the mylohyoid line resting closely beneath the mucous membrane of third molar.

**Flowchart 17.6:** Divisions of maxillary nerve.

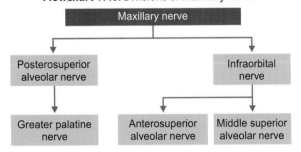

**Flowchart 17.7:** Divisions of mandibular nerve.

The following structures derive its nerve supply from the lingual nerve.
- The lingual gingiva of the entire mandibular arch
- The dorsum and ventral surface of two-thirds of the tongue
- The mucosa of the inner surface of the mandible in the sublingual region.

### Inferior Alveolar Nerve

Inferior alveolar nerve is the largest division of the mandibular nerve. It runs downward between sphenomandibular ligament and ramus of the mandible. It enters mandibular foramen through the mandibular canal, where it gives off mylohyoid nerve.

### Mylohyoid Nerve

Mylohyoid nerve is an efferent type. It runs forward and downward in the mylohyoid groove and then into the digastric triangle where it supplies the mylohyoid muscle and anterior belly of the digastric muscle.

### Mental Nerve

The mental nerve exits from the mandible through the mental foramen and supplies to the facial gingival of the mandibular incisors, canines and premolars, and the mucosa and the skin of the lower lip.

### Incisive Nerve

Incisive nerve continues forward within the body of the mandible in the mandibular canal and supplies the pulp of the mandibular incisors and canine teeth, the periodontal ligament, and the alveolar process of the incisors and canines.

### Auriculotemporal Nerve

This nerve originates from the main trunk of the mandibular nerve below the base of the skull turning backward beneath the lateral pterygoid muscle to supply pain and proprioception fibers to the TMJ and also to the outer ear, the skin of the lateral aspect of the skull, cheek, and the parotid gland.

## INNERVATION OF MAXILLA

The maxillary nerve gives off posterosuperior alveolar nerve and infraorbital nerve. The posterosuperior alveolar nerve supplies maxillary posterior teeth, alveolar mucosa, interdental septa, and periodontal tissues. The infraorbital nerve divides into middle superior alveolar nerve and anterosuperior alveolar nerve. Both the branches of infraorbital nerve run downward to supply premolars and anterior teeth. Middle superior alveolar nerve supplies maxillary premolars and their supporting soft tissues (alveolar mucosa, labial gingiva, lingual gingiva, and periodontal membrane). Anterosuperior alveolar nerve supplies anterior teeth (incisors and canine) and their surrounding structures.

## INNERVATION OF MANDIBLE

The mandible nerve gives off inferior alveolar nerve which enters the mandibular foramen accompanying with inferior alveolar artery. Mandibular teeth and their surrounding structures including soft and hard tissues derive nerve supply from the inferior alveolar nerve, which is the branch of mandibular nerve. This inferior alveolar nerve gives off mental nerve and enters the mental foramen, while incisive branch enters the incisive foramen. These two branches collectively supply mandibular teeth and their supporting hard and soft tissue structures.

## INNERVATION OF PALATE AND LIPS

Greater palatine nerve supplies the palate and superior labial nerve supplies to upper lip, and inferior labial nerve supplies to lower lip.

## BIBLIOGRAPHY

1. Ash MM, Nelson SJ (Eds). Wheeler's Dental Anatomy, Physiology and Occlusion, 8th edition. St Louis: Saunders; 2003.
2. Clemente CD (Ed). Gray's Anatomy of the Human Body, 30th edition. Philadelphia: Lea and Febiger; 1985.
3. Kraus B, Jordan R, Abrams L. Dental Anatomy and Occlusion. Williams and Wilkins; Baltimore: 1969.
4. Osborn JW (Ed). Dental Anatomy and Embryology. Oxford: Blackwell Scientific Publications; 1981.
5. Sicher H, DuBrul EL (Eds). Oral Anatomy, 7th edition. St Louis: CV Mosby; 1975.
6. Woelfel JB, Scheid RC (Eds). Dental Anatomy: Its Relevance to Dentistry, 5th edition. Williams and Wilkins: Baltimore; 1997.

## MULTIPLE CHOICE QUESTIONS

1. The ramus of the mandible join the body of the mandible at an_____
   a. Acute angle
   b. Obtuse angle
   c. Right angle
   d. 20 degree
2. The maxilla is:
   a. Dense
   b. Hollow or porous
   c. Mixed
   d. None
3. The incisive fossa of the mandible is located at _____
   a. Above the alveolar border of the central and lateral incisors and anterior to the canine
   b. Immediately below the alveolar border of the central and lateral incisors and anterior to the canine
   c. Below the alveolar border of the maxillary central incisors
   d. Below the alveolar border of the canine
4. The maxillary sinus is also called as:
   a. Antrum of maxilla
   b. Antrum of mandible
   c. Antrum of highmore
   d. Antrum of lowmore

5. The strongest portion of the mandible, which gives greatest strength to the mandible is _____
   a. Inferior border
   b. Superior border
   c. Medial border
   d. Lateral border
6. Which of the following is correct regarding the frontal process of the maxilla?
   a. Superiorly, it articulates with frontal bone
   b. Medially, it forms part of the lateral wall of the nasal cavity
   c. Anteriorly, it articulates with nasal bone
   d. All of the above
7. The maxilla articulates with:
   a. The nasal bone
   b. The frontal bone
   c. Lacrimal bone
   d. All of the above
8. Which of the following is correct regarding the maxillary sinus?
   a. The maxillary sinus lies within the body of the bone and is of corresponding pyramidal form, the base is directed toward the nasal cavity
   b. Sinus is closed in laterally and above by the thin walls that forms the anterolateral, posterolateral, and orbital surface of the body
   c. A layer of sinus mucosa is also always between the root tips and the sinus cavity
   d. All of the above
9. The shape of the mandible is:
   a. Horseshoe shaped
   b. "U" shaped
   c. "V" shaped
   d. Triangular shaped
10. The only movable bone of the skull is:
    a. Maxilla
    b. Mandible
    c. Cranial bone
    d. Hyoid bone

**Answers**

| | | | | | | | |
|---|---|---|---|---|---|---|---|
| 1. b | 2. b | 3. b | 4. c | 5. a | 6. d | 7. d | 8. d |
| 9. a | 10. b | | | | | | |

# 18

# Temporomandibular Joint

## INTRODUCTION

The temporomandibular joint (TMJ) **(Fig. 18.1)** connects the mandibular jawbone to the skull. Left and right synovial joints of TMJ form a bicondylar articulation between the temporal bone of the skull above and the mandible below; it is from these bones that its name is derived.

The TMJ is also a *ginglymoarthrodial* joint, a term that is derived from ginglymus, meaning a hinge joint, allowing motion only backward and forward in one plane, and arthrodia, meaning a joint of which permits a gliding motion of the surfaces.

The features exhibited by the TMJ common to synovial joints include a disk, bone, fibrous capsule, fluid, synovial membrane, and ligaments. However, there are several features that differentiate and make this joint unique. Its articular surface is covered by fibrocartilage instead of hyaline cartilage; it permits both hinge and gliding/translatory movements;

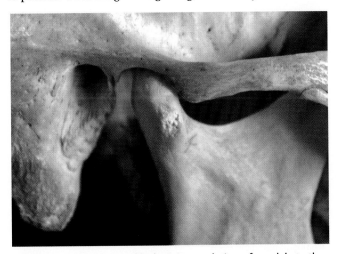

**Fig. 18.1:** Temporomandibular joint—relation of condyle to the glenoid fossa.

the movement is not only guided by the shape of the bones, muscles, and ligaments but also by the occlusion of the teeth, since both the joints are joined by a single mandibular bone and cannot move independently of each other.

The most important functions of the TMJ are mastication and speech. This chapter briefs the TMJ and its surrounding structures.

## ARTICULAR SURFACES (FIGS. 18.2A AND B)

The joint has superior and inferior articular surfaces. The superior or upper articular surface is formed by articular eminence and anterior part of the mandibular fossa/glenoid fossa **(Fig. 18.2A)**. The inferior articular surface is formed by the head of the condyle of the mandible **(Fig. 18.2B)**.

## INTRA-ARTICULAR DISK (FIG. 18.3)

The most important feature of the TMJ is the articular disk. It is a biconcave fibrocartilaginous structure located between the mandibular condyle and the temporal bone component of the joint. Its function is to accommodate a hinging action as well as the gliding actions between the temporal and mandibular articular bone.

The articular disk is a roughly oval, firm, and fibrous plate with its long axis being transversely directed. It is shaped like a peaked cap that divides the joint into a larger upper compartment and a smaller lower compartment. Hinging movements take place in the lower compartment and gliding movements take place in the upper compartment.

The superior surface of the disk is said to be saddle-shaped to fit into the cranial contour, while the inferior surface is concave to fit against the mandibular condyle. The disk is thick, round to oval all around its rim, divided into an *anterior band* of 2 mm thickness, a *posterior band of* 3 mm thickness, and thin *intermediate band* of 1 mm thickness in the center. More posteriorly there is a *bilaminar or retrodiskal region*. The disk is attached all around the joint capsule except for the strong straps that fix the disk directly to the medial and lateral condylar poles, which ensure that the disk and condyle move together in protraction and retraction.

The anterior extension of the disk is attached to a fibrous that supports the joint. The two minor ligaments, the capsule

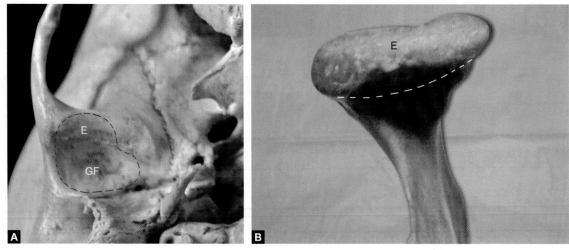

**Figs. 18.2A and B:** Articular surfaces of temporomandibular joint (TMJ). (A) Glenoid fossa (GF) and articular eminence (E); (B) Condyle.

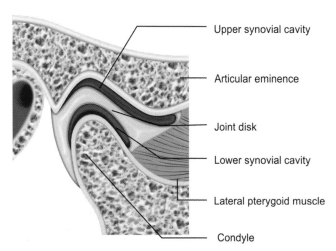

**Fig. 18.3:** Intra-articular disk.

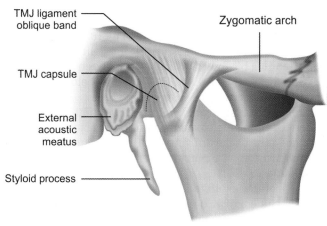

**Fig. 18.4:** Fibrous capsule. (TMJ: temporomandibular joint)

superiorly and inferiorly. In between, it gives insertion stylomandibular and sphenomandibular ligaments are to the lateral pterygoid muscle, accessory and are not directly attached to any part of the joint.

## FIBROUS CAPSULE (FIG. 18.4)

The fibrous capsule is a thin sleeve of tissue completely surrounding the joint. It extends from the circumference of the cranial articular surface to the neck of the mandible. The synovial membrane lining the capsule covers all the intra-articular surfaces except the pressure-bearing fibrocartilage.

## LIGAMENTS OF TEMPOROMANDIBULAR JOINT (FIG. 18.5)

The TMJ has one major and two minor ligaments. The temporomandibular ligament is the major ligament, while the

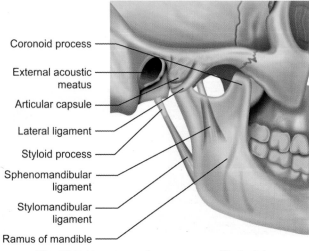

**Fig. 18.5:** Ligaments of temporomandibular joint.

sphenomandibular ligament and stylomandibular ligament are minor ligaments.

## Temporomandibular Ligament/Lateral Ligament

The joint capsule is strengthened by the temporomandibular ligament. It is in fact the thickened lateral portion of the capsule and cannot be readily separated from the capsule. This ligament provides the main means of support for the joint, resists dislocation during functional movements by restricting distal and inferior movements of the mandible.

## Sphenomandibular Ligament

The sphenomandibular ligament is a remnant of the dorsal part of Meckel's cartilage. It is attached superiorly to the spine of the sphenoid, and inferiorly to the lingual of the mandibular foramen.

## Stylomandibular Ligament

It is a reinforced lamina of the deep cervical fascia. It is attached above to the lateral surface of styloid process and below to the angle and posterior border of the ramus of the mandible.

## BLOOD AND NERVE SUPPLY TO TEMPOROMANDIBULAR JOINT

The TMJ derives blood supply from superficial temporal and maxillary artery. The TMJ derives nerve supply from auriculotemporal and masseter nerves.

## MUSCLES OF THE JOINT

The masticatory muscles surrounding the joint are groups of muscles that contract and relax in harmony so that the jaws function properly. When the muscles are relaxed and flexible and are not under stress, they work in harmony with the other parts of the TMJ complex. The muscles of mastication produce all the movements of the jaw. They are involved in the activity of mastication and speech.

Different set of muscles are required for the opposite movements of the mandible. The muscles of mastication are *adductors (jaw closers/elevators) and abductors (jaw openers/ depressors)*. The temporalis, masseter, and medial pterygoid muscles are adductors, while the lateral pterygoid muscles are the primary abductors of the jaw. The muscles that produce forward movement (protrusive) are also used alternately to move the jaw from side to side (laterally).

## Masseter Muscle (Fig. 18.6)

The principal and strongest muscle of mastication is the masseter, which stems from the temporal bone and extends downward on the outer surface of the mandible to its lower angle. It consists of two overlapping heads.

## Origin

### Superficial head

- It originates from anterior two-thirds of the lower border of the zygomatic arch and adjoining the zygomatic process of maxilla.
- Fibers of this layer of masseter pass downward and backward at 45°.

**Deep head:** It originates from deep surface of the zygomatic arch.

## Insertion

- The superficial layer is inserted at lower part of the ramus of the mandible.
- The middle layer of masseter muscle is inserted into the middle part of the ramus of the mandible.
- The deep layer is inserted at the upper part and coronoid process of the mandible.

## Nerve Supply

The masseter muscle derives nerve supply from masseter nerve which is an anterior division of mandibular nerve, which in turn is a division of trigeminal nerve.

## Action

- It is a powerful elevator of the mandible.
- It also helps in ipsilateral excursion.

## Temporalis Muscle (Fig. 18.6)

Temporalis muscle is a fan-shaped muscle and the largest masticatory muscle that fills the temporal fossa.

## Origin

This muscle originates from the floor of temporal fossa and from overlying temporal bone.

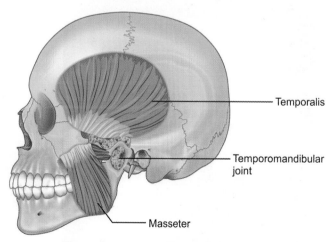

**Fig. 18.6:** Masseter and temporalis muscles.

*Insertion*

Temporalis muscle is inserted at margins and deep surface of coronoid process and anterior border of ramus of the mandible.

*Nerve Supply*

The temporalis muscle derives nerve supply from temporal branch of mandibular nerve.

*Action*

- Its anterior fibers help in elevation of the mandible.
- Its posterior fibers retract the protruded mandible.
- It also helps in lateral/side-to-side grinding movement of the mandible.

### Medial Pterygoid Muscle (Fig. 18.7A)

The medial pterygoid runs parallel to the masseter but on the inside of the jaw. It originates at a wing-shaped protrusion of the cranium. The medial pterygoid and the masseter muscles form a sling around the back end of the mandible and work together to pull it shut.

It is a quadrilateral muscle, has a small superficial and a large deep head.

*Origin*

- Its superficial head originates from the tuberosity of the maxilla and adjoining bone.
- Its deep head, which is larger, originates from the medial surface of the lateral pterygoid plate and the adjoining process of the palatine bone.

*Insertion*

- The fibers run downward, backward, and laterally.

- It is inserted on the medial surface of the angle and the adjoining ramus of the mandible, below and behind the mandibular foramen, and the mylohyoid groove.

*Nerve Supply*

It derives its nerve supply by the nerve to medial pterygoid, a branch of the main trunk of mandibular nerve.

*Action*

- It elevates the mandible.
- It protrudes the mandible along with the lateral pterygoid muscle.
- Medial and lateral pterygoids of two sides contract alternatively to produce side-to-side lateral movement of the mandible.

### Lateral Pterygoid Muscle (Fig. 18.7B)

Lateral pterygoid muscle is short conical muscle and has upper and lower heads.

*Origin*

- The upper head of the lateral pterygoid muscle is small and originates from infratemporal surface of the greater wing of sphenoid bone.
- The lower head is large and originates from lateral surface of the lateral pterygoid plate of the sphenoid bone.

*Insertion*

- The fibers of superior head are inserted into the capsule and medial part of the intra-articular disk of TMJ.
- The fibers of inferior head insert into pterygoid fovea on the anterior surface of the neck of the mandible.

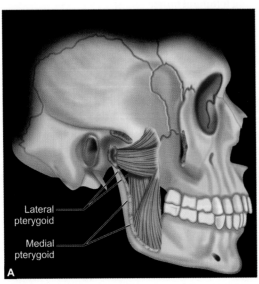

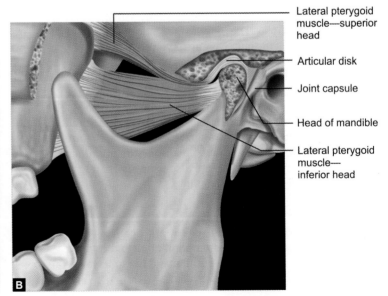

**Figs. 18.7A and B:** Medial and lateral pterygoid muscles.

### Nerve Supply

The lateral pterygoid muscle derives nerve supply from a branch from anterior division of the mandibular nerve.

### Action

- Depress mandible to open mouth with suprahyoid muscles.
- Lateral and medial pterygoid muscles protrude the mandible.
- Left lateral pterygoid and right medial pterygoid produce lateral grinding movements.

### Accessory Muscles of Mastication

Along with the four muscles of mastication, some accessory muscles are also involved in the process of mastication. They mainly include buccinator, orbicularis oris, digastric, genioglossus, mylohyoid, geniohyoid, tensor tympani, and palatine muscles.

## MANDIBULAR MOVEMENTS AND MUSCLE ACTIVITY

Mandibular movements involve complex neuromuscular patterns, originating in part, in a pattern generator in the brainstem and modified by influences from higher centers (cerebral cortex and basal ganglia) and from peripheral influences (the periodontium, muscles, etc.).

Radiographs in **Figures 18.8A and B** show the TMJ in open and closed positions of the mandible.

The main muscles involved in activities of jaw opening and closing, protrusion, retrusion, and lateral movements are listed here.

### Elevation of Mandible

- Right and left temporalis (anterior fibers)
- Right and left masseter
- Right and left medial pterygoid muscles.

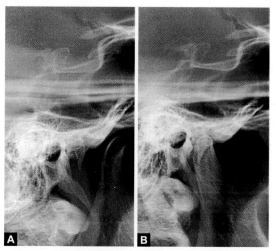

**Figs. 18.8A and B:** Radiographs showing temporomandibular joint (TMJ) in (A) open; and (B) closed position of mandible.

### Depression of Mandible

Opening of mandible is mainly affected by lateral pterygoid muscle.

- Right and left lateral pterygoids (inferior heads)
- Right and left suprahyoid and infrahyoid muscles
- Anterior belly of digastric and mylohyoid.

### Protrusion

Protrusion occurs by the lateral and medial pterygoid and masseter and suprahyoid group of muscles.

- Right and left lateral pterygoids (inferior heads)
- Right and left medial pterygoids
- Right and left superior heads of masseter.

### Retrusion

- Right and left posterior fibers of temporalis
- Right and left deep heads of masseter.

### Lateral Movements

#### Movement to the right side (right lateral excursion)

- Right masseter
- Right temporalis
- Left medial and lateral pterygoids.

#### Movement to the left side (left lateral excursion)

- Left masseter
- Left temporalis
- Right medial and lateral pterygoids.

## BIBLIOGRAPHY

1. Ahlgren J. Mechanisms of mastication. Acta Odontol Scand. 1966;24:109.
2. Beyron H. Occlusal relations and mastication in Australian aborigines. Acta Odontol Scand. 1964;22:597-678.
3. Hickey JC, Allison ML, Woelfel JB, et al. Mandibular movement in three dimensions. J Prosthet Dent. 1963;13:72-92.
4. Hjortsjö CH. The mechanism in the temporomandibular joint. Acta Odontol Scand. 1953;11:5-23.
5. Lavelle LB. Applied Oral Physiology, 2nd edition. London: Wright Butterworths and Copublications; 1988.
6. McNamara JA. The independent functions of the two heads of the lateral pterygoid muscle. Am J Anat. 1973;138:197-205.
7. Owall B, Moller E. Tactile sensibility during chewing and biting. Odont Revy. 1974;25:327.
8. Posselt U. The physiology of occlusion and rehabilitation. Oxford: Blackwell; 1963.

## MULTIPLE CHOICE QUESTIONS

1. The stylomandibular ligament of temporomandibular joint (TMJ) is attached:
   a. Above to the lateral surface of the styloid process
   b. Below the angle and posterior border of the ramus of the mandible

c. Both of the above
d. None of the above.

2. Which of the following is incorrect regarding the ligaments of the TMJ?
   a. Stylomandibular ligament is attached above to the lateral surface of the styloid process
   b. Sphenomandibular ligament is attached superiorly to the spine of mandibular foramen
   c. Lateral ligament is attached to articular tubercle
   d. Fibrous capsule is attached below to the articular tubercle.

3. The TMJ gets its blood supply from:
   a. Braches from superficial temporal and maxillary arteries
   b. Braches from mandibular arteries
   c. External carotid artery
   d. Mental artery.

4. TMJ gets its innervations from:
   a. Auriculotemporal nerve
   b. Masseter nerve
   c. Both of the above
   d. None of the above.

5. The muscle responsible for protrusive movement of the mandible:
   a. Lateral pterygoid and medial pterygoid muscles
   b. Superior heads of masseter.
   c. Temporalis muscle
   d. Both a and b

6. Elevation of the mandible is brought about by:
   a. Masseter muscle
   b. Temporalis muscle
   c. Medial pterygoid muscle
   d. All of the above.

7. Retrusive mandibular movement is produced by:
   a. Posterior fibers of temporalis
   b. Deep heads of masseter.
   c. Medial and lateral pterygoid muscles
   d. Both a and b

8. Left lateral mandibular movement is produced by:
   a. Left lateral pterygoid and right medial pterygoid muscles
   b. Right lateral pterygoid muscle left medial pterygoid muscles
   c. Lateral pterygoid muscle only
   d. Medial pterygoid muscle only.

9. Depression of the mandible is produced by:
   a. Mainly the lateral pterygoid muscle
   b. Digastric, geniohyoid, and mylohyoid muscles
   c. Both of the above
   d. None of the above.

10. Which of the following muscle is not an antigravity muscle?
    a. Masseter muscle
    b. Temporalis muscle
    c. Medial pterygoid muscle
    d. Lateral pterygoid muscle.

**Answers**

1. c    2. d    3. a    4. c    5. d    6. d    7. d    8. a
9. c    10. d

# 7

## SECTION

# Occlusion

# 19

**CHAPTER**

# Occlusion

---

> **💡 Did you know?**
>
> ✎ **Monoplane posteriors** with flat cusps are given in complete denture patients with bruxism and poor neuromuscular control.
> ✎ In recent decades, it has been speculated that there is a relationship between occlusion of teeth and whole body posture.

## INTRODUCTION

Occlusion, in simpler terms, means contact between the teeth. More technically, it is the relationship between the maxillary and mandibular teeth when they approach each other, as occurs during chewing or at rest. Occlusion has both static and dynamic aspects. Static occlusion refers to contact between teeth when the jaw is closed and stationary, while dynamic occlusion refers to occlusal contacts made when the jaw is moving, as with chewing.

It is essential to understand that the masticatory (or stomatognathic) system is generally considered to be made

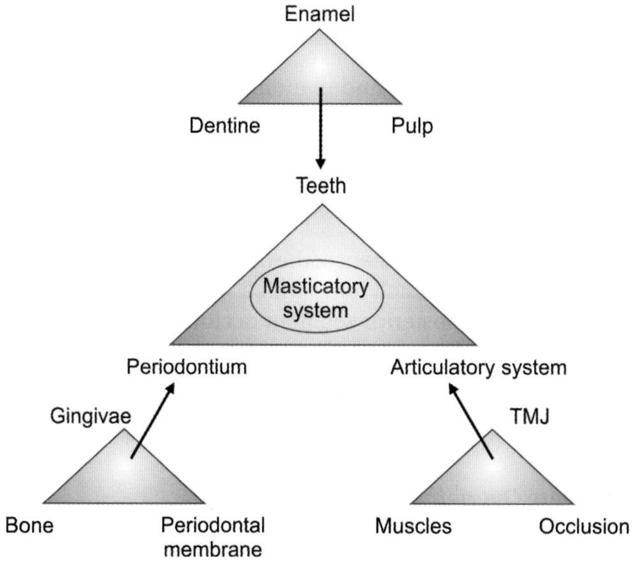

**Fig. 19.1:** The masticatory system.
(TMJ: temporomandibular joint).

up of three interdependent parts—(1) the teeth, (2) the periodontal tissues, and (3) the articulatory system (**Fig. 19.1**). The importance of occlusion in dental practice is based primarily upon the relationships that it has within these interconnected biomechanical systems. When one considers how almost all forms of dental treatment have a potential for causing occlusal change, the need to understand the concepts of normal occlusion becomes quite obvious.

Most dental procedures involve occlusal surfaces of teeth. Knowledge of occlusal norms and how to properly examine stomatognathic system is a key to prevent uncontrolled changes in interarch relationships and development of temporomandibular disorders. Analysis of occlusion should be performed before, during, and after every dental procedure that changes vertical dimension and occlusal surfaces.

Several concepts of an "ideal" or optimal occlusion of the natural dentition have been suggested by Angle, Schnyler, Beyron, D'Amico, Friel, Hellman, Lucia, Stallard Stuart and Ramfjord and Ash. Concepts of ideal occlusion are primarily used in orthodontics and conservative dentistry.

## TERMS COMMONLY USED IN DISCUSSIONS ABOUT OCCLUSION AND MALOCCLUSION

### Ideal Occlusion

It is a preconceived theoretical concept of occlusal structural and functional relationship that includes idealized principles and characteristics that an occlusion should be.

### Normal Occlusion

Normal occlusion is a class-I relationship of the maxillary and mandibular first molars in centric occlusion. Normal occlusion is an absence of large or many facets, bone loss, closed vertical dimension, crooked teeth, bruxing habit, loose teeth, and freedom from joint pain.

### Physiological Occlusion

Physiological occlusion refers to an occlusion that deviates in one or more ways from ideal yet it is well adapted to that particular environment, is esthetic, and shows no pathological manifestations or dysfunctions.

## Functional Occlusion

Functional occlusion is defined as an arrangement of teeth, which will provide the highest efficiency during the excursive movements of the mandible, which is necessary during function.

## Balanced Occlusion

An occlusion in which balanced and equal contacts are maintained throughout the entire arch during all excursions of the mandible.

## Therapeutic Occlusion

It is an occlusion that has been modified by appropriate therapeutic modalities in order to change a nonphysiological occlusion to one that is at least physiological, if not ideal.

## Traumatic Occlusion

Traumatic occlusion is an abnormal occlusal stress, which is capable of producing or has produced an injury to the periodontium.

## Trauma from Occlusion

It is defined as periodontal tissue injury caused by occlusal forces through abnormal occlusal contacts.

## Centric Occlusion

It is the maximum intercuspation or contact attained between maxillary and mandibular posterior teeth.

## Centric Relation

Centric relation is the most posterior position of the mandible relative to the maxilla at a given vertical dimension.

## Centric Relation Occlusion

Centric relation occlusion (when centric relation and centric occlusion coincide) is the simultaneous even contact between maxillary and mandibular teeth into maximum interdigitation with the mandible in centric relation (most retruded position).

## DEVELOPMENT OF OCCLUSION

Dental occlusion undergoes significant changes from birth until adulthood and beyond. This continuation of changes in the dental relationship during various stages of the dentition can be divided into four stages:
1. *Gum pad stage*: 0–6 months
2. *Deciduous dentition*: 6 months to 6 years
3. *Mixed dentition*: 6–12 years
4. *Permanent dentition*: 12 years and beyond.

## GUM PAD STAGE (0–6 MONTHS)

The jaws are devoid of teeth at birth. Gum pad stage extends from birth up to the eruption of first primary tooth usually the lower central incisors at around 6 months of age. The gum

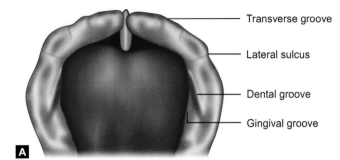

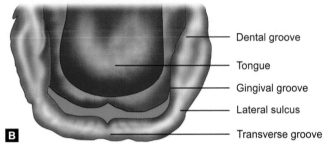

**Figs. 19.2A and B:** The gum pads: (A) Maxillary; (B) Mandibular.

pads are pink in color and firm in consistency. The maxillary gum pad is horseshoe shaped, and the mandibular gum pad is U/square shaped **(Figs. 19.2A and B)**.

The gum pads develop in two portions—buccal and lingual portions, which are separated by the *dental groove*. The gum pads in both the arches show certain elevations and grooves that outline the portion of various primary teeth that are still developing in the alveolar ridges.

These grooves are called as *transverse grooves*. The prominent transverse groove separating canine and first deciduous molar segments in both the arches is called the *lateral sulcus*. The lateral sulci are often used to judge the interarch relationship at a very early stage. The *gingival groove* separates the maxillary and mandibular gum pads from the palate and floor of the mouth, respectively.

### Characteristic Features of Gum Pad Stage

#### Infantile Open Bite

Usually the anterior segment of the upper and lower gum pads do not approximate each other with a space created between them, while the posterior segment occlude with each other at molar region **(Fig. 19.3)**. The tongue is positioned in this space between the upper and lower gum pads during suckling. This infantile open bite is transient and gets self corrected with the eruption of deciduous incisors.

#### Complete Overjet

The maxillary gum pad is usually larger and overlaps the mandibular gum pad both horizontally and vertically with a complete overjet all around. In this way, the opposing surface of the pads provide for a very efficient way of squeezing milk during breastfeeding.

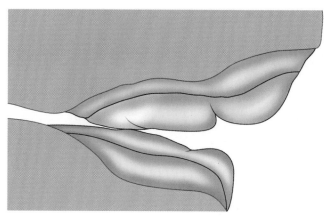

**Fig. 19.3:** Relationship between upper and lower gum pads in infants.

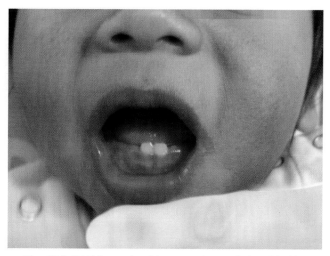

**Fig. 19.5:** Deciduous dentition stage is usually heralded by eruption of mandibular central incisors.

### Anteroposterior Relationship

In general, the mandibular lateral sulci are more posterior to the maxillary lateral sulci.

### Precocious Eruption of Primary Teeth

***Natal and neonatal teeth:*** Usually, jaws are devoid of teeth at birth. However, occasionally infants are born with one/two erupted teeth, usually the mandibular incisors. Such teeth present at birth are called as *natal teeth* (Fig. 19.4). Teeth that erupt within 30 days of life are called as the *neonatal teeth.* Familial tendency is observed in this condition and such premature eruption of tooth may cause problems during feeding. It is advised to retain them unless they are too mobile.

## DECIDUOUS DENTITION STAGE
## (6 MONTHS TO 6 YEARS)

The deciduous dentition stage spans from the time of eruption of primary teeth until the eruption of the first permanent tooth around 6 years of age.

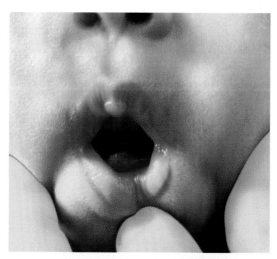

**Fig. 19.4:** Natal tooth in a newborn child.

### Eruption Chronology of Primary Teeth

Eruption of the primary teeth begins by 6 months of age when primary mandibular incisors erupt into oral cavity **(Fig. 19.5)**. Eruption of all the primary teeth is generally complete by two and half years by which age the deciduous dentition is in full function. Root formation of primary teeth is usually completed by 3 years of age.

Although considerable variation is seen in the eruption timing of deciduous teeth, there appears to be no significant gender differences. The chronology of primary teeth is presented in Chapter 3, Table 3.1.

The sequence of eruption of primary teeth may also show some variation. However, in most of the cases, the lower central incisors are the first teeth to erupt, followed by the upper central incisors. Usually, the lateral incisor, first molar, and canine tend to erupt earlier in maxilla than in the mandible. Deciduous dentition generally shows the following order of eruption:

$$\frac{\text{AB} \quad\quad \text{D} \quad\quad \text{C} \quad\quad \text{E}}{\text{A} \quad\quad \text{B} \quad\quad \text{D} \quad\quad \text{CE}}$$

- Central incisors
- Lateral incisors
- First molars
- Canines
- Second molars.

By 3 years of age, the occlusion of deciduous dentition is completely established and dental arches remain relatively constant with no significant changes up to 6 years of age.

### Characteristics of Occlusion of Deciduous Dentition

#### Interdental Spacing

Interdental spacing, when present in permanent dentition, is considered abnormal. However, presence of interdental spacing is an important and normal feature of deciduous dentition **(Figs. 19.6A to C)**, which is required for the accommodation of larger permanent teeth at a later stage.

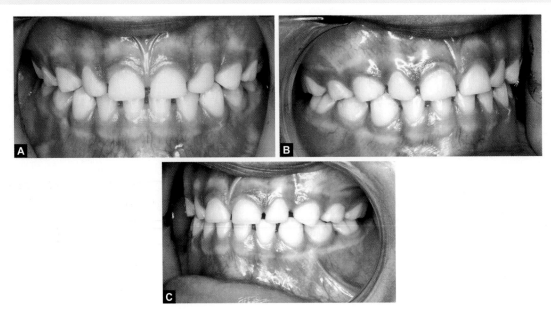

**Figs. 19.6A to C:** Presence of interdental spacing in primary dentition is physiological and a desirable feature, which aids in accommodation of larger successor teeth. Figure shows adequate physiological spacing in a 4-year-old child.

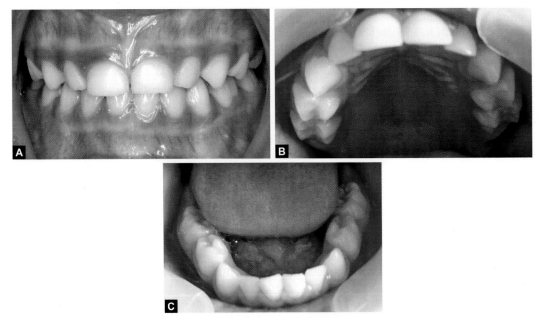

**Figs. 19.7A to C:** Insufficient interdental spacing in a 5-year-old child. Inadequate interdental spacing in primary dentition often leads to crowding in permanent dentition.

Spaces present between deciduous teeth are often referred to as *physiological or developmental spaces.* Sufficient interdental space is needed for the permanent teeth to erupt into an uncrowded position and for establishment of their proper alignment. Malocclusion with crowding of teeth can be expected in case of unspaced primary dentition (**Figs. 19.7A to C**). Leighton BC (1969) has given the probability of crowding of permanent dentition based on the amount of interdental spacing available in the primary dentition (**Table 19.1**).

**Table 19.1:** Probability of crowding of permanent teeth based on available spaces between primary teeth—Leighton BC (1969).

| Space in primary teeth | Chances of crowding of permanent teeth |
|---|---|
| >6 mm | None |
| 3–5 mm | 1 in 5 |
| <3 mm | 1 in 2 |
| No spacing | 2 in 3 |
| Crowded primary teeth | 1 in 1 |

Physiological/developmental spacing in deciduous dentition includes: Generalized spacing between teeth primate spaces.

### Generalized Spacing

According to Foster (1982), generalized spacing occurs in almost 75% of the individuals in the primary dentition stage. Generalized spacing between the teeth are seen in both the dental arches and helps in accommodation of larger successor teeth.

### Primate Spaces/Anthropoid Spaces/Simian Spaces

In addition to the generalized spacing, localized spacing are often present mesial to the upper canine and distal to the lower canine. Such spaces, originally described by Lewis and Lehman (1929), are a normal feature of the permanent

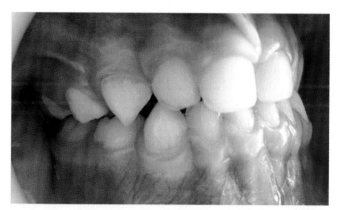

**Fig. 19.8:** Primate/anthropoid/simian spaces—developmental spaces present mesial to upper canines and distal to lower canines.

dentition in the higher apes (primates) and in the human primary dentition, and are usually referred to as the anthropoid spaces. Anthropoid spaces appear to be a more constant feature of deciduous dentition **(Fig. 19.8)**.

***Significance of anthropoid spaces:*** Following eruption of primary first molars, when canine teeth erupt and reach occlusion, the primate spaces facilitate proper interdigitation of the opposing canines into class-I canine relationship.

### Incisor Relationship

Incisor relationship in deciduous dentition normally shows:
- Increased overbite (deep bite)
- Increased overjet.

***Deep bite:*** An increased overbite is usually seen in the initial stages of development with the deciduous mandibular incisors contacting the cingulum area of the deciduous maxillary incisors in centric occlusion **(Figs. 19.9A to C)**. Deep bite may be due to the fact that the primary incisors are more vertically placed than the permanent incisors.

The ideal position of the deciduous incisors has been described as being more vertical than the permanent incisors, with a deeper incisal overbite.

This deep bite later gets self-corrected by:
- Attrition of incisors
- Eruption of deciduous molars
- Differential growth of the alveolar processes of the jaws.

***Increased overjet:*** Excessive incisal overjet is often observed in deciduous dentition. About 72% of children exhibited an increased overjet in a study conducted by Foster. Excessive overjet usually gets corrected later by the forward growth of the mandible.

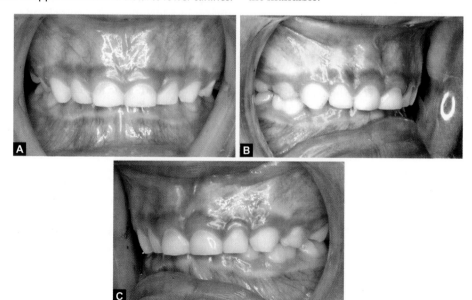

**Figs. 19.9A to C:** Increased overbite (deep bite) is a normal feature of deciduous dentition. It may be due to the fact that the primary incisors are more vertically placed than the permanent incisors.

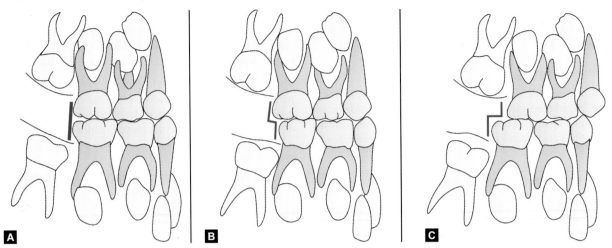

**Figs. 19.10A to C:** Terminal plane relationships: (A) flush/straight terminal plane—the distal surfaces of maxillary and mandibular second deciduous molars are in same vertical plane; (B) mesial step—distal surface of mandibular deciduous second molar is more mesial to the distal surface of the maxillary deciduous second molar (mandibular primary second molar is ahead of the maxillary deciduous second molar); (C) distal step—maxillary second deciduous molar is ahead of the mandibular second deciduous molar.

### Molar Relationship

The anteroposterior molar relationship in deciduous dentition is described in terms of the *terminal planes*. The terminal planes are the distal surfaces of the maxillary and mandibular second primary molars.

Moyers described three possible kinds of primary molar relationships **(Figs. 19.10A to C)**:
1. Straight/flush terminal plane
2. Mesial step
3. Distal step.

#### Flush terminal plane:

- *Straight/flush terminal plane:* The distal surfaces of the maxillary and mandibular deciduous molars are in same vertical plane **(Fig. 19.10A)**.

  It is of significance to note that the mandibular second primary molar has a greater mesiodistal diameter than the primary maxillary second molar. This difference in the dimensions makes the distal surfaces of both maxillary and mandibular deciduous second molars to fall in same vertical plane in centric occlusion. Such an arrangement is called as *flush terminal plane*. Flush terminal plane is considered to be the ideal kind of molar relationship in the primary dentition.
- *Mesial step*: In this terminal plane relationship, the distal surface of the mandibular deciduous second molar is more mesial to the distal surface of the maxillary deciduous second molar **(Fig. 19.10B)**.
- *Distal step*: Here, the distal surface of the mandibular deciduous second molar is more distal to the distal surface of the maxillary deciduous second molar. In other words, the maxillary second deciduous molar is ahead of the mandibular second deciduous molar **(Fig. 19.10C)**.

*Significance of terminal plane relationship:* Determining the terminal plane relationship in the primary dentition stage is of great importance, because the erupting first permanent molars are guided by the distal surfaces of the second primary molars as they erupt into occlusion. Thus, the terminal plane relationship of primary dentition largely determines the type of molar relationship in the permanent dentition.

## MIXED DENTITION STAGE (6–12 YEARS)

Mixed dentition stage is a transition stage when primary teeth are exfoliated in a sequential manner, followed by the eruption of their permanent successors. This stage spans from 6 years to 12 years of age, beginning with the eruption of the first permanent tooth, usually a mandibular central incisor or a first molar. It is completed at the time when the last primary tooth is shed. Significant changes in occlusion are seen in mixed dentition period due to the loss of 20 primary teeth and eruption of their successor permanent teeth. Most malocclusions develop at this stage.

Mixed dentition stage can be divided into the following phases:
- Early/first transitional period
- Intertransitional period
- Late/second transitional period.

### Early Transitional Period (6–8 Years)

Early transitional period is concerned with the replacement of the primary incisors by their successors and the addition of four permanent molars to the dentition. This usually occurs in the age range of 6–8 years.

### Emergence of the First Permanent Molars

The first permanent molars erupt at 6 years of age with mandibular molar preceding the maxillary in most cases. The first molars are considered to play an important role in the establishment of occlusion in the permanent dentition

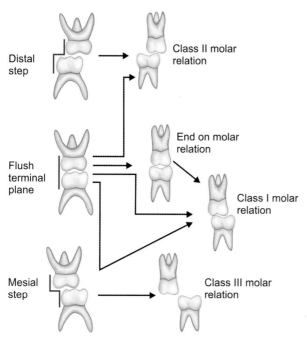

**Fig. 19.11:** The possible effects of terminal plane relationship on permanent dentition.

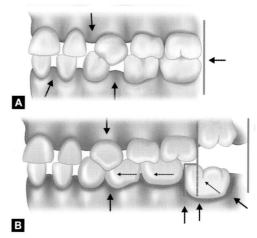

**Figs. 19.12A and B:** Early mesial shift: Erupting lower permanent first molars shift mesially utilizing the primate spaces in early mixed dentition period to establish class-I molar relationship.

and class-I molar relationship is considered as the normal anteroposterior molar relationship. The location and relationship of first permanent molars is influenced by the presence of interdental spacing and the terminal plane relationship of the primary molars.

The erupting first permanent molars are guided by the distal surfaces of the second primary molars as they erupt into occlusion. Thus, the terminal plane relationship of primary dentition largely determines the type of molar relationship in the permanent dentition, among other factors.

The possible effects of terminal plane relationship on permanent dentition are described in **Figure 19.11**.

*Effects of flush terminal plane:* Flush terminal plane usually develops into class-I molar relationship in the permanent dentition. Some cases of flush terminal plane may also develop into class-II molar relationship when forward mandibular growth is not sufficient.

In the presence of flush terminal plane, the first permanent molars initially assume a cusp-to-cusp or end-on molar relationship, as they erupt distal to the second primary molars. The lower first permanent molar has to move 2–3 mm anteriorly in relation to the upper first permanent molar in order to transform the end-on relation to class-I molar relation. This transformation from end-on to class-I molar relation occurs in two ways designated as *early and late mesial shifts.*

*Early mesial shift:* Early mesial shift of lower permanent molars occur by utilization of the interdental physiological spaces present between primary teeth including the primate spaces.

The eruptive force of permanent molars pushes the deciduous molars forward into the spaces, thereby establishing class-I molar relationship. As this change occurs in early mixed dentition, the shift is called the *"early mesial shift"* (**Figs. 19.12A and B**).

*Late mesial shift:* In the absence of sufficient developmental spaces in primary dentition, the erupting permanent first molars may not be able to establish class-I relationship in early mixed dentition period. In such cases, class-I molar relationship can be established following the exfoliation of primary second molars; by utilizing Leeway space (Leeway space is explained later in this chapter). As this occurs in late mixed dentition, it is called as the "late mesial shift" (**Fig. 19.13**).

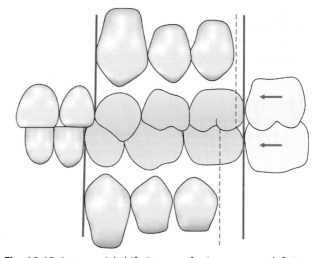

**Fig. 19.13:** Late mesial shift: In case of primate space deficiency, class-I molar relationship can be achieved in late mixed dentition period following exfoliation of primary second molars, utilizing the leeway space.

***Effects of mesial step:*** When deciduous second molars are in mesial step, the first permanent molars directly erupt into class-I molar relationship. Few cases may also progress to class-III molar relations, if forward growth of the mandible persists.

***Effects of distal step:*** Distal step in primary dentition usually leads to Angle's class-II molar relationships in the permanent dentition. A few cases may go into class-I molar relationship.

### Eruption of Permanent Incisors

Permanent incisors erupt lingual to the primary incisors and mandibular central incisors are often the first to erupt. How the larger permanent incisor teeth are accommodated is described here.

### Incisal Liability

It can be readily appreciated that the mesiodistal crown dimensions of permanent incisors are considerably greater than that of the primary incisors. This difference in the mesiodistal crown dimension between the primary and permanent incisors is termed as *incisal liability* by Warren Mayne.

According to the average tooth size given by Black:
- Incisal liability in maxillary arch is about 7.6 mm, i.e. the maxillary permanent incisors are larger than their predecessors by 7.6 mm.
- Incisal liability in mandibular arch is about 6.0 mm, i.e. mandibular permanent incisors are 6.0 mm larger than their predecessors.

Thus, the amount of space available in the arch following exfoliation of the primary incisors is far less than the amount of space needed for accommodation of their permanent successors. Some degree of transient crowding may occur due to incisal liability at about 8–9 years of age, and persist until the emergence of canines when the space for teeth may again be adequate.

During the course of mixed dentition period, nature makes some adjustments to achieve the fit and maintain the dynamic balance. The incisal liability is overcome by the following factors:
- *Utilization of interdental spacing between primary anterior:* Incisal liability is partly compensated by the developmental spaces that exist in the primary dentition. Anterior crowding of permanent dentition may develop in the absence of interdental spacing.
- *Increase in the intercanine arch width:* Continuing growth of the jaws often results in an increase in the intercanine arch width during the mixed dentition period. This may significantly contribute to accommodation of the bigger permanent incisors in the arches.
- *Change in incisor inclination:* As stated previously, the deciduous incisors are more vertically positioned than the permanent incisors. Permanent incisors exhibit a more

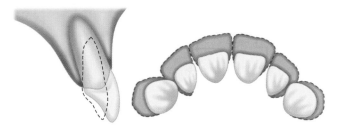

**Fig. 19.14:** Relationship of primary and permanent incisors over basal plane: Deciduous incisors are vertically placed over basal bone, while permanent incisors exhibit more labial inclination that tends to increase the dental arch perimeter.

labial inclination, which tends to increase the dental arch perimeter. The change in the labiolingual inclination of incisors also contributes to overcome the incisal liability by adding 2–3 mm to the arch **(Fig. 19.14)**.

### Intertransitional Period

After permanent first molars and incisors establish occlusion, there is an interim period of 1–2 years before the commencement of second transitional period in which little changes in the occlusion are seen. This phase of mixed dentition stage is relatively stable with only minor changes taking place and is referred to as intertransitional period.

### Second Transitional Period (10–13 Years)

The second transitional period involves replacement of molars and canines by the premolars and permanent canines, respectively, and the emergence of permanent second molars. Exfoliation of mandibular primary canine at around 10 years of age usually makes the beginning of second transitional period.

### Eruption of Permanent Canines

Mandibular canine erupts following the eruption of the incisors at around 9 years, while the maxillary canine usually erupts after the eruption of one or both the premolars, around 12–13 years.

### Ugly Duckling Stage (Figs. 19.15A to C)

A transient malocclusion is often observed to develop in the maxillary anterior region during 8–12 years of age. This corresponds to the eruption of permanent maxillary canines. Clinicians need to recognize it as a self-correcting malocclusion and the anxious parents and children may have to be reassured. The courses of events in the development of ugly duckling stage are discussed in **Flowchart 19.1**.

Broadbent described this stage of development as the ugly duckling stage as the children appears ugly with crooked teeth during this phase of development. The condition resolves by itself as the continuously erupting canines shift the pressure from roots of lateral incisors to their crowns. By the time,

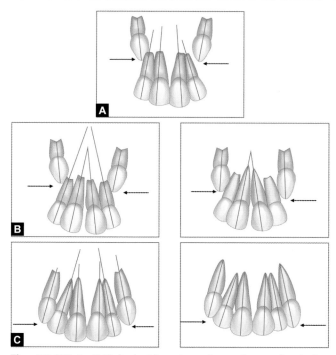

**Figs. 19.15A to C:** Ugly duckling stage: A transient malocclusion observed during 8–12 years corresponds to eruption of permanent maxillary canines and resolves after their complete eruption. It requires no treatment.

**Flowchart 19.1:** The development of ugly duckling stage.

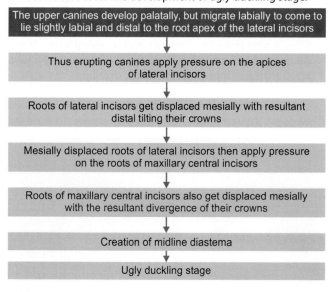

canines are fully erupted the midline diastema is closed and laterals are realigned along the arch.

## Eruption of the Premolars

The important portion of the dental arch in the development of occlusion is the premolar segment.

This is because the erupting premolars are significantly smaller in mesiodistal dimension than the primary molars which they replace. Thus, major changes in occlusion are observed during the premolar emergence.

### *Leeway Space of Nance (Fig. 19.16)*

In general, the combined mesiodistal crown dimension of the primary canine and primary first and second molars is larger than the combined mesiodistal crown dimension of their successor namely, permanent canine and first and second premolars. The amount of space gained by their difference in the posterior segments is termed as the leeway space of *Nance* and is present in both the arches.

Measurement of leeway space for maxillary and mandibular arches is given here.

### *In maxilla:*
- Leeway space in maxilla in each quadrant is about 0.9 mm
- The total leeway space in maxilla is 1.8 mm.

### *In mandible:*
- Leeway space in each quadrant of the mandible is about 1.7 mm
- The total leeway space in the mandible is 3.4 mm.

*Significance of leeway space of Nance:* Presence of excessive leeway space is a favorable feature, which provides for the mesial movement of the permanent molars. Leeway space in

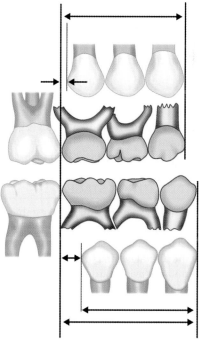

**Fig. 19.16:** Leeway space of Nance: Space gained by the difference between the mesiodistal widths of primary canine, molars and permanent canine, and premolars. Relatively greater space gained in the mandibular arch helps in establishment of class-I permanent molar relationship.

the mandibular arch is more than that of the maxillary arch. This is because the primary mandibular molars are wider than the primary maxillary molars. The leeway space between the two arches causes the mandibular first premolar to move relatively more than the maxillary first premolar in a mesial direction. Such an arrangement causes a change in the molar relationship from end-on in the early mixed dentition period to class-I relation at the late mixed dentition period (late mesial shift).

Leeway space deficiency may be seen in some individuals when size of unerupted premolars and permanent canine are larger than the space available.

### Eruption of Permanent Second Molars

Emergence of second permanent molars ideally should follow the eruption of the premolars. If the second molars erupt before the premolars erupt fully, a significant shortening of the arch perimeter occurs and malocclusion may be more likely to occur.

### Change in the Anteroposterior Molar Relationship in Mixed Dentition

To begin with newly erupted permanent first molar occlude in a cusp-to-cusp relation, especially when deciduous dentition exhibit flush terminal plane. End-on molar relationship is considered normal in early mixed dentition stage, changes to class-I molar relationship, which is considered normal in permanent dentition stage by the following factors:
- Leeway space of *Nance*
- Differential mandibular growth.

### Differential Mandibular Growth

During growing period, both the maxilla and the mandible grow downward and forward.

However, the mandible grows relatively more forward than the maxilla during this developmental stage. Such differential mandibular growth is thought to contribute to the transition from end-to-end to class-I molar relationship.

## PERMANENT DENTITION STAGE

Permanent dentition stage is pretty well established by about 13 years of age, with the eruption of all permanent teeth except the third molars. Permanent successors develop from lingual extension of the dental lamina (successional lamina) and the permanent molars develop from the posterior extension of the dental lamina. The permanent incisors develop lingual to the primary incisors and move labially as they erupt. The premolars develop below the divergent roots of the primary molars.

Permanent dentition begins to form at birth, during which, calcification of the first permanent molars becomes evident.

Chronology of permanent dentition is depicted in Chapter 3, Table 3.2.

Sequence of eruption of permanent dentition is more variable than that of the primary dentition. In addition, there are significant differences in the eruption sequences between the maxillary and the mandibular arch.

Most common eruption sequence in maxilla:
- 6-1-2-4-3-5-7-8
- 6-1-2-4-5-3-7-8

Most common eruption sequence for mandibular arch:
- (6-1)-2-3-4-5-7-8

These are also the most favorable sequences for the prevention of malocclusion. It must be noted that, there is a difference in eruption timing of the canines in the two arches. In the mandibular arch, the canine erupts before the premolars, whereas in the maxillary arch the canine generally erupts after the premolars.

When second molars erupt before the premolars are fully erupted significant shortening of the arch perimeter occurs, increasing the likelihood of malocclusion.

### Characteristics of Occlusion in Permanent Dentition

Some of the characteristics of the normal occlusion in the permanent dentition stage are listed below:
- *Overlap:* The arch form of maxilla tends to be larger than that of the mandible. Thus, the maxillary teeth overlap the mandibular teeth both in labial and buccal segments in centric occlusion **(Fig. 19.17)**. Such overlapping of upper teeth over the lower teeth has a protective feature—the cheeks, lips, and tongue are less likely to be caught between the teeth during opening and closing movements of the jaws.

  Cheek biting is often seen in molar region after dental restorations of second molars giving end-to-end occlusal relationship without any horizontal overlap.
- *Intra-arch tooth contacts*: With the exception of the maxillary third molars and mandibular central incisors, each permanent tooth occludes with two teeth from the

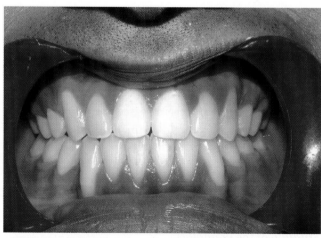

**Fig. 19.17:** Maxillary teeth overlap mandibular teeth in labial as well as buccal segments in centric occlusion.

opposite arch. In other words, each permanent tooth has two antagonistic teeth.

- *Angulations*: Permanent teeth have buccolingual and mesiodistal angulations, whereas the primary teeth are generally vertically positioned in the alveolar bone.
- *Arch curvatures*: The anteroposterior curvature exhibited by the mandibular arch is called the curve of Spee. The corresponding curve in the maxillary arch is called the compensating curve. The buccolingual curvature from one side of the arch to the others is called the curve of Wilson.
- *Incisor relationship*: The vertical overlap of the maxillary incisors over the mandibular incisors is called as *overbite*. It is about 1–2 mm. The horizontal overlap is called the *overjet* and is generally between 1 mm and 3 mm **(Figs. 19.18A and B)**.
- *Molar relationship*: In permanent dentition stage, the class-I molar relationship is the ideal relationship. In class-I molar relationship, the mesiobuccal cusp of the maxillary first

molar is in the buccal groove of the mandibular first molar **(Figs. 19.19A and B)**.

## Occlusal Contacts and Intercuspal Relations between Arches

### Types of Cusps

The human dentitions present two types of cusps and are as follows:

*1. Supporting cusps/centric holding cusps/stamp cusps:* The lingual cusps of the maxillary posterior teeth and the buccal cusps of the mandibular posterior teeth are referred to as supporting cusps/centric holding cusps or stamps cusps. Supporting cusps occlude in the central fossa and marginal ridges of opposing teeth **(Fig. 19.20)**.

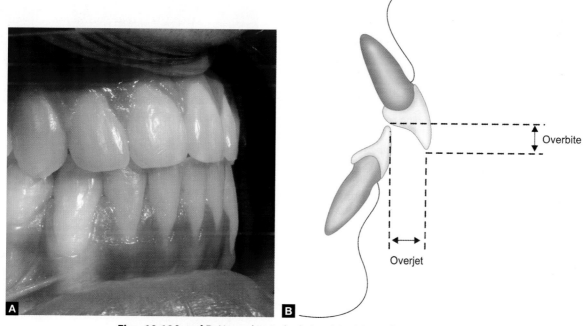

**Figs. 19.18A and B:** Normal incisal relationship: (A) Overbite; (B) Overjet.

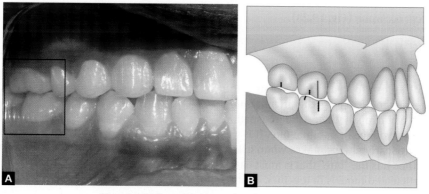

**Figs. 19.19A and B:** Normal molar relationship.

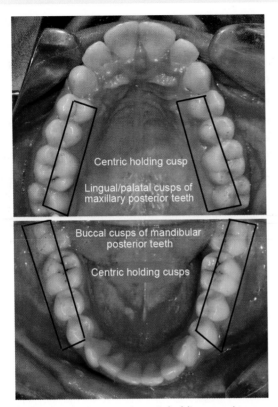

**Fig. 19.20:** Supporting cusp/centric holding cusp/stamp cusp.

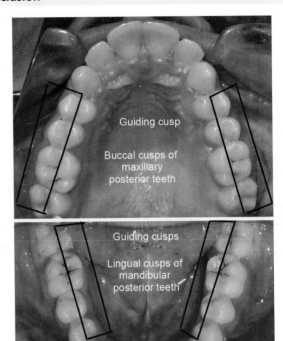

**Fig. 19.21:** Nonsupporting cusp/guiding cusp/shear cusp.

*2. Nonsupporting cusps/guiding cusps/shear cusps:* The buccal cusps of the maxillary posterior teeth and the lingual cusps of the mandibular posterior teeth are called nonsupporting cusps/ guiding or shear cusps. They guide the mandible during lateral excursions and shear food during mastication **(Fig. 19.21)**.

### Cusp–Fossa and Cusp–Marginal Ridge Relations

The supporting cusps of molars and premolars occlude in the fossae or marginal ridges of the opposing teeth.

When a supporting cusp of one tooth occludes in a single fossa of a single opposing tooth, it is referred to as *cusp–fossa occlusion* or *tooth-to-tooth arrangement* **(Fig. 19.22)**.

When a supporting cusp occludes with two opposing two teeth on their marginal ridges, it is called *cusp–embrasure occlusion* or *tooth-to-teeth occlusion* **(Fig. 19.23)**.

### Movements in Centric

#### Centric Occlusion

Centric occlusion can be described as the occlusion the patient makes when they fit their teeth together in *maximum intercuspation*. Common synonyms for this are intercuspation position (ICP), bite of convenience or habitual bite. It is the occlusion that the patient nearly always makes when asked to close their teeth together. It is the "bite" that is most easily recorded. It is how unarticulated models fit together. Finally,

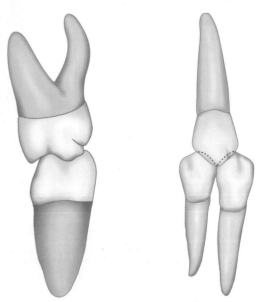

**Fig. 19.22:** Cusp–fossa occlusion (tooth-to-tooth).

**Fig. 19.23:** Cusp–embrasure occlusion (tooth-to-teeth).

it should be remembered that it is the occlusion to which the patient is accustomed, i.e. the habitual bite.

Thus, centric occlusion can be defined as the relationship of the mandible to the maxilla when the teeth are in maximum occlusal contact, irrespective of the position or alignment of the condyle-disk assemblies.

### Centric Relation (Fig. 19.24)

Centric relation is not an occlusion at all. It has nothing to do with teeth because it is the only "centric" that is reproducible with or without teeth present. Centric Relation is a jaw relationship: it describes a conceptual relationship between the maxilla and mandible.

It is the position of the mandible when the condyles are in an orthopedically stable position. Centric relation can be described as that position of the mandible relative to the maxilla, with the articular disk in place, when the muscles that support the mandible are at their most relaxed and least strained position. This position is independent of tooth contact.

***Significance of centric relation:*** There may be arguments about the exact position of centric relation and on how that position is clinically best found. There is, however, a broad agreement between dentists who have studied this subject that there exists a *reproducible* position of the mandible relative to the maxilla, and that this position is reproducible irrespective of the guidance that the occlusal surfaces of the teeth may provide. Patients with no teeth still have a centric relation. Furthermore, there is inter- and intraoperator reliability in finding it.

It is important to record centric occlusion and centric relation for the success of any dental prosthesis such as complete dentures.

### Centric Occlusal Contacts

According to Hellman, there are 138 points of possible occlusal contacts for 32 teeth **(Figs. 19.25A and B)**. Concepts of ideal occlusion are used primarily in orthodontics and even in restorative dentistry. Centric occlusal contacts are classified into anterior centric occlusal contacts and posterior centric occlusal contacts.

***Anterior centric occlusal contacts:*** Anterior centric occlusal contacts consist the labial and lingual range of contacts of maxillary and mandibular anteriors and are in line with the buccal range of posterior centric contacts.

Anterior centric occlusal contacts are listed below:
* Lingual surfaces of maxillary incisors and canines; 6
* Labial surfaces of mandibular incisors and canines; 6.

***Posterior centric occlusal contacts:*** Posterior centric occlusal contacts consist of the buccal range of contacts and the lingual range of contacts of maxillary and mandibular posteriors.

Posterior centric occlusal contacts are listed below:
Triangular ridges of lingual cusps of mandibular premolars and molars; 16
* Triangular ridges of buccal cusps of premolars and molars; 16

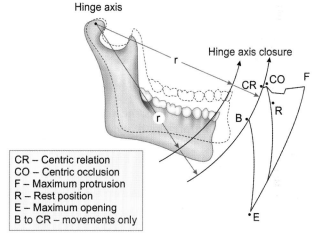

CR – Centric relation
CO – Centric occlusion
F – Maximum protrusion
R – Rest position
E – Maximum opening
B to CR – movements only

**Fig. 19.24:** Mandibular movements projected on sagittal plane.

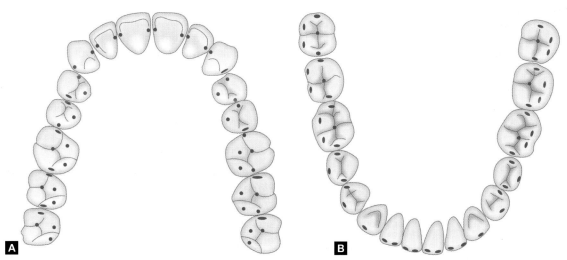

**Figs. 19.25A and B:** Occlusal contacts: (A) Maxillary arch; (B) Mandibular arch.

- Buccal embrasure of mandibular premolar and molars; 8
- Lingual embrasure of maxillary premolars and molars (including the canine and first premolar embrasure accommodating the mandibular premolar); 10
- Lingual cusp points of maxillary premolars and molars; 16
- Buccal cusp points of mandibular premolars and molars; 16
- Distal fossae of premolars; 8
- Central fossae of the molars; 12
- Mesial fossae of the mandibular molars; 6
- Distal fossae of the maxillary molars; 6
- Lingual grooves of the maxillary molars; 6
- Buccal grooves of the mandibular molars; 6.

### Movements away from Centric/Eccentric Movements (Fig. 19.26)

All occlusal contact relations away from the centric occlusion involve eccentric jaw movements. Eccentric movements include:
- Protrusive movement—maximal forward movement
- Retrusive movement—maximal posterior movement
- Lateral movements—left or right movement
- Maximal mouth opening.

During right lateral movement, the mandible is depressed, the dental arches are separated, and the jaw moves to the right of the centric occlusion on *right working side*. The left side is now called *nonworking side*.

During protrusive movements, the mandible is depressed and then moves forward, bringing the anterior teeth together at points most favorable for the incision of food. After protrusive movement, a retrusive movement to centric occlusion occurs.

Retrusive movement from centric occlusion to retruded contact position seems to occur in bruxism and sometimes during swallowing.

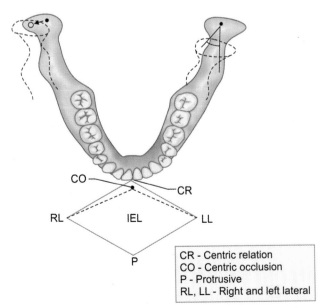

CR - Centric relation
CO - Centric occlusion
P - Protrusive
RL, LL - Right and left lateral

**Fig. 19.26:** Mandibular movements projected on sagittal plane.

### Dynamic Occlusion

The dynamic occlusion refers to the occlusal contacts that are made while the mandible is moving relative to the maxilla. The mandible is moved by the muscles of mastication and the pathways along which it moves are determined not only by these muscles but also by two guidance systems—*posterior guidance* and *anterior guidance*.

#### Condylar Guidance

Condylar guidance refers to the downward movement of both the condyles along the slopes of the articular eminence during protrusive movements leading to separation of the posteriors. This guidance during jaw movements is provided by the temporomandibular joints (TMJ). As the head of the condyle moves downwards and forwards, the mandible is moving along a guidance pathway, which is determined by the intra-articular disk and the articulatory surfaces of the glenoid fossa, all of which is enclosed in the joint capsule.

#### Tooth Guidance (Anterior guidance)

If teeth are touching during a protrusive or lateral movement of the mandible then those (touching) teeth are also providing guidance to mandibular movement. This is the anterior guidance and this is provided by *whichever* teeth touch during eccentric movements of the mandible. In the natural dentition, a variety of contact relations may be found, including group function, cuspid disocclusion only, or some combination of canine, premolar and molar contacts in lateral movements.

*Group function (Fig. 19.27A):* Multiple contacts occur between the maxillary and mandibular teeth on the working side during lateral movements.

*Canine/cuspid guidance (posterior guidance) (Fig. 19.27B):* Canine guidance refers to a dynamic occlusion that occurs on the canines during a lateral excursion of the mandible. A canine protected occlusion refers to the fact that the canine guidance is the only dynamic occlusal contact during this excursive movement. In other words, only maxillary and mandibular canines are in contact during lateral/eccentric mandibular movements.

*Incisal guidance (Fig. 19.27C):* Incisal guidance refers to guidance provided by the surfaces of maxillary incisors during protrusive movements of the mandible.

### Compensatory Curves

#### Curve of Spee (Anteroposterior Curve/the Curve Occlusal Plane)

First described by Von Spee of Germany in 1890, the curve of Spee refers to the anteroposterior curvature of the occlusal surfaces, beginning at the tip of the mandibular cuspid and following the buccal cusps of premolars and molars continuing as an arc through the condyle (**Fig. 19.28**).

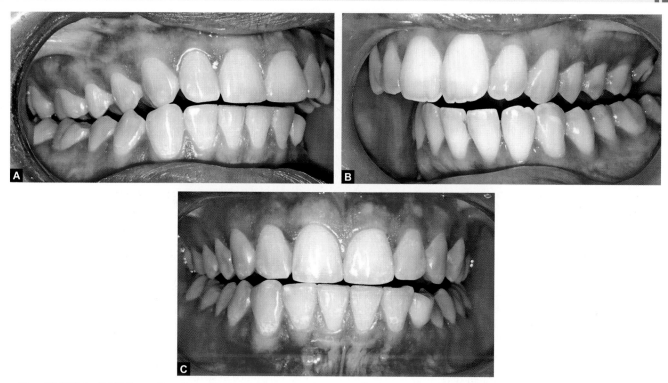

**Figs. 19.27A to C:** (A) Group function with multiple contacts between the posterior teeth during right lateral movement; (B) Canine guided occlusion with only upper and lower canines in contact during left lateral movement; (C) Incisal guidance during protrusion

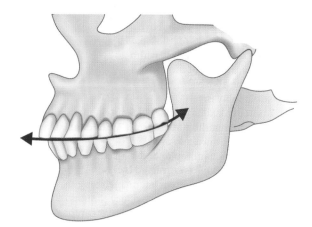

**Fig. 19.28:** Curve of Spee.

If the curve is extended, it would form a circle of about 4-inch diameter. Optimum curve of Spee allows for normal protrusive movements of the mandible.

### Curve of Wilson (Side-to-Side Curve)

The curve of Wilson is the mediolateral curve that contacts the buccal and lingual cusps of each side of the arch **(Fig. 19.29)**. It results from inward inclination of the lower posterior teeth, making lingual cusps lower than the buccal cusps on

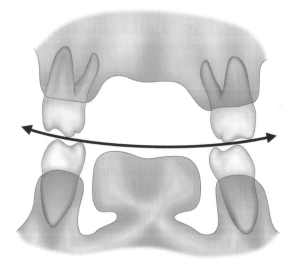

**Fig. 19.29:** Curve of Wilson.

mandibular arch, and an outward inclination of maxillary posterior teeth.

Curve of Wilson allows exquisite lateral movements used in during chewing. It helps in two ways:
1. Teeth are aligned so as to have optimum resistance masticatory forcers.

2. The elevated buccal cusps prevent food from going past the occlusal table.

### Curve of Monson

The curve of Monson is obtained by extending the curve of Spee and **Curve of Wilson** to all cusps and incisal edges. It is suggested that the mandibular arch adopted itself to the curved segment of a sphere of a 4-inch radius.

### Occlusal Stability

The stability of the occlusion and maintenance of tooth position are dependent on all of the forces that act upon the teeth. Occlusal forces, eruptive forces, lip and cheek pressure, periodontal support, and tongue pressure are important in maintaining the position of teeth. Tooth position and occlusion will remain stable as long as these forces are balanced.

### BIBLIOGRAPHY

1. Bishara SE, Hoppens BJ, Jakobsen JR, et al. Changes in molar relationship between the deciduous and permanent dentition: a longitudinal study. Am J Orthod Dentofac Orthoped. 1988;93:19.
2. Friel S. The development of ideal occlusion of the gum pads and teeth. Am J Orthodont. 1954;40:1963.
3. Howe RP, McNamara JA Jr, O'Conner KA. An examination of dental crowding and its relationship to tooth size and arch dimension. Am J Orthod. 1989;83:363.
4. McNamara JA Jr, Brudon WL. Orthodontics and Dentofacial Orthopedics, 1st edition. Ann Arbor: Needham Press; 2001.
5. Morrees C, Chadha JM. Available space for the incisors during dental development—a growth study based on physiologic age. Angle Orthod. 1965;35:12.
6. Moyers RE. Handbook of Orthodontics, 3rd edition. Chicago: Yearbook; 1973.
7. Ramfjord SP, Ash MM. Occlusion. ; Philadelphia: WB Saunders; 1966.

### MULTIPLE CHOICE QUESTIONS

1. Physiological spaces seen mesial to maxillary canine and distal to mandibular canines are:
   a. Primate space
   b. Simian space
   c. Anthropoid space
   d. All of the above
2. Curve of Spee is _____
   a. Cusp tips of the posterior teeth follows a gradual curve from left to right side
   b. Cusp tips of the posterior teeth follows a concave curve anteroposteriorly
   c. Highest point of a curve or greatest convexity or bulge
   d. None of the above
3. Flush terminal plane is:
   a. Normal feature of deciduous dentition
   b. Plane where distal surface of upper and lower second deciduous molar are in same plane
   c. Maxillary deciduous molar is ahead of mandibular
   d. Both (a) and (b)
4. First transition period in mixed dentition is:
   a. Characterized by emergence of first permanent molar
   b. Eruption of permanent canines
   c. None of the above
   d. All of the above
5. Shift in molars from a flush terminal plane to a class-I relation occurs by:
   a. Early shift
   b. Late shift
   c. Mesial shift
   d. Early and late shift
6. Leeway space is utilized by:
   a. Early shift
   b. Late mesial shift
   c. Mesial shift
   d. Distal shift
7. Incisal liability is:
   a. Difference in space between maxillary and mandibular incisors
   b. Difference in space between primary and permanent incisors
   c. Both (a) and (b)
   d. None of the above
8. Incisal liability is corrected by:
   a. Utilization of interdental spaces
   b. Increase in intercanine width
   c. Change in incisor inclination
   d. All of the above
9. Incisor liability is:
   a. 7 mm in maxillary arch and 5 mm in mandibular arch
   b. 5 mm in mandibular arch and 7 mm in maxillary arch
   c. 5–7 mm in maxillary arch
   d. 5–7 mm in mandibular arch
10. Ugly duckling stage is corrected by:
    a. Eruption of permanent lateral incisors
    b. Eruption of permanent maxillary canines
    c. Eruption of permanent mandibular canines
    d. Eruption of second molar

**Answers**

| 1. d | 2. b | 3. d | 4. a | 5. d | 6. b | 7. b | 8. d |
|------|------|------|------|------|------|------|------|
| 9. a | 10. b | | | | | | |

# 8

## SECTION

# Oral Physiology

## Section Outline

# Functions of Teeth, Phonetics, Mastication and Deglutition

## INTRODUCTION

Oral physiology mainly concentrates on the research on biological processes in the oral and maxillofacial regions. Teeth, along with other oral apparatus, participate and fulfill the important physiological functions such as mastication (chewing), deglutition (swallowing), taste, and speech.

## FUNCTIONS OF TEETH

- *Mastication of food*: Digestion of food begins in the oral cavity. Food is broken down and chewed before entering the digestive system so that our body can easily absorb nutrients from them. Different types of teeth are used to bite, shear, and grind the food so as to make a bolus that can be easily swallowed.
- *Speech*: Human beings are social animals and speech is one of the important means of communication. The human speech is highly complex and teeth play a very crucial role in helping to form correct pronunciations. We make certain phonetic sounds using a combination of our vocal chords, lips, teeth, and the tongue.
  Although vowels can be uttered without using our teeth or lips, certain sounds rely entirely on the contact between the teeth and the lips or the teeth and the tongue. The sounds that will be most affected if the teeth are missing are F, V, S, and T.
- *Facial aesthetics*: Teeth, especially the anterior teeth provide the elasticity and facial appearance and give a good facial profile to the person. Any discoloration, fracture, malalignment or missing of front teeth adversely affect one's facial appearance and thus may also affect his or her self-esteem.

- *Function of incisors*:
  - Mainly used for biting, cutting, and shearing the food during mastication process
  - Plays a pivotal role in esthetics and phonation.
- *Function of canines*:
  - Assist the permanent incisors and premolars in the mastication
  - Mainly used for tearing the food
  - Helps in seizing, slicing, and chewing food
  - In carnivorous animals, the canine teeth are used for pretension (seizing) of their prey and act as important tools during hunting and in self-defense.
- *Function of premolars*:
  - They grind the food along with the molars
  - They support the cheeks and reinforce the esthetics during smile.
- *Function of molars*:
  - Molars have widest occlusal tables and are the main teeth used for trituration and comminution of food
  - They also support the cheeks.

## IMPORTANCE OF PRIMARY TEETH

The deciduous dentition is very much essential for the normal growth and development of the jaws and establishment of normal occlusion of permanent dentition. Well-cared primary teeth ensure proper alignment of the permanent teeth by "preserving" space for the latter until they erupt. Malocclusion with severe crowding can occur when primary teeth are lost prematurely.

Importance of primary teeth can be listed as follows:

### Efficient mastication of food:

- With the establishment of primary occlusion, child learns to masticate the food efficiently.
- Neuromuscular coordination required for masticatory process is established at primary dentition stage itself.

### Maintenance of a proper diet and good nutrition:

- Primary teeth are the only teeth present until 6 years of age and thus it is important to provide the child with a comfortable functional occlusion of primary teeth.

- A child with missing or grossly decayed primary teeth may reject food that is difficult to chew.

***Maintenance of normal facial appearance:***
- A well-cared set of deciduous dentition contributes to establishment and maintenance of the normal facial appearance during the tender age of childhood.
- It contributes to normal psychological and cognitive development of the child. Prematurely lost or rampantly carious front teeth may hamper a child's self-confidence due to mocking from their peers.

***Development of clear speech:***
- Teeth, especially the anteriors, are essential for normal pronunciation of consonants
- Speech is developed in early childhood and congenital absence or premature loss of anterior primary teeth can hamper the development of clear speech.

***Maintenance of normal eruption schedule of permanent successors:*** Normal eruption schedule of permanent teeth is disturbed when primary teeth are lost prematurely due to caries or trauma. As a consequence malocclusion may develop.

***Maintenance of space for eruption of permanent successor teeth:***
- Primary teeth serve a very important function of "preserving" the space for eruption of their permanent successor teeth. They act as natural space maintainers.
- Maintenance of space is especially important in canine and molar regions since their successors, the permanent canines, and premolars erupt relatively later in life.
- When primary teeth are lost prematurely, the adjacent teeth migrate into the available space leading to a decrease in the arch length. This causes a lack of space in the arch for the erupting permanent successors and results in the development of malocclusion.

## MASTICATION

Mastication is a complex rhythmical activity that requires coordination of the neuromusculature. It is the cutting down of the food substances into small particles and grinding them into a soft bolus.

Mastication is a repetitive sequence of jaw opening and closing with a profile in the vertical plane called the chewing cycle **(Flowchart 20.1)**.
The human chewing cycle consists of three phases:
1. *Opening phase*: The mouth is opened and the mandible is depressed.
2. *Closing phase*: The mandible is raised toward the maxilla.
3. *Occlusal or intercuspal phase*: The mandible is stationary and the teeth from both upper and lower arches approximate.

Each chewing cycle lasts approximately for 0.8–1.0 second. During normal function, 7–15 kg force occurs during swallowing and chewing.

### Jaw Reflexes

The reflexes associated with mastication are:
- Jaw—closing reflex
- Jaw—opening reflex
- Tooth contact reflex
- Jaw—unloading reflex
- Horizontal jaw reflex.

### Factors Affecting Mastication

- Saliva facilitates mastication, moistens the food particles, makes a bolus, and assists swallowing. The neuromuscular control of chewing plays an important role in the comminution of the food.
- Characteristics of the food, e.g. water and fat percentage and hardness, are known to influence the masticatory process.
- Food hardness is sensed during mastication and affects masticatory force, jaw muscle activity, and mandibular jaw movements.

## DEGLUTITION

Swallowing of food is known as deglutition. It occurs in three phases **(Fig. 20.1)**:
1. Phase I: Oral stage
2. Phase II: Pharyngeal stage
3. Phase III: Esophageal stage.

**Flowchart 20.1:** Masticatory cycle.

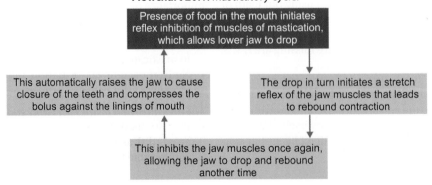

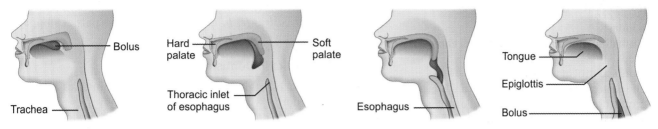

**Fig. 20.1:** Stages of deglutition.

## Phase I: Oral Stage

It occurs after mastication. Phase I is a voluntary stage. The food moves from mouth to pharynx. The bolus is placed over the posterodorsal surface of tongue. Soft palate is raised and seals the nasopharynx, to prevent nasal regurgitation.

Respiration is reflexly stopped.

## Phase II: Pharyngeal Stage

It is an involuntary stage. Bolus is pushed from pharynx into esophagus. Its entry back into the mouth, upward into the nasopharynx and down into the larynx is prevented by a number of defensive mechanisms and thus the bolus enters straight into the esophagus due to:
- Stretching of the opening of the esophagus due to upward movement of the larynx
- Simultaneous relaxation of the upper esophageal sphincter
- Peristaltic contractions in the pharynx
- Elevation of larynx.

During this phase, the epiglottis is transversely deflected and vocal cords are closed.

Respiration remains inhibited throughout this phase.

## Phase III: Esophageal Stage

It is also an involuntary stage. In this stage, the bolus is transported from pharynx to the stomach by the peristaltic movement. Peristalsis is a rhythmic movement of contraction followed by relaxation of the muscles of the gastrointestinal tract. As the bolus reaches the end of the esophagus, lower esophageal sphincter relaxes and the bolus enters the stomach.

## Deglutition Reflex

Deglutition begins as a voluntary act but becomes involuntary during the pharyngeal and esophageal stages. This is because of the activation of the deglutition center.

## Applied Physiology

- Due to inefficiency of the lower esophageal sphincter, there is reflux of the gastric contents into the esophagus. In healthy persons, it is called gastroesophageal reflux. If it is too frequent, it is called *gastroesophageal reflux disease* (GERD).

- It can also cause heart burn by reflux into the respiratory tract causing choking during sleep, mimicking angina pain.
- Persistent gastroesophageal disease may lead to Barrett's esophagitis which can eventually progress to esophageal cancer.
- If the lower esophageal sphincter fails to relax properly, the bolus of the food is held up in the esophagus, a condition known as *achalasia*.

## SPEECH

The development of higher centers in humans is reflected in the ability to communicate with each other not seen in any other species. It is an art that requires both sensory analysis as well as motor control.

Speech is a combination of phonetic sounds created using a combination of vocal cords, teeth, lips, and tongue. There are certain sounds such as the vowels that can be made without using teeth or lips. However, certain sounds rely entirely on the contact between the teeth and the lips or the teeth and the tongue. The sounds that will be most affected if the teeth are missing are F, V, S, and T. There are other factors that will determine how we speak and make phonetic sounds such as the physical structure of our mouth and teeth and even the length of the tongue.

The following examples emphasize the importance of teeth in the speech formation:
- To make "TH" sound, your tongue must make contact with the upper row of your teeth.
- For you to make an "F" or a "V" sound, the upper teeth must make contact with the lower lips.

Speech has two aspects:
1. *Sensory aspect*: Language input involving ears and eyes.
2. *Motor aspect*: Language output involving vocalization and its control.

### Sensory Aspect

Destruction of portions of auditory or visual association areas in the cortex results in inability to understand the written or spoken word and may lead to word blindness or word deafness—dyslexia.

## Motor Aspect

It includes:
- Formation of thoughts in mind with choice of words to be used
- Motor control of vocalization.
- The centers associated with speech are Broca's area (speech production), Wernicke's area, and angular gyrus (primary auditory area, primary visual area).

Sounds are produced in the larynx initially with the help of abdominal, thoracic, and laryngeal muscles. Final meaningful speech is produced in the pharyngeal, oral, and nasal cavities by the activities of organs such as the lips, tongue, and soft palate.

## Classification of Sounds

Sounds may be:
- Voiced (i.e. vocal folds in the larynx vibrate for sound production)
- Breathed (i.e. vocal folds do not vibrate)

Two main groups of speech sound are:
1. Vowels
2. Consonants.

### Vowels

All vowels are voiced, produced without interruption of air flow, are modified by resonance, and are created by high amplitude waves.

### Consonants

These are produced when air is impeded before it is released. They may be voiced (e.g. b, d, z) or breathed (e.g. p, t, s) and are of low amplitude.

Classified based on:

### Place of articulation:
- Bilabial (e.g. *b, p, m*): Two lips are used
- *Labiodental:* Lower lip meets maxillary incisors (e.g. *f, v*)
- *Linguodental:* Tip of tongue contacting incisors and hard palate (e.g. *d, t*)
- *Linguopalatal:* Tongue meets palate away from incisor (e.g. *g, k*)
- Glottal sound.

### Manner of articulation:
- *Plosives (p, b, t, d, g, k):* Require complete stoppage of air
- *Fricatives (f, v, th):* Require only partial stoppage
- *Affricatives (c, h, j):* Although involves partial stoppage require rapid release of air.

## Phonetics in Dentistry

Speech is vital to human activities. Phonetics must be considered with mechanics and aesthetics as a cardinal factor that contributes to the success of dental prosthesis. Thus phonetics plays a pivotal role in complete, removable, and fixed denture rehabilitation as well as has high impact on smile designing and esthetic dentistry.

## MULTIPLE CHOICE QUESTIONS

1. This phase of deglutition is a voluntary phase..
   a. oral stage
   b. pharyngeal stage
   c. esophageal stage
   d. Both a and b
2. Heart burn may mimic:
   a. tooth ache
   b. angina pain
   c. neuralgia pain
   d. none of the above
3. Tongue must make contact with the upper row of teeth to produce the sound..
   a. all vowels
   b. "v"
   c. "p"
   d. "th"
4. The upper teeth must make contact with the lower lips to produce the sound..
   a. all vowels
   b. "f' and "v"
   c. "p"
   d. "th"
5. Respiration remains inhibited throughout this phase of deglutition.
   a. oral stage
   b. pharyngeal stage
   c. all the stages
   d. Both a and b

**Answers**

1. a    2. b    3. d    4. b    5. b

# 9 SECTION

# Tooth Carving

## Section Outline

# Tooth Carving—Rationale, Armamentarium and Step-by-Step Procedure

## INTRODUCTION

The importance of knowing tooth morphology and its application in clinical dentistry cannot be overemphasized. Tooth carving is one of the best methods for learning tooth morphology. Carving gives a three-dimensional understanding of details of tooth form, right from the simple design of an incisor to the complex anatomy of the molar.

This chapter gives the rationale, armamentarium, general principles of carving, and step-by-step carving procedure.

## RATIONALE OF TOOTH CARVING

It is no secret that good carving skills come handy in clinical practice, especially during restoration of lost tooth structure, tooth recontouring, and laboratory procedures such as fabrication of metal/ceramic crowns and veneers. Restoration of anterior teeth using tooth-colored material such as composite also requires carving skills to bring about the natural contour of teeth conductive to esthetic appeal.

Accurate reproduction of the occlusal anatomy when restoring part/whole tooth structure is very much essential in order to maintain the normal occlusal harmony. Improper finishing or under carving may lead to microleakage, while overfilled restoration may cause discomfort and pain due to high points. Overhanging proximal restoration often leads to food impaction and periodontal problems.

Though some are born with artistic hand, with practice anyone who systematically follows the steps of carving should be able to carve a reasonably good tooth form out of a wax block.

## ARMAMENTARIUM (FIG. 21.1)

### Wax Blocks

Wax blocks made of paraffin wax are used for carving teeth. The blocks come in various colors (e.g. white, blue, pink, and yellow). They usually measure about 4.00 cm × 1.25 cm × 1.25 cm.

An ideal wax block should be:
• Tough and not very soft in room temperature
• Free of air bubbles and impurities
• Should not flake or chip off during manipulation
• Allow/amenable to polishing.

### Lecron Carver (Fig. 21.2)

Lecron carver is a double-ended instrument made of stainless steel.

Carvers come in various designs and dimensions, thus carry different model numbers by the manufacturer.

It has a handle/shaft with two working ends attached to the shaft with neck/shank. The handle is generally serrated to facilitate firm grip of the instrument. The working end of the carver should be sharp and free of any nicks/scratches on them.

### *Knife-shaped Working End (Fig. 21.3)*

The knife-shaped working end has a straight part and a curved part. The straight part is used for most steps of carving unless otherwise specified. The curved part is used for occlusal carving, and for obtaining concavity of lingual fossa.

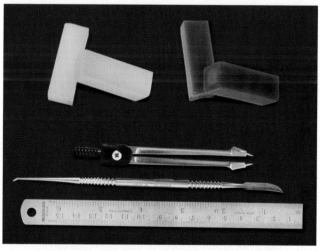

**Fig. 21.1:** Materials required for tooth carving.

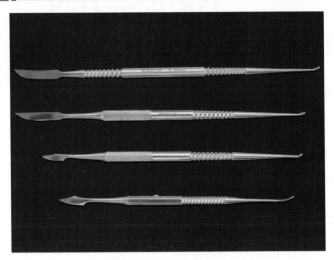

**Fig. 21.2:** Lecron carver.

### Spoon-shaped Working End (Fig. 21.4)

The spoon-shaped working end is generally used for carving lingual grooves of anteriors and developmental depression on roots.

### Ruler with Millimeter Markings

It is used for measuring.

### Divider

It can be used for measuring the carved tooth specimen especially the curved parts.

### Cotton or a Piece of Soft Silk Cloth

It is used for polishing the finished carving. However, overzealous polishing must be avoided as the anatomic details carved may get faded.

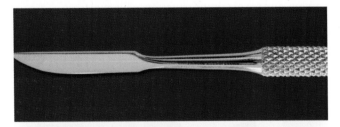

**Fig. 21.3:** Knife-shaped working end of the carver.

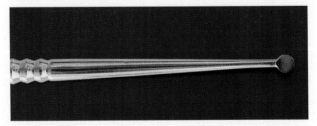

**Fig. 21.4:** Spoon-shaped working end of the carver.

## GENERAL PRINCIPLES OF CARVING

One must know the detailed anatomy of the tooth before attempting to carve. Extracted teeth specimen devoid of caries and gross attrition serve as ideal models for carving. The average measurement of the tooth to be carved (refer Table 1.8 in Chapter 1) should be used to reproduce the exact form of the tooth.

Proper method of handling the carver and the wax block is the first step in learning the skills of carving.

### Instrument Grasp

We use the pen grasp while writing **(Fig. 21.5A)**. For tooth carving, the carver should be held using the *modified pen grasp*, which gives flexibility and allows for optimum force application **(Fig. 21.5B)**. In the modified pen grasp, the carver is held at its neck using the thumb, index finger, and the middle finger. The middle finger is held closer to the working end of the carver and index finger is bent at its second joint.

The *palm and thumb* grasp is usually used while sharpening an instrument **(Fig 21.5C)**.

### Instrument Stabilization

While giving strokes, the carver is stabilized by finger rests using the ring and little fingers of the operating hand.

- *Finger on finger rest* **(Fig. 21.6A)**: Support is gained by resting the ring and little finger of the operating hand on the finger(s) of the nonoperating hand holding the block.
- *Finger on block rest* **(Fig. 21.6B)**: The ring and little finger of the operating hand are placed on wax block held with the nonoperating hand.

Either of these finger rests are used depending on the operator's ease and situation. Carving should never be done without using finger rest.

## PRELIMINARY STEPS

Before carving any tooth, some preliminary steps have to be followed:

- *Smoothening of wax block*: Before carving, wax block should be checked for any porosities/irregularities. All the surfaces of the block should be smoothened.
- *Preliminary markings* **(Fig. 21.7)**:
  - The block is divided into three parts—(1) crown, (2) root, and (3) base. The length of crown and root is measured and marked on the block. The remaining part of the block serves as a base.
  - It is a good practice to mark midline on all the surfaces of the block, so that the carved tooth will be properly centered over the base.
  - The crown portion is divided into three parts—(1) cervical, (2) middle, and (3) incisal/occlusal third.
  - An attempt should be made to preserve the base as the carving is best displayed along with an intact base.

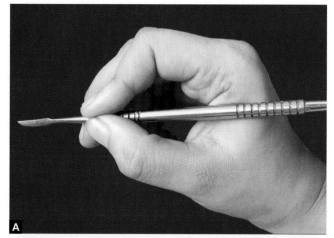

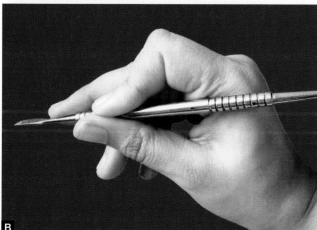

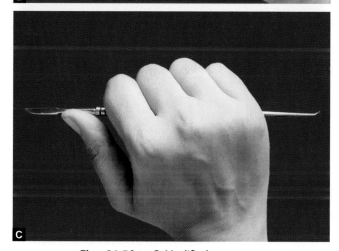

**Figs. 21.5A to C:** Modified pen grasp.

## Carving of Maxillary Central Incisor
## (Figs. 21.8 and 21.9)

The procedure of carving a permanent maxillary central incisor is described below. The basic steps of carving remain same for all other incisor with only minor changes required.

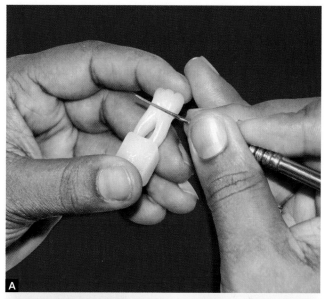

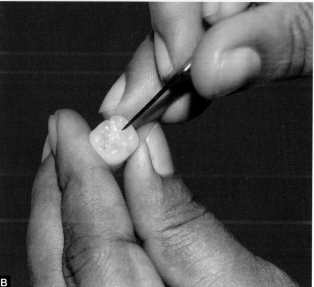

**Figs. 21.6A and B:** (A) Finger on finger rest; (B) Finger on block rest.

*Note:* The longer and straight part of working end is used for most steps in carving unless otherwise specified.

### Crown Carving

- *Step 1*: Obtaining triangular proximal form of incisor
  - 1A: Marking triangle with conserving wax at cervical third—crest of labial and lingual contour at cervical third.
  - 1B: Removal of excess wax outside the triangular marking.
- *Step 2*: Obtaining convex labial surface—both cervicoincisally and mesiodistally
- *Step 3*: Obtaining concavoconvex lingual surface
  - Obtaining concave lingual fossa
  - Obtaining convex cingulum

- *Step 4:* Obtaining trapezoid facial form
  - *4A:* Marking trapezium on the labial surface
  - *4B:* Reduction of wax outside trapezoid marking
- *Step 5:* Obtaining lingual convergence of crown
- *Step 6:* Carving developmental grooves in lingual fossa
  - Spoon-shaped working end is used

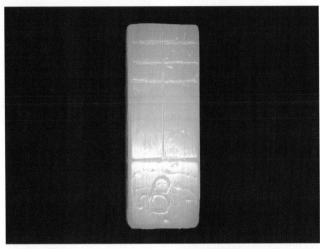

**Fig. 21.7:** Preliminary markings on the wax block.

- *Step 7:* Giving finishing touches to crown
  - Rounding the distoincisal angle
  - All line angles are rounded.

### Root Carving

- *Step 8:* Obtaining conical root form from labial and lingual aspects
- *Step 9:* Obtaining conical root form from proximal aspects
- *Step 10:* Cervical line carving and finishing.

Finished carving from all aspects is shown in **Figure 21.9**.

## Carving of Maxillary Lateral Incisor (Figs. 21.10A to E)

The procedure of maxillary lateral incisor carving is essentially similar to that of maxillary central incisors except following feature:

- Tooth dimension smaller
- Both mesioincisal and distoincisal angles of the crown are rounded with the latter being more so
- Root is slender and has distal curvature at apical third.

## Carving of Mandibular Central Incisor (Figs. 21.11A to E)

The basic steps remain same as that of the maxillary central incisor.

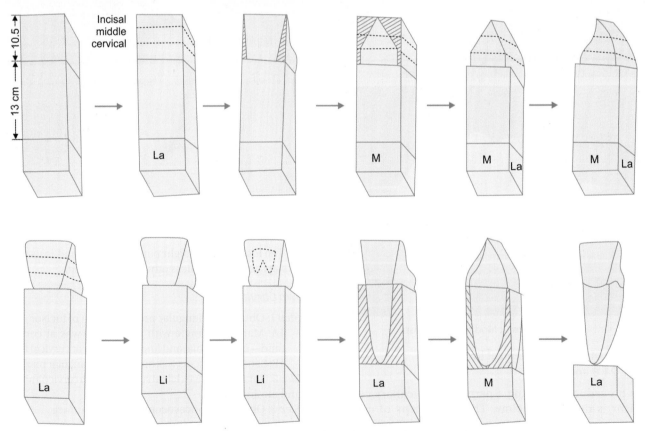

**Fig. 21.8:** Schematic representation of maxillary central incisor carving steps.

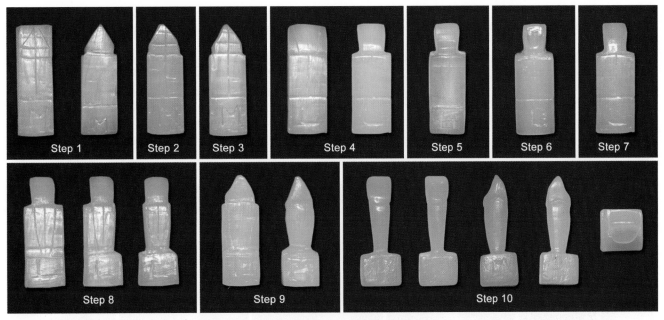

**Fig. 21.9:** Step-by-step procedure for carving a maxillary central incisor and finished carving from all the aspects (See text for details of the procedure).

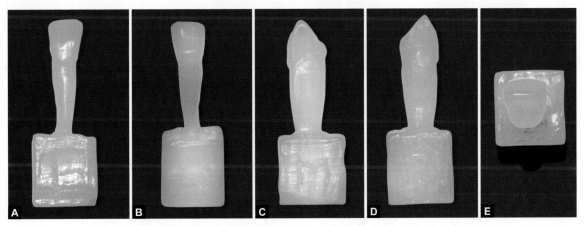

**Figs. 21.10A to E:** A specimen carving of maxillary lateral incisor.

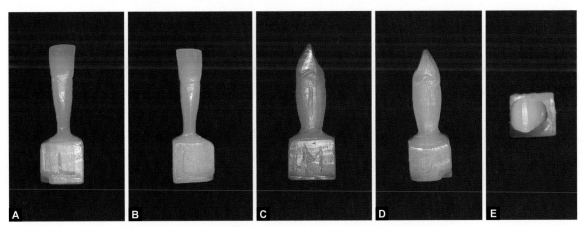

**Figs. 21.11A to E:** A specimen carving of mandibular central incisor.

*Facts to keep in mind:*
- Crown is smaller mesiodistally and bilaterally symmetrical
- Both incisal angles are sharp
- From incisal view, the labial ridge is perpendicular to the labiolingual bisecting line.

## Carving of Mandibular Lateral Incisor (Figs. 21.12A to E)

All steps similar to that of the mandibular central incisor, except that:
- Crown dimension is more

- Crown is bilaterally asymmetrical
- From incisal view, incisal ridge is at an angle to the labiolingual bisecting line and curved distally.

## Carving of Maxillary Canine (Figs. 21.13 and 21.14)

All the anteriors including canine essentially have a triangular/wedge-shaped proximal form. Thus the initial steps of canine carving aimed at obtaining the proximal form are similar to the technique employed for maxillary central incisor carving.

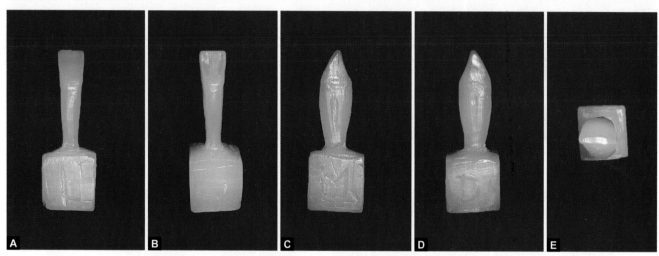

**Figs. 21.12A to E:** A specimen carving of mandibular lateral incisor.

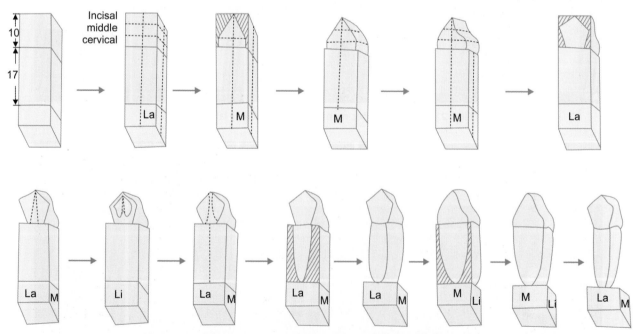

**Fig. 21.13:** Schematic representation of maxillary canine carving steps.

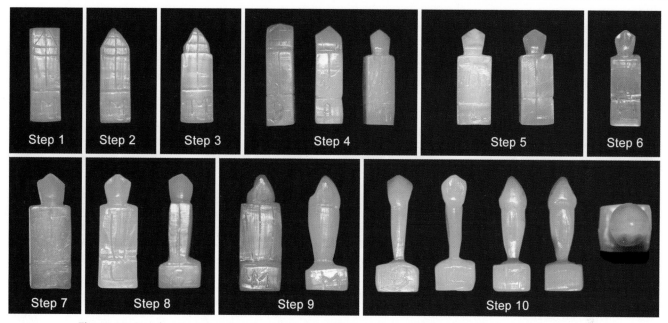

**Fig. 21.14:** Step-by-step procedure for carving a maxillary canine and finished carving from all the aspects
(See text for details of the procedure).

## Crown Carving

- *Step 1:* Obtaining triangular proximal form
  - 1A: Marking triangular outline with conserving maximum at the cervical third for prominent cingulum
  - 1B: Reduction of excess wax outside the marking
- *Step 2:* Obtaining convex labial surface
- *Step 3:* Obtaining concavoconvex lingual surface
  - Concave lingual fossa
  - Convex and prominent cingulum
- *Step 4:* Obtaining pentagonal facial form
  - Marking pentagon on labial surface with distal cusp slope longer
  - Wax reduction outside the marking
- *Step 5:* Obtaining lingual convergence of crown
- *Step 6:* Lingual fossae carving
  - Lingual ridge divides lingual fossa into mesial and distal lingual fossae
  - Spoon-shaped working end used
- *Step 7:* Finishing touches the crown
  - Rounding the line angles
  - Mesial cusp slope made concave.

## Root Carving

- *Step 8:* Obtaining long conical root form from labial and lingual aspects
- *Step 9:* Obtaining broad conical root form from proximal aspects
- *Step 10:* Cervical line carving and finishing
  - Lingual convergence of root
  - Developmental depression on mesial and distal root surface
  - Distal root curvature.

## Carving of Mandibular Canine (Figs. 21.15A to E)

The basic steps are same as that of maxillary canine, except the following:

- The labial and lingual ridges are not so prominent
- The crown is narrow but long.

## Carving of Maxillary First Premolar (Figs. 21.16 and 21.17)

Carving procedure of posterior teeth differs from that of the anteriors in that, the occlusal surface has to be carved with all the details including the cusps, cusp ridges, triangular fossa, etc.

Premolars appear pentagonal from buccal aspect and their buccal and lingual surfaces have ridges analogs to the labial ridge found on canines. Thus, the steps used for obtaining pentagonal form; buccal and lingual ridges bear resemblance to canine carving technique.

The maxillary first premolar has two roots. The crown is hexagonal from the occlusal view. It has two cusps; lingual cusp being smaller.

## Crown Carving

- *Step 1:* Reduction of crown height lingually toward smaller lingual cusp
- *Step 2:* Obtaining pentagonal buccal and lingual crown form
  - 2A: Marking a pentagon on labial surface with mesial cusp slope longer
  - 2B: Reduction of excess wax outside the marking
- *Step 3:* Obtaining lingual convergence of crown (occlusal view)
- *Step 4:* Obtaining buccal and lingual contours of crown with crests of contour at cervical and middle thirds, respectively

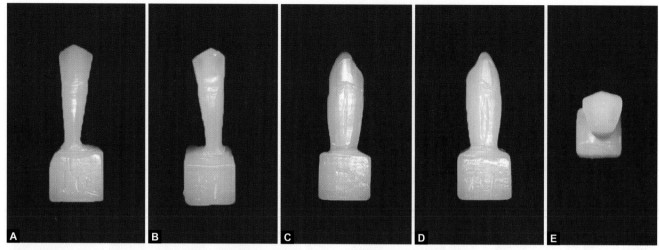

**Figs. 21.15A to E:** A specimen carving of mandibular canine.

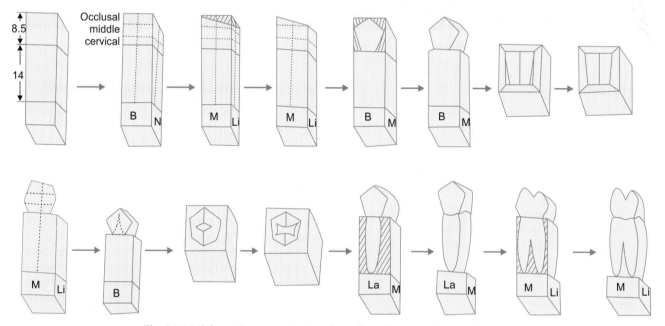

**Fig. 21.16:** Schematic representation of maxillary first premolar carving steps.

- *Step 5:* Obtaining buccal and lingual ridges by removing the wax on either side of the midline on each surface
- *Step 6:* Occlusal carving
  - 6A: Making a "V"-shaped notch on occlusal surface with larger area for buccal cusp
  - 6B: Carving the cusp slopes and triangular ridges of the cusps.

Using the distal end of the knife-shaped working end, strokes are given in an oblique direction from the buccal cusp toward the mesial and distal margins alternatively. This will form the inclined slopes and triangular ridge of the buccal cusp simultaneously. Same is repeated to form the lingual cusp.

Mesial and distal triangular fossae are carved, their base toward marginal ridges.

### Root Carving

- *Step 7:* Obtaining conical root form from the buccal and lingual aspects
- *Step 8:* Obtaining bifurcated root from the proximal aspects
- *Step 9:* Mesial marginal developmental groove carving
- *Step 10:* Cervical line carving and finishing

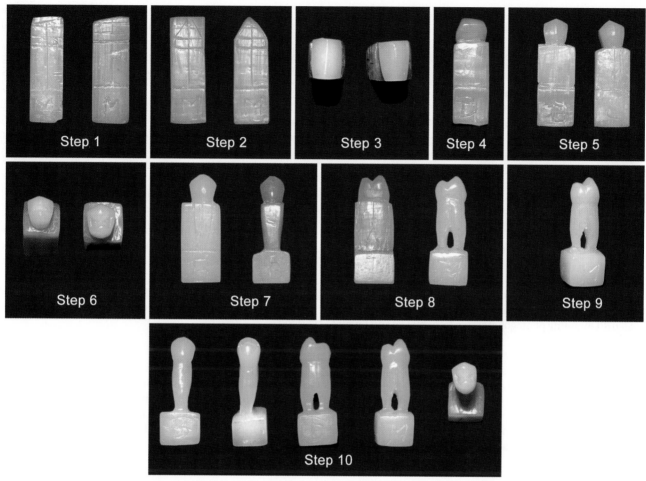

**Fig. 21.17:** Step-by-step procedure for carving a maxillary first premolar and finished carving from all the aspects (See text for details of the procedure).

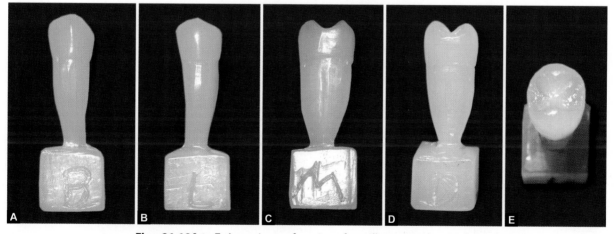

**Figs. 21.18A to E:** A specimen of carving of maxillary second premolar.

## Maxillary Second Premolar Carving (Figs. 21.18A to E)

Carving technique for maxillary second premolar is similar to that of maxillary first premolar with following changes:

- Both the cusps are same in height, so the occlusal slope is carved
- Single root

- Crown oval and not angular, and has many supplemental grooves giving a wrinkled appearance.

## Carving a Mandibular First Premolar (Figs. 21.19 and 21.20)

Carving technique for mandibular premolars differs from that of maxillary premolars in that, the mandibular premolars have their crowns lingually inclined over the root base.

The mandibular premolar has a small lingual cusp and its buccal cusp tip is in line with the vertical root axis.

### Crown Carving

- *Step 1:* Obtaining rhomboidal proximal form
  - 1A: Marking a rhombus on the mesial surface with lingually slanting occlusal table. Buccal cusp tip should come at midline
  - 1B: Removal of excess wax outside the margin
- *Step 2:* Obtaining crests of buccal and lingual contours at cervical and middle thirds, respectively
- *Step 3:* Obtaining pentagonal crown from buccal and lingual aspects
  - 3A: Marking a pentagon on buccal surface of the crown
  - 3B: Reduction of excess wax outside the marking
- *Step 4:* Obtaining buccal and lingual ridges
- *Step 5:* Obtaining lingual convergence of crown
- *Step 6:* Occlusal carving
  - 6A: Marking "V"-shaped notch on the occlusal surface with three-fourth area toward the buccal cusp portion

- 6B: Carving the cusp slopes, inclined planes, and the triangular ridges of cusps. Triangular ridge of the lingual cusp is not prominent.
- *Step 7:* Carving the mesiolingual developmental groove.

### Root Carving

- *Step 8:* Obtaining conical root form from buccal and lingual aspects
- *Step 9:* Obtaining broad conical root form from proximal aspects
- *Step 10:* Cervical line carving and finishing.

## Carving of Mandibular Second Premolar (Fig. 21.21)

Mandibular second premolar has a slight lingual crown tilt over the root base. The crown may have three cusps or two cusps. Lingual cusp is sharp, well developed and lingual crown convergence is not marked.

Basic procedure is similar to that of mandibular first premolar carving, with some differences in the occlusal carving.

### Crown Carving

- *Step 1:* Obtaining rhomboid proximal crown form with slight lingual crown tilt over the root base
- *Step 2:* Obtaining crest of the buccal and lingual contours at the cervical third and middle third, respectively
- *Step 3:* Obtaining pentagonal crown form from the facial aspect

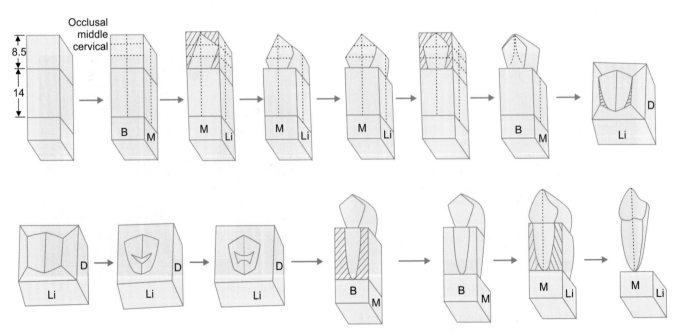

**Fig. 21.19:** Schematic representation of mandibular first premolar carving steps.

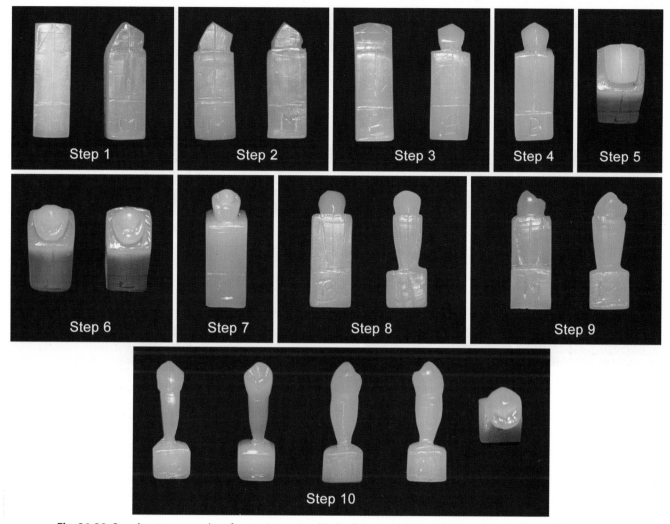

**Fig. 21.20:** Step-by-step procedure for carving a mandibular first premolar and finished carving from all the aspects (See text for details of the procedure).

- *Step 4:* Obtaining the buccal and lingual ridges
- *Step 5:* Occlusal carving
  - 5A: Marking a "Y"-shaped notch on the occlusal surface dividing the lingual portion into two parts for mesiolingual and distolingual cusps.
  - 5B: Carving cusp slopes, inclined planes, and the lingual ridges of each cusp.

### Root Carving

*Root carving is similar to that of the mandibular first premolar:*
- *Step 6:* Obtaining conical root form from buccal and the lingual aspects
- *Step 7:* Obtaining conical root form from the proximal aspects
- *Step 8:* Cervical line carving and finishing.

Figure 21.22 shows occlusal view of two cusp type of the mandibular second premolar with "U"- and "H"-shaped

occlusal groove pattern; and three cusp type with "Y"-shaped groove pattern.

### Carving a Maxillary First Molar (Figs. 21.22 and 21.23)

Molars have broad occlusal table with four to five cusp. Maxillary first molar has five cusps and three roots.

### Crown Carving

- *Step 1:* Obtaining crest of curvature on buccal (at cervical third), lingual (at middle third), and proximal (at occlusal third) surfaces
  - At the end of this step, we get a proximal trapezoidal form
- *Step 2:* Obtaining rhomboidal occlusal form with two acute and two obtuse angles
- *Step 2A:* Rounding off mesiolingual and distobuccal line angles to make them obtuse
- *Step 2B:* Tapering the buccal surface toward distal.

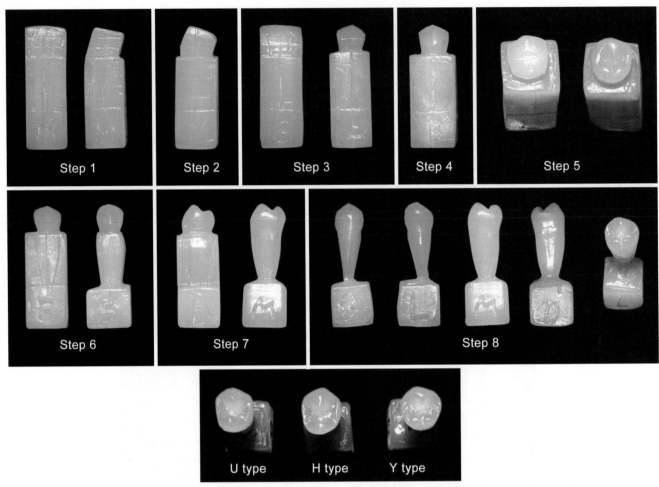

**Fig. 21.21:** Step-by-step procedure for carving a mandibular second premolar and finished carving from all the aspects (See text for details of the procedure).

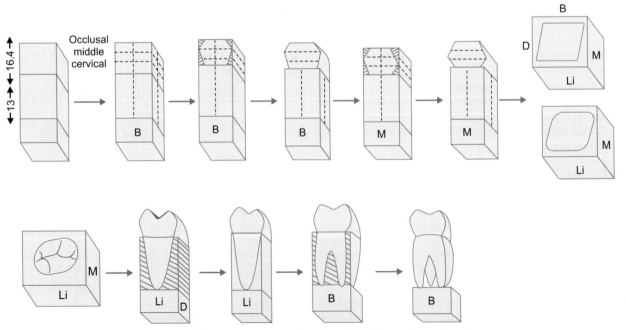

**Fig. 21.22:** Schematic representation of maxillary first molar carving steps.

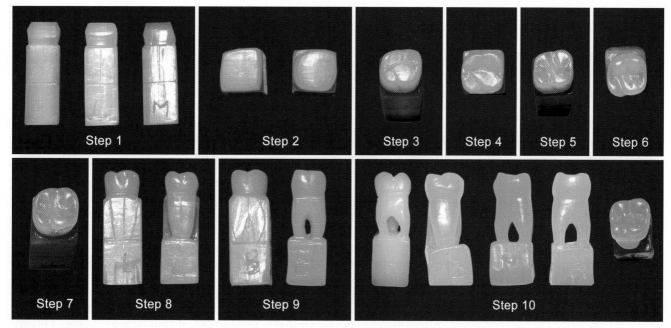

**Fig. 21.23:** Step-by-step procedure for carving a maxillary first molar and finished carving from all the aspects
(See text for details of the procedure).

## Occlusal Carving

- *Step 3:* Marking of the developmental grooves on occlusal surface
- *Step 4:* Division of occlusal table into buccal and lingual portions, which slope toward the center
- *Step 5:* Carving four major cusps with their inclined planes and triangular ridges.
  This is done by giving obliquely directed strokes on either side of each cusp tip using the distal end of the carver's knife-shaped working end.
- *Step 6:* Carving the oblique ridge by merging distal cusp ridge of mesiolingual cusp and triangular ridge of distobuccal cusp
- *Step 7:* Cusp of Carabelli carving and finishing the crown with highlighting all grooves, triangular fossae, and ridges.

## Root Carving

- *Step 8:* Division of the root portion into buccal and palatal halves. Obtaining the conical lingual root form from the lingual aspect
- *Step 9:* Obtaining two buccal roots from the buccal aspect
- *Step 10:* Finishing the carving with cervical line marking and rounding all the line angles.

### Carving of Maxillary Second Molar (Figs. 21.24A to E)

The carving procedure differs from that of the maxillary first molar in that:
- No cusp of Carabelli
- Oblique ridge is less prominent
- Distolingual cusp is smaller

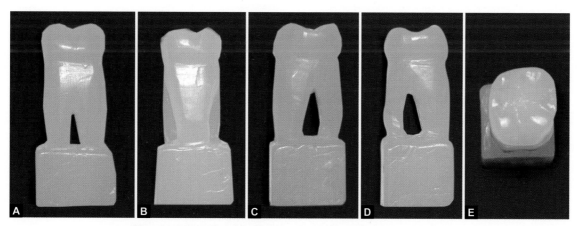

**Figs. 21.24A to E:** A specimen carving of maxillary second molar.

• Roots are parallel, less divergent, and curve more distally. **Figures 21.24A to E** show a specimen carving.

## Carving a Mandibular First Molar (Figs. 21.25 and 21.26)

Mandibular first molar is bifurcated and has five cusps.

### Crown Carving

• *Step 1*: Obtaining the crest of curvature on buccal (at cervical third), lingual (at middle third), and proximal (at occlusal third) surfaces
• *Step 2*: Obtaining rhomboidal proximal form by slanting the buccal surface above the cervical ridge
• *Step 3*: Obtaining mandibular occlusal form by rounding all the line angles and lingual convergence of the crown
• *Step 4*: Division of the occlusal table into buccal and lingual halves, which slopes toward the central developmental groove
• *Step 5*: Division of occlusal table into five portions for five cusps and marking the developmental grooves and triangular fossae
• *Step 6*: Carving the five cusps with their inclined planes and triangular ridges

• *Step 7*: Finishing the crown by deepening the developmental grooves and carving the triangular fossae.

### Root Carving

• *Step 8*: Obtaining the conical root form from the proximal aspects
• *Step 9*: Obtaining bifurcated roots from the buccal and lingual aspects
• *Step 10*: Finishing the carving by rounding the line angles and carving the cervical lines.

## Carving of Mandibular Second Molar (Figs. 21.27A to E)

While carving the mandibular second molar, the following differences are to be considered:
• No distal cusp
• Crown has a rectangular occlusal form
• There is a bulge at the mesiobuccal line angle cervically
• Roots are less spaced.
**Figures 21.27A to E** show a specimen carving.

The finished carvings can be preserved and displayed by arranging them in dental arch form as shown in **Figure 21.28**.

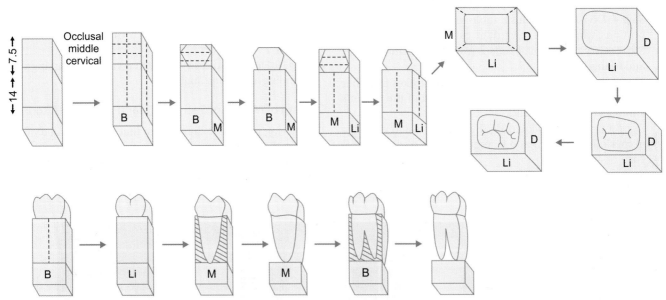

**Fig. 21.25:** Schematic representation of mandibular first molar carving steps.

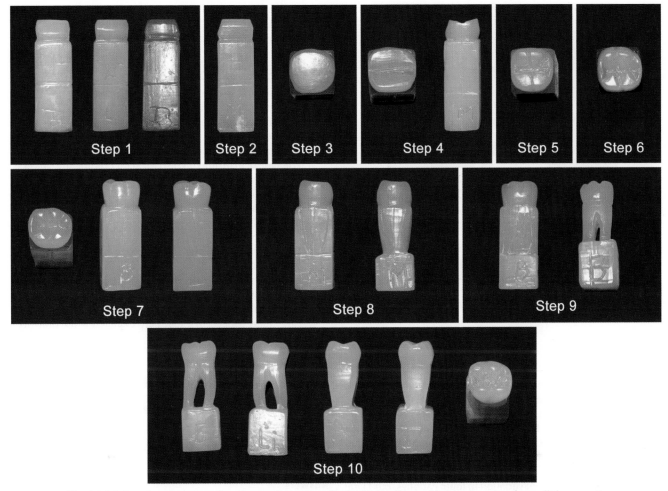

**Fig. 21.26:** Step-by-step procedure for carving a mandibular first molar and finished carving from all the aspects (See text for details of the procedure).

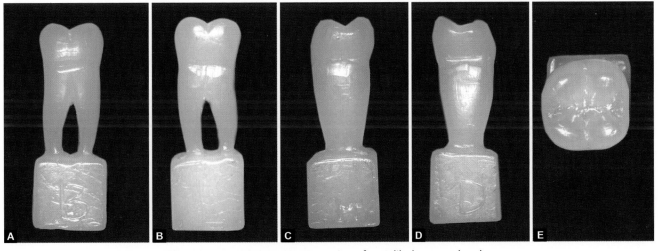

**Figs. 21.27A to E:** A specimen carving of mandibular second molar.

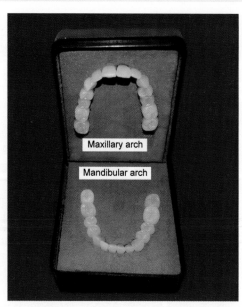

**Fig. 21.28:** Preservation and display of tooth carvings.

## BIBLIOGRAPHY

1. Kataoka S, Nishimura Y, Sadan A. Nature's Morphology: An atlas of tooth shape and form. (IL), USA: Quintessence Publishing; 2002. p. 1.
2. Lucas PW. Dental Functional Morphology: How Teeth Work (Cambridge Studies in Biological and Evolutionary Anthropology). Cambridge, UK: Cambridge University Press; 2004. p. 1.
3. Rantanen AV. A study of variation in tooth carvings. Eur J Oral Sci. 1970;78(1-4):28-33.
4. Siésseree S, Vitti M, de Sousa LG, et al. Educational Material of Dental Anatomy Applied to Study the Morphology of Permanent teeth. Braz Dent J. 2004;15(3):238-42.

## MULTIPLE CHOICE QUESTIONS

1. The methods used for tooth carving include:
   a. Wax reduction method
   b. Wax addition method
   c. Both A and B
   d. None of the above
2. The type of instrument grasp ideal for holding the carver is:
   a. Pen grasp
   b. Modified pen grasp
   c. Palm and thumb grasp
   d. Any of the above
3. Tooth carving exercises help in:
   a. Understanding the morphology of teeth in three dimensions
   b. Improves hand dexterity
   c. Improves clinical practice
   d. All of the above
4. How many aspects of a tooth are depicted while drawing a tooth?
   a. 2 aspects
   b. 3 aspects
   c. 4 aspects
   d. 5 aspects
5. The material commonly used to carve the tooth is:
   a. Modeling wax block
   b. Paraffin wax block
   c. Modeling clay
   d. Impression compound

**Answers**

1. c    2. b    3. d    4. d    5. b

# Index

Page numbers followed by *b* refer to box, *f* refer to figure, *fc* refer to flowchart, and *t* refer to table.